Neonatal Immunity

Contemporary Immunology

Series Editor: *Noel R. Rose,* MD, PhD

Neonatal Immunity

by

Constantin Bona, MD, PhD

Mount Sinai School of Medicine,
New York, NY

Foreword by

Noel R. Rose, MD, PhD

The Johns Hopkins University Schools of Medicine and Public Health,
Baltimore, MD

HUMANA PRESS ✳ TOTOWA, NEW JERSEY

© 2005 Humana Press Inc.
999 Riverview Drive, Suite 208
Totowa, New Jersey 07512

www.humanapress.com

This publication is printed on acid-free paper. ∞
ANSI Z39.48-1984 (American National Standards Institute) Permanence of Paper for Printed Library Materials.

Production Editor: Mark J. Breaugh.

Cover design by Patricia F. Cleary.

For additional copies, pricing for bulk purchases, and/or information about other Humana titles, contact Humana at the above address or at any of the following numbers: Tel.: 973-256-1699; Fax: 973-256-8341; E-mail: humana@humanapr.com or visit our Web site: http://www.humanapress.com

Printed in the United States of America. 10 9 8 7 6 5 4 3 2 1

E-ISBN:1-59259-825-0

Library of Congress Cataloging in Publication Data

Neonatal immunity / edited by Constantin Bona ; foreword by Noel R. Rose.
    p. ; cm. -- (Contemporary immunology)
  Includes bibliographical references and index.
  ISBN 1-58829-319-X (alk. paper)
  1. Infants (Newborn)--Immunology. 2. Maternally acquired immunity.
  [DNLM: 1. Immunity, Maternally-Acquired. 2. Animals, Newborn--immunology. 3. Antibody-Producing Cells--Infant, Newborn. 4. Autoimmune Diseases--Infant, Newborn. QW 553 N438 2004]
  I. Bona, Constantin A. II. Series.
  QR184.5.N46 2004   2005
  616.07'9--dc22

                    2004007841

Foreword

Recently, Arthur Silverstein *(1)*, a pioneer in studies of prenatal and neo-natal immunity, published an historical article, entitled "The Most Elegant Immunological Experiment of the XIX Century." In it, he described some extraordinary experiments carried out by Paul Ehrlich between 1892 and 1894. These experiments can truly be cited as the genesis of today's developmental and neonatal immunology. The story, in brief, started after the demonstration by Behring and Kitasato in 1890 of specific antitoxins circulating in the blood of animals immunized against diphtheria or tetanus. These experiments were quickly translated into the use of antitoxins to prevent or treat these diseases in human patients. Intrigued by reports that babies from immune mothers were protected from disease, Paul Ehrlich undertook a series of studies, using the plant toxins ricin and abrin as model antigens. He mated ricin- or abrin-immunized male mice with non-immune females and mated immunized females with non-immune males. The offspring of these matings were tested for protection by a challenge injection of the appropriate toxin. He found that only the offspring of immunized females were protected. Protection was specific but only temporary. Pups of immune fathers showed no protection. Thus, for the first time, Ehrlich demonstrated protective passive immunity by maternal transfer. Realizing that antitoxin transfer could occur across the placenta or through milk, Ehrlich next set up experiments in which the offspring of immunized mothers were given to suckle on non-immune foster mothers or, conversely, offspring of non-immune mothers to suckle on immune foster mothers. In the first case, the antitoxic antibody initially present declined rapidly. In less than 3 wk all of the newborn were susceptible to the toxin challenge. In contrast, in the offspring of non-immune mothers fed by immune wet nurses, a high degree of immunity was established, which persisted for more than 6 wk. The milk of immune mothers, Ehrlich concluded, is an ideal source of protective antibody for the newborn. Finally, Ehrlich passively immunized nursing mice with a horse antitoxin and found that the antibodies in milk could traverse the intestinal wall of the newborn.

It can rightly be said that in these simple, elegant experiments, Ehrlich laid down the basic principles of contemporary neonatal immunology. His fundamental experiments have been repeated in many forms and confirmed many times. For example, Fig. 34 in the present volume nicely recapitulates Ehrlich's principal findings. It relates, moreover, to some of the urgent practical questions of our time. Group B streptococcal infections are a frequent cause of sepsis and meningitis during the first 2 mo of life. There might be great value in immunizing mothers with the appropriate antigen of Group B streptococci in order to protect their newborns during this critical, vulnerable period. The experiments of Martin, Rioux, and Gagnon described on page 163 of this book essentially reproduce Ehrlich's experiments, using Group B streptococcal infection rather than a toxin, and confirm the potential value of maternal immunization in protecting the newborn.

Our knowledge of immunology has expanded greatly since the final decade of the 19th century and, with it, has come newer understanding of neonatal and developmental immunology. One half of a century after he first proposed it, Ehrlich's concept that adaptive immunity depends upon specific receptors represented as side chains on cells was resurrected by Burnet *(2)* in his clonal selection theory. The basic concept that antigen is a selective rather than an instructive agent still underlies today's immunologic thought. Burnet's original view was that the interaction of an antigen with a quiescent, mature, receptor-bearing immunocyte (i.e., lymphocyte) leads to cell proliferation and a positive immune response. A similar interaction with an immature immunocyte, on the other hand, provokes death of the antigen-specific lymphocyte. Thus exposure to an antigen during fetal life when most lymphocytes are immature is likely to lead to deletion rather than proliferation and a positive response. We now recognize that the immunologic unresponsiveness of the fetus is relative and time related, and that in many species a robust immune response is possible in late fetal and neonatal periods. This volume describes classical studies in which the progressive maturation of the early immune response is clearly described. Yet, we know that the newborn human is still unable to manage many infections on its own and requires passively acquired antibody from its mother. Moreover, passively acquired immunity in the newborn is largely, if not completely, antibody-born. Cell-mediated protection is not transferred from mother to offspring. It is, in fact, paradoxical that recent investigations have suggested that maternal lymphocytes can pass through the placenta and establish themselves in the newborn to form immunologic chimeras. There is evidence that this chimeric state may result years later in a graft-vs-host reaction that is interpreted as autoimmune disease.

Burnet's original premise that contact of an immature lymphocyte with its corresponding antigen would lead to cell elimination rather than proliferation is represented in our present view of central tolerance of self. Expression of self-antigens in the thymus during early stages of T-lymphocyte generation leads to negative selection and deletion of self-reactive clones. The ability to express self-antigens in the thymic environment is genetically controlled and at least one of the genes responsible has recently been identified in humans and mice as belonging to the >AIRE= family of genes. This is certainly only the first of many genes with similar functions and is of the greatest importance in understanding the construction of the neonatal immune response.

We now realize that clonal deletion of T cells in the thymus is an incomplete process and self-reactive T cells are often present in peripheral locations. Post-thymic mechanisms are required to keep such self-reactive T cells in check. A number of regulatory mechanisms are engaged in avoiding the onset of pathogenic autoimmune responses and maintaining physiologic homeostasis.

With that thought in mind, a number of years ago, we *(3)* proposed that clonal balance rather than clonal selection is a more appropriate term for describing the development of the immune response. The term clonal balance suggests that the immune response depends on the ratio of factors promoting or retarding the immune response. The balance between positive and negative vectors is very delicate and the outcome is determined by the genetics of the host as well as the manner of antigen presentation. In practical terms, it is the context of the presentation of an antigen that dictates the quality and quantity of the immune response. It depends upon the signals passed by the cells presenting antigen to the initial T cells and by the T cells interacting with other cells. These signals depend, among other factors, on the degree of maturity of the host.

If we accept the notion of clonal balance, developmental and neonatal immunology is the study of the context in which antigen is presented to immunocompetent cells. The context is a dynamic one and depends on the maturity of the many cells that direct the immune response. It determines the cellular basis of both the adaptive immune response and of the earlier innate immune response.

The present volume sets out the issues of neonatal immunology in terms of our contemporary appreciation of the changing dynamics of the clonal balance. Many enigmatic phenomena of the past now become more understandable; yet, the basic principles laid down by Ehrlich in 1892 are still applicable.

REFERENCES

1. Silverstein AM. The most elegant immunological experiment of the XIX century. Nat Immunol 2000;1:93–94.
2. Burnet FM. The Clonal Selection Theory of Acquired Immunity. Cambridge, Cambridge University Press, 1959.
3. Rose NR. Current concepts of autoimmune disease. Transplant Proc 1988; 20 (Suppl 4):3–10.

Noel R. Rose, MD, PhD
The Johns Hopkins University Schools of Medicine and Public Health

Preface

The field of classical neonatal immunology has been dominated over the past 50 years by two theories. The first theory is that lymphocytes specific for self-antigens are deleted during fetal development. Current research carried out in transgenic mice supports this hypothesis, with continual evidence of the deletion of self-reactive clones during fetal development. The second long-held theory is that the immune system of neonates is highly susceptible to developing immune tolerance, leading to unresponsiveness to immunization. This theory became a paradigm based on an experiment performed in mice showing that the injection of newborns with allogeneic bone marrow cells prevented the rejection of an allogeneic skin graft.

Commonly, a paradigm built on a widely accepted finding becomes an eternal truth; an established paradigm generally leads to its temporal dominance and an apparent intellectual rigor. Scientists frequently differentiate into several groups with respect to a given paradigm. One group of scientists searches for new findings aimed at strengthening the paradigm, and these findings sometimes result in a beneficial practical application. For example, the paradigm of neonatal tolerance was instrumental in advancing our knowledge of the mechanism of tolerance. Currently, the reconstitution of the immune system of immune-deficient patients with cord blood stem cells is considered less harmful than reconstitution with bone marrow. A second group of scientists continues to look for new findings that cannot always be explained by the current paradigm. The accumulation of new findings that do not fit within the currently accepted paradigm leads to an intellectual crisis. This is a critical point in the evolution of science in which the competition between old and new findings may then lead to the formulation of a new paradigm. The cycle paradigm–crisis–paradigm is repeated until a new theory or a universal model is formulated or accepted.

In the last several decades there has been remarkable progress in our understanding of neonatal immunity. Advances in cellular immunology, molecular biology, recombinant DNA and proteins, and the function of cytokines and chemokines have changed our understanding of the immunity of neonates and infants. New discoveries have revolutionized the study of neonatal immune responsiveness, facilitating the development of efficient vaccines for newborns, a greater understanding of impaired immune response in neonates afflicted by immunodeficiency or genetic defects, and a clearer knowledge of the developing immune system. New experimental findings and clinical observations have shown that neonates, and in some species fetuses, respond to

foreign antigens in a manner consistent with the existence of both quantitative and phenotypic differences between newborn and adult lymphocytes.

The aim of *Neonatal Immunology* is to present classical and current
information and discuss cutting-edge discoveries that will hopefully lead to
new horizons in biological research and result in scientific progress in such
areas as vaccination of infants, stem cells, gene therapy, and transplantation.

I wish to express my thanks for the support of my wife, Alexandra, and
my daughter Monique for their help in editing some of the chapters. Thanks
also to Cristina Stoica for her help in gathering references and composing
figures, to Dr. T. Brumeanu for valuable information and discussion regarding Chapter 9, and to Dr. Sunil Thomas for proofreading the manuscript.

Constantin Bona, MD, PhD

Contents

1

Structure and Function of the Immune System in Vertebrates

1. INTRODUCTION

During evolution, vertebrates developed an immune system able to cope with the universe of foreign antigen represented by approx 1 billion different structurally defined antigenic determinants (epitopes). The word "immune" (from the Latin *immunis* meaning except or free from taxes) defines the function of the immune system, which is endowed with intricate defense mechanisms to neutralize aggressive foreign molecules or to overcome microbial infectious agents. The immune system has a limited reactivity to self-antigen by virtue of its ability to discriminate self from nonself.

The vertebrate immune system comprises two major arms: innate immunity (natural, nonspecific) and adaptive immunity (specific, acquired). Cells of the immune system and soluble factors mediate the interaction between these two arms. Germline genes selected by evolutionary forces encode the function of the immune system, and the replicative genetic material is inherited by offspring. Although the information contained in the genetic material that encodes innate immunity is quite stable, that which encodes the adaptive immunity can be modified throughout life by subtle changes in germ line gene repertoire and in various vertebrate species by changes during evolution through Darwinian selection pressure.

2. INNATE IMMUNITY

Innate immunity is mediated by two defense reactions: constitutive and inducible by self-altered cells or by macromolecules and microbes.

The constitutive mechanisms include physical barriers (e.g., skin and mucosal epithelia) and chemical factors endowed with antibacterial properties present within the skin or in secretion of mucosal tissues (saliva, tears), such as lysozyme and defensins. These molecules exhibit destructive properties against bacteria, and fungal cell walls are not active against a host's cells or self-molecules. Similarly, macromolecules endowed with antimicrobial properties are present in various cells or tissues and are recruited in the defense reactions.

From: *Contemporary Immunology: Neonatal Immunity*
By: Constantin Bona © Humana Press Inc., Totowa, NJ

One of the effector molecules of innate immunity is the complement. The liver constitutes the primary site of complement synthesis during ontogenetic development and in adults. Complement is an effector system of host defense reactions, which acts against pathogens contributing to phagocytosis of bacteria and the release of inflammatory mediators at the site of inflammation. Other factors include lysins, agglutinins, antibacterial peptides, and acute phase proteins. All of these molecules that mediate innate immunity are germline-gene encoded, and their presence and activity do not depend on stimulation by foreign antigen.

The cells involved in innate immune defense reaction are the polymorphonuclear leukocytes (PMNs) (neutrophils, eosinophils, basophils), monocyte macrophages, dendritic cells, natural killer (NKs), and γ/δ T cells. These cells are able to clear the microbes or the toxins from the body and secrete cytokines, which form a functional network that enables crosstalk between the cells that mediate innate and adaptive immunity.

Innate immunity in vertebrates has an ancestral origin. This concept originated from the discovery by Metchnikoff of phagocytosis in invertebrates, including the transparent larvae of starfish and the water flea Daphnia *(1)*. Soon after Metchnikoff's discovery, the phagocytosis of bacteria was demonstrated in other invertebrates (insects and flies) and in vertebrates. In vertebrate species, the neutrophils, eosinophils, mast cells, macrophages, and dendritic cells are able to phagocytize not only bacteria and foreign cells but also aged or apoptotic self cells *(2)*. We demonstrated that the neutrophils and macrophages are also able to internalize both exotoxins (Dick toxin, diphtheria toxin, and *Escherichia coli* neurotoxin) and endotoxins *(3–5)* by fluid phase pinocytosis.

There is a large body of information demonstrating the presence of components that are characteristic of innate immunity in invertebrates (reviewed in ref. *6; see* Table 1). Some of these molecules are constitutively expressed and others are induced subsequent to infection with bacteria *(6)*.

The ancestral origin of innate immunity in vertebrates is also illustrated by the fact that Toll-like receptors that are expressed in the effector cells of vertebrates were found in Drosophila *(7,8)*. The Drosophila Toll proteins play an important role in flies' defense reactions against infection caused by fungi *(8)*.

There are various target molecules that are recognized by the effector cells that mediate innate immunity. The target molecules could be classified into two major categories: (a) molecules involved in the phagocytosis process, and (b) molecules that are recognized by receptors, which trigger signaling pathways that result in the activation of genes that are involved in the immune processes.

Table 1
Molecules Characteristic of Innate Immunity in Invertebrates

Species	Molecule Acute phase proteins
Insects	Pentraxin, complement, macroglobulin
Crustaceans	C-reactive protein, LPS binding protein
	Antimicrobial peptides
Tunicates	Clavanin, stylelin, lumbricin
Drosophila	Defensin (cecropin, transferrin)
Mytilus	Defensin (mytilin, myticin)
	Lysines
Earthworm (*Eisenia fetida*)	Fetidin, lysenin, eiseniapore, CCF-1
	Complement-like proteins
Sea urchin	C3

Abbreviations: LPS, lipopoly saccharide.

2.1. Molecules Recognized by Receptors Mediating Internalization

The effectors of innate immunity—neutrophils, macrophages, and dendritic cells—can recognize and internalize microbes and altered self-macromolecules and cells.

In early studies, we showed that the pinocytosis of human immunoglobulins and sheep red blood cells in the absence or presence of specific serum was significantly reduced after treatment of guinea pig neutrophils with periodic acid and neuraminidase (Table 2). These results suggest that the glycoprotein molecules associated with the surface of neutrophils are involved in the internalization process (9). These results also showed that the phagocytic process and the internalization of immune complexes is significantly enhanced by opsonins, because the internalization via FcR (10) is more efficient than the phagocytosis mediated by nonspecific opsonins such as histones or other proteins (11).

Scavenger receptors, which are associated with the membranes of endothelial cells and macrophages located in liver (Kupfer cells) and spleen, are involved in recognizing numerous physiological waste macromolecules and clearing them from the blood. Such molecules are self-polysaccharides and proteins that result from hydrolysis of extracellular matrix glycoproteins, altered serum proteins, or foreign macromolecules caused by the degradation of bacterial and fungal proteins or colloidal dyes. Seternes et al. (12) showed that the presence of scavenger

Table 2

Alteration of the Uptake of Foreign Matter Subsequent to Treatment of Guinea Pig Neutrophils With Chemical or Enzymatic Agents

| | Pinocytosis index of Igs % | | Phagocytosis index of SRBC% + Anti-SRBC | |
Agents	Nil	+ Anti-Ig serum	Nil	serum
Control	34.6±2.48	38.9±4.54	1.1± 0.38	12.4±1.08
Periodic acid	11.2 ±2.71	9.9± 2.62	1.2±0.58	1.6±1.01
Neuraminidase	21± 2.3	24.77±3.1	0.25±0.13	1.72±0.48
Trypsin	34.5± 6.24	34.77±4.27	0.71±0.25	2.69±0.7.8

Data published from ref. *9*.
Abbreviations: SRBC, sheep red blood cells.

receptors are common to cells from seven different vertebrate species: lamprey, fish, frogs, lizards, chickens, mice, and rats. The scavenger function that induces the clearing of physiological waste molecules is mediated by at least five types of receptors: (a) hyaluronan receptors that recognize hyaluronan and condroidin sulfate *(13)*; (b) the collagen receptor for several α collagen chains *(14)* and N-terminal peptides of procollagen *(14)*; (c) the mannose receptor for C-terminal peptides derived from collagen *(15)*; (d) the receptor for modified lipoproteins *(16)*; and (e) FcR for immune complexes *(10)*.

The C-type lectins play a role in the phagocytosis of apoptotic cells, such as rodent thymocytes induced to undergo apoptosis by glucocorticoids. The C-lectins probably recognize galactose-rich glycoproteins because the phagocytosis of apoptotic cells can be inhibited by preincubation of macrophages with N-acetyl galactosamine or galactose *(17)*.

The recognition of altered self is poorly understood but could be related to the alteration in the surface glycoproteins or the phospholipid component of the membrane *(17)*. This hypothesis is strongly supported by our previous studies, which demonstrate an increased phagocytosis of guinea pig macrophages of autologous red blood cells treated with periodic acid or lecithinase *(18)*. The results presented in Table 3 show that the rate of phagocytosis of autologous red blood cells (RBC) is negligible. However, it was significantly increased after artificial alteration of glycoproteins subsequent to oxidation (with periodic acid) of hydroxy or α-amino alcohol groups of polysaccharides or the hydrolysis of lecithin, which is a major component of the RBC membrane. The internalization of the altered cells may be mediated by the phosphatidyl serine receptor. This receptor binds red-cell ghosts and sickled red cells, which have lost normal asymmetry of membrane phospholipid leaflets by unmasking anionic phospholipids such as phosphotidylserine contained in the inner monolayer *(17)*.

Table 3
Effect of Enzymatic Pretreatment of Phagocytosis
of Autologous RBC by Guinea Pig Macrophages

Pretreatment of RBC with	Mean rate of phagocytosis
Nil	0.3±0.1
Cathepsin-C	0.93±0.2
Periodic acid	21.6±8.45
Lecithinase	22.1±1.61

Data published from ref. *19*.
Abbreviations: RBC, red blood cells.

2.2. Molecules Recognized by Toll Receptors Involved in Signaling Pathways and the Activation of Various Genes

The molecules recognized by Toll-like receptors (TLRs) that trigger signaling pathways are refereed to pathogen-associated molecule patterns (PAMPs) *(17)*.

Toll proteins that were originally described in Drosophila were considered to play a role in controlling the development of the dorsal patterning of the fly embryo and antifungal defense reaction *(8,19)*. In Drosophila, four members of the TLR family have been identified. Structural studies demonstrated that the cytoplasm tail domain of the Drosophila Toll protein exhibits a high homology with the mammalian interleukin (IL)-1 receptor *(20)*. Activation of Toll receptors plays a role in innate immune reaction and has been demonstrated in transfection experiments. Transfection of Schneider insect cells with plasmid-containing Drosophila Toll protein activated the transcription of genes that encode antimicrobial peptides such as diptericin, attacin, and defensin *(21)*. Genetic complementation studies have suggested that the secreted protein Spatzle is the natural ligand for TLR in Drosophila *(22)*.

Later, homologs of Drosophilla Toll proteins were rapidly identified in humans *(23,24)*. The effector cells mediating innate immunity (e.g., monocytes; macrophages; and intestinal, dendritic, and NK cells) express TLRs.

In vertebrates, numerous ligands for the nine TLRs were identified (Table 4). The major characteristic of the binding of ligands recognized by cells that mediate innate immunity is that the recognition process is not clonal restricted since the ligands bind to TLRs expressed on a variety of cells.

The TLR recognized PAMPs, conserved molecular macromolecules, essential for the survival of bacteria.

The IL-1 receptor/Toll-like receptor represents a superfamily of receptors found in many vertebrate species. This family includes IL-1R, IL-1R Acp, IL-18R, IL-18R Acp, and the orphan receptor. Although IL-1 and IL-18 are the

Table 4
Toll Receptors and Their Ligands

Toll receptor	Ligand
TLR IL-I	IL-1, IL-18, LPS
TLR 2	Clindrical *E. coli* LPS, yeast zymosan
	Lipoproteins (mycoplasma, mycobacteria, OspA Borrelia burgdoferi)
	Lipopeptide (*Treponema pallidum*)
	Peptidoglycan (*Staphylococcus aureus, B.subtilis* Streptoccocus)
	Arabinofuranos (Mycobacteria)
TLR 3	Viral dsRNA
TLR 4	Conical *Pseudomones gingivalis*, leptospira LPS, Lipoteichoic acid (*S. aureus*), HSP60
TLR 5	Flagellin
TLR 6	Neisseria LPS
TLR 7	Imiquimod
TLR 9	CpG motif

Abbreviations: TLR, toll receptor; IL, interleukin; LPS, lipopolysaccharide, dsRNA, double-stranded ribonucleic acid.

ligands of IL-1 and IL-18 receptors, the ligand for the orphan receptor is unknown. The TLRs signal pathways that lead to the activation of multiple genes, which encode proteins involved in host response to infectious agents or injuries *(25)*.

TLR 2 recognizes mainly bacterial, mycoplasmal lipoproteins and glycolipids (reviewed in ref. *26*). Lipoproteins bind to TLR by their lipoylated N-termini. Most lipoproteins are triacylated at the N-termini, with the exception of mycoplasma lipoprotein, which is diacylated. TLR 2 also recognizes mycobacterium cell wall glycolipids such as lipoarabinomannan (LAM), which contains arabinofuranosyl sidechains. Interestingly, the receptor can distinguish subtle structural differences in LAM. For example, it does not recognize AraLAM from *M. tuberculosis* or bacillus Calmette-Guerin (BCG), which contain LAM that is terminally capped with mannose. Macrophages produce proinflammatory cytokines in response to zymosan, which binds to TLR 2. It was proposed that TLR 2 subsequent to the binding of various ligands is recruited in phagosomes and participates in receptor-mediated phagocytosis and, therefore, may discriminate between structurally different ligands. This concept is supported by cytological data, which demonstrate that after phagocytosis of zymosan by macrophages the TLR 2 is enriched around the phagosome *(27)*.

TLR 3 recognizes viral double-stranded RNA (dsRNA) that is synthesized during the replication process by various viruses. The recognition of dsRNA by TLR 3 was elegantly demonstrated in an experiment showing that although poly (I:C) stimulates human cells expressing TLR 3, it failed to activate production of IL-6, IL-12 and tumor necrosis factor (TNF) by macrophages from TLR 3–/– mice *(28)*.

TLR 4 mainly recognizes LPS from various gram-negative bacteria, lipoteichoic acid from *Streptococcus aureus*, and HSP60, which is an endogenous protein. The role of TLR 4 in the recognition of LPS is strongly supported by two sets of observations: (a) the presence of an mis-sense point mutation within the TLR 4 gene-encoding cytoplasm tail of the receptor in C3H/HeJ mice, which are unresponsive to LPS *(29)*, and (b) lipopolysaccharide (LPS) hyporesponsiveness of TLR4–/–mice resembles the defective LPS response of C3H/HeJ mice *(30)*. The recognition of HSP60 endogenous protein by TLR 4 was demonstrated by the inability of macrophages from C3H/ HeJ—but not C3H/HeN—mice to induce the synthesis of TNF-α and nitric oxides after exposure to HSP60 protein *(31)*.

TLR 5 recognizes flagellin, the major component of the flagella, which extends from the outer membrane of gram-negative and gram-positive bacteria *(32)*. This was demonstrated by studying the ability to stimulate cells incubated with flagellated and nonflagellated *Listeria moncytogenes* of *E. coli* and a mutant *Salmonella typhimurium* strain bearing the deleted flagellin gene.

TLR 9 recognizes CpG-rich bacterial DNA. This was demonstrated by a lack of production of cytokines by macrophages and the maturation of dendritic cells in TLR9-/- mice following exposure to CpG containing DNA *(33)* (Table 4).

Studies carried out in Drosophila showed that the signaling via Toll proteins involves an adaptor protein tube that transmits the signal to Pele, a serine-threonine kinase, which, in turn, signals the dorsal-Cactus complex equivalent to mammalian NF-κB *(34–36)*. The signaling pathways through mammalian TLR 1,2,3, and 4 are quite common and resemble those described in Drosophila, suggesting a highly phylogenetically conserved system. The intracellular domain (TIR) of TLR 2,3, and 4 is similar to IL-1R domain. In the case of IL-1R, the ligand engagement recruits the MyD88 adaptor protein, equivalent of Drosophila tube protein, that associates to IL-1R protein by direct TIR–TIR domain interaction. The death domain of MyD88 recruits IL-1R-associated protein kinases, (IRAK4) that is related to the Pele kinase of Drosophila. After phosphorylation, IRAK 4 dissociates from the receptor and associates with the TNF receptor activation factor 6 (TRAF6). TRAF6 then activates NF-κB, p38 mitogen-activating protein kinase (MAPK), and Jien kinase (JNK), leading to activation of transcription factors c-Jun and AP-1 *(37)*. ECSIT protein identified both in Drosophila and humans appears to bridge TRAF6 to MAPK activation via MEKK1 *(21)*.

There are some subtle differences in the signaling pathways triggered by TLRs. Thus, in the case of TLR 4, a MyD88 independent pathway exists in which the binding of LPS to receptor recruits Mal-TIRAP, which then activates IRAK4 *(38)*. The MyD88 independent signaling pathway was demonstrated in a study showing that the LPS induced NF-κB activation in MyD88-deficient cells (reviewed in ref. *38*).

Signaling pathways mediated by TLR 2 and 4 leads to the activation of the p38-MAPK pathway and of AP-1, NF-κB, and c-Jun transcription factors *(38)*. The signaling pathway via TLR 3 by dsRNA induces MyD66-dependent activation of IL production, whereas the maturation of dendritic cells and the activation of NF-κB, c-Jun, and p38MAPK are induced via MyD88-independent pathway *(28)*.

2.3. NK Cells and Innate Immunity

NK cells play an important role in innate immunity, particularly in earlier stages of the invasion of the body by infectious agents or aberrantly differentiated cells subsequent to oncogenic transformation. Like the response of monocytes and dendritic cells to pathogens, the NK response is not clonally restricted. This results from the monomorphic nature of NK receptors. One type of receptor represented by Fcγ receptor mediates Antibody-dependent cell-mediated cytotoxiated (ADCMC) reaction, a process in which the antibody specific for a target antigen bridges the target cell with NK cells. A second group of receptors is involved in lysing virus-infected and tumor cells that lack major histocompatibility complex (MHC) molecules. The second group of receptors can be divided into three families. The first family contains killer-cell inhibitory receptors (KIR) expressed on human NK cells. The second family consists of receptors that display high homology to the C-type lectin receptors expressed on the surface of other effector cells involved in innate immunity. This receptor is a heterodimer composed of CD94/NKG2 that is expressed in both human and murine NK cells. In humans, these receptors recognize HLA-E, a minor MHC antigen and in mouse Qa-1^b, a nonclassical MHC antigen *(39)*. In mice, whereas CD94 is monomorphic, the NKG2 is polymorphic. The third family of inhibitory receptors, Ly49, is expressed only in some murine strains. This receptor family is polymorphic, because it consists of 14 highly related genes (Ly49 A–N). The inhibitory effect results from the binding of Ly49 to the α1/α2 domain of MHC class I molecules *(40)*.

In humans, NK cells constitute 10–15% of peripheral blood lymphocytes (PBL) and mediate cytotoxic activity against cells infected with viruses or against tumor cells irrespective of their antigen specificity. Similarly to mice, human NK cells express three types of receptors: (a) the Fcγ receptors that mediate ADCMC; (b) the inhibitory receptors that belong either to the Ig superfamily (KIR and ILTC) or to the C-type lectin family (NKG2A/CD94); and (c) the activating receptor group composed of several molecules, including NKp30, NKp44, and NKp46 *(41)*.

3. ADAPTIVE IMMUNITY

Adaptive immunity represents the specific immune response of individuals who have been exposed to foreign antigen or, in some pathological conditions, to self-antigen. The effectors of adaptive immunity include B lymphocytes, which are derived from bone marrow or bursa of Fabricius, and T lymphocytes, which are derived from the thymus.

B lymphocytes mediate humoral immune response by virtue of their ability to produce antibody identical to the Ig receptor that is associated with their membrane. The Ig receptor is able to recognize epitopes on the surface of native or partially degraded antigenic macromolecules. T cells mediate cellular immune reactions. In contrast to B cells, T cells, via their T-cell receptor (TCR), do not recognize epitopes on the surface of native antigen. They are able to recognize peptides of various lengths resulting from the degradation of macromolecules taken up by antigen-presenting cells (monocytes, macrophages, dendritic cells, and B cells). They can recognize the peptides only in association with MHC class I molecules, such as a subset of T cells that display CD8 marker or MHC class II and CD1 molecules by T cells that display the CD4 marker.

Adaptive immunity can be divided into two major categories: (a) active adaptive immunity induced by natural exposure to foreign antigen or subsequent to vaccination, and (b) passive immunity resulting from passive transfer of antibodies from mother to newborn (natural, passive immunity) subsequent to parenteral administration of specific antibodies (artificial, passive immunity) or infusion of lymphocytes (adoptive transfer immunity).

Adaptive immunity is characterized by three major features. First, the immune response is specific for 1 billion structurally different antigens, borne by protein, glycoprotein, polysaccharide, lipoprotein, and glycolipid macromolecules. The receptor of the lymphocyte recognizes a single epitope of a macromolecule even if a given macromolecule bears a multitude of epitopes. Each lymphocyte recognizes a given epitope by its receptor: Ig receptor in the case of B cells and TCR in the case of T cells. Antigen-specific lymphocytes exist in the body before exposure to antigen, and the specificity of their receptors was selected during species history by evolutionary Darwinian forces, namely, antigen-selection pressure.

The second main feature of adaptive immunity is the ability of lymphocytes to discriminate self from nonself. This remarkable property is related to the elimination (deletion) or functional inactivation (anergy) of lymphocytes expressing receptors that are specific for self-antigen during fetal development.

The third feature is immunological memory. Subsequent to the exposure to antigen, the pre-existing lymphocytes are activated and differentiate either into effector cells or memory cells. After a new exposure to antigen, the memory cells are rapidly activated, proliferate, and make a prompt specific response, enabling the body to respond specifically and rapidly to antigen. Therefore, the memory cells are lymphocytes that were previously activated by antigen. These cells have a long half-life. Obviously, the prompt response of memory cells to a new exposure to antigen (challenge) represents a beneficial mechanism of adaptive immunity in defense reactions against infectious agents. It is noteworthy that in certain conditions this can be deleterious when the tolerance of lymphocytes to self-antigen is broken down and leads to the occurrence of autoimmune diseases.

The concept of adaptive immunity was derived from three revolutionary discoveries: the discovery of the anti-smallpox vaccine by Jenner, the discovery of the anti-anthrax and rabies vaccines by Pasteur, and the demonstration of passive acquired immunity through injection of anti-diphtheria toxin antibodies by von Behring and Kitasato *(42)*.

The demonstration that antitoxin antibodies prevent diphtheria led to the concept of humoral theory of adaptive immunity, namely, that substances present in body fluids mediate the immune response. Ehrlich *(43)* proposed that these substances actually represented receptors expressed on the surface of cells that are able to interact with antigen based on a chemical complementarity.

The discovery of phagocytosis by Metchnikoff *(1)* provided the framework for cellular theory of the immune response. This theory emerged from the observation that the cells that are able to phagocytize microbes are the major players in the defense reactions. Both theories were proposed in a period when the immunologists ignored the function of lymphocytes. Gowans *(44)* demonstrated later that the lymphocytes are the effectors of specific adaptive immune responses.

However, these theories failed to explain two major features of the adaptive immunity: specificity and tolerance.

The properties of adaptive immunity were explained by Burnet, who proposed the clonal theory *(45)*.

The clonal theory is based on the concept that each lymphocyte is genetically programmed to recognize a single antigenic specificity. Thus, the immune system represents a collection of clones derived from precursors that are able to recognize a single epitope by its receptor. Evolutionary forces during phylogeny selected the genes that encode the specificity of the lymphocyte receptors. The antigen represents the Darwinian selective pressure, and the diversity of the immune response results from a random rearrangement of genes that encode the lymphocyte receptor, which diversify may be amplified further by the somatic hypermutation process throughout life. Therefore, once the antigen enters into the body, it selects the clone that bears a complementary receptor for a given epitope.

A unifying element of clonal theory is the ability of lymphocyte clones to discriminate self from nonself. Burnet proposed that the clones that are able to recognize self-antigen are deleted during ontogeny. Thus, clonal theory proposed that both the randomization of specificity for foreign antigen and tolerance susceptibility for self-antigen are limited to the ontogenetic and perinatal period of the development of the immune system.

Clonal theory became a paradigm for the immunologists since a large body of experimental evidence supported it. Thus, the following was demonstrated:

(a) The lymphocytes belonging to the same clone bind a single antigen and lymphocytes could be eliminated if the antigen is labeled with a radioactive element.
(b) In a heterozygous animal, a B cell makes antibodies by carrying a single allotype and idiotype genetic marker. The allotypes are antigenic markers of heavy or light chains of Ig molecules that are shared by all individuals of a genotypically identical, inbred strain or by groups of individuals of outbred species. The idiotypes are phenotypic markers of V genes that encode the Ig receptor of B cells or TCR receptor of T cells.
(c) All the progenitors of a clone share identical genes that encode the specificity of their receptor (ref. *49*).

Burnet *(45)* postulated that unresponsiveness to self-antigen results from the process of deletion of self-reactive clones during ontogeny (clonal deletion), which leads to central tolerance. Central tolerance occurs as a result of negative selection in central lymphoid organs—in bone marrow where B cells are generated and in the thymus where T cells develop. The concept of negative selection of B cells is well supported by studies carried out in transgenic mice. Thus, in mice, it has been shown that B cells that express V_H and V_L genes, which encode antibodies specific for allogeneic MHC class I molecules *(46)* or hen egg lysozyme (HEL), have been deleted *(47)*.

Clonal theory views the immune system as disconnected clones that are waiting to encounter an antigen, which induces their expansion and differentiation into effector cells.

Jerne *(48)* proposed a theory that pictured the immune system as a network in which the clones speak to each other using idiotype dictionary. The idiotype expressed on the receptor of a clone can be recognized by the receptor of a different clone, and this type of recognition of self-structures ensures the connectivity of clones that make up the immune system.

The network theory is based on the following three major postulates:

(a) The idiotypes expressed on the receptors of lymphocytes function as links between clones exhibiting various specificities, and as a target for regulatory mechanisms, which control expansion of clones in various stages of the ontogenetic development of the immune system and in various stages of the immune response.

(b) Idiotypes are internal images of antigen and, therefore, represent links between the external universe of foreign antigen and the inner immune system.

(c) Through a self-recognition process, idiotypes can activate a cascade of complementary clones (operationally called anti-idiotypes), which display regulatory functions. The activation of clones by anti-idiotypic antibodies can replace the stimulation by foreign antigen. The idiotype-mediated suppression shall prevent overwhelming of the immune system by a clone that is expanded subsequent to antigen stimulation (reviewed in ref. *49*).

4. CELLS OF THE IMMUNE SYSTEM

4.1. Phenotypic Characteristics of Mature Cells Involved in Innate Immunity

The cells mediating innate immunity, an important first line of defense, are the granulocytes (neutrophils, eosinophils, and basophils), monocyte-macrophages, and dendritic and NK cells. Each type of cells exhibits different phenotypes based on cell structure, the expression of different membrane cytodifferentiation antigen and receptors, enzyme content, and the display of different functions.

4.1.1. Neutrophils

Neutrophils represent approx 60% of total white blood cells (WBCs). These cells are 10–15 μm in diameter, with slightly basophilic cytoplasm and indented nuclei, which characterize the young (band) cells, and with polylobated nuclei, which are characteristic for older (segmented) cells. Within the cytoplasm, three types of granules can be observed: (a) primary, or azurophilic, granules, which stain purple with Giemsa; (b) secondary granules, which stain faintly pink with Giemsa; and (c) peroxisomes. Primary and secondary granules are typical lysosomes, which fuse with endosomes containing phagocytized particles that are degraded by the enzymes contained in these granules (Fig. 1).

Primary granules contain various types of hydrolyzes that have an optimal activity at pH 5.0, including lysozyme and cationic proteins. Secondary granules contain lysozyme, collagenase, cytochrome, vitamin B_{12}-binding protein, and lactoferrin. The peroxisomes contain myeloperoxidase, which reduces oxygen and hydrogen peroxide (Table 5).

The neutrophils express some cytodifferentiation antigen, which are shared with other WBCs and various receptors. Some of these receptors bind to growth factors that are essential for the differentiation of myeloid cells. Another set of receptors is involved in the internalization of immune complexes and bacteria covered with IgG opsonins and complement. The neutrophils express receptors that bind to chemokines or to chemoatractans formyl peptides (FPR, mFPR1, mFPR2). These receptors play an important role in the migration of

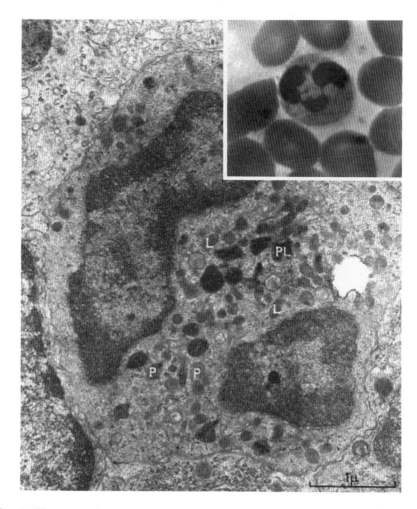

Fig. 1. Electron micrograph and light microscopy of a neutrophil. Multilobated nucleus with predominant heterochromatin. The cytoplasm is packed with an abundant variety of granules: lysosome (L); phagolysosomes (PL), which are mostly clear; peroxisome (P); and azurophilic granules, which are the darkest.

neutrophils from the blood to tissue and, in particular, toward inflammatory foci caused by pathogens. In general, the movements of neutrophils are random. However, when the local medium contains formyl peptides derived from bacteria, the neutrophils move toward the source of peptides, a phenomenon called chemotaxis. The chemotaxis allows for the accumulation of leukocytes at the site of microbial infection and inflammation. The FPRs expressed in human neutrophils have an important role in innate immunity. For example, dysfunctional FPR alleles were associated with juvenile peridontitis *(50)*. There

Table 5
Proteins and Enzymes Contained Within Neutrophils
Granules Primary, Azurophilic Granules

Enzymes

PRIMARY GRANULES
    Cathepsins, collagenases, proteinas-3, elastases, lysosyme,
    α-manno-sidase, β-galactosidase, β-glucuronidase,
    β-glycerphosphatase N-acetyl-β-glucoseaminidase,
    meyloperoxidase lipase, α-amylase, phosphlipases,
    nucleases

Proteins

Cationic proteins, α-defensin

SECONDARY GRANULES   Enzymes

    Collagenases, lysozyme

Proteins

    Lactoferrin, cytochrome b, vitamin B12-BP
    Peroxisomes

Enzymes

Peroxydases

are also receptors for various cytokines, such as CD118 binding to IFN-α and -β and CD132 binding to IL-2 and receptors for IL-4, IL-7, and IL-14 cytokines (Table 6).

The main function of neutrophils is to internalize particulate antigen by phagocytosis and soluble macromolecules by pinocytosis. Figures 2 and 3 show neutrophils phagocytizing autologous red blood cells (RBCs) treated with lecithinase and the pinocytosis of fluoresceine-labeled Dick erythrotoxin.

The opsonin antibodies that bind complement enhance phagocytosis. This was clearly demonstrated in the phenomenon of immunoadherance *(51)*. Figure 4 shows the kinetics of phagocytosis using neutrophils of *Staphylococci* that are bound to RBC covered with antibacterial opsonins and complement. Recent studies showed that endosomes bearing vesicle-associated protein 3 (VAMP3) fuse with the plasma membrane at the site where phagocytosis is initiated, and subsequently, the phago-endosome is internalized. This process contributes to the preservation of the cell membrane during phagocytosis, avoiding loss and preserving the integrity of the membrane *(52)*. Phagocytosis induces the activation of Ras-ERK MAPK module in neutrophils. In contrast, phagocytosis that is initiated by FcγR recruits Syk (reviewed in ref. *53*).

Table 6
CD Antigens and Receptors Associated With Neutrophil's Membrane

CD antigens	
CD65 (poly-*N*-acetyllactose amine), CD69 CD165 (sialomucine), CD94 (C-type lectin)	

Receptor	Ligand
α-integrin family	
CD11a	ICAM-1.3
CD11b	ICAM-1
CD11c	Fibrinogen, iC3b
β-integrin family	
CD18	ICAM-1-3, fibrinogen, iC3b
CD29	Collagen, Laminin, fibronectin
Complement receptors	
CD35	C3b, C4b
CD46	C3b,C4b
CD48	Cb2
CD88	C5a
Fc receptors	
CD23	Ig Fcε
CD64 (FcγRI, CD32 FcγRII)	Ig Fcγ
Growth factor receptors	
CD114	G-CSF
CD116	GM-CSF
Interleukin receptors	
CD118	IFNα and β
CD132	IL-2, IL-4, IL-7, IL-14, IL-15
CD153	TNF-α
Chemokine receptors	
CD128	IL-8
CXCR2	CXCL2,CXCL3, CXCL5
CXCR1	CXCL7, CXCL8, CXCL9, CCl24
Chemotactic receptors	
FFR, mFR1, mFPR2, FPRL1	Formyl-peptides

Abbreviations: ICAM, intercellular adhesion molecule; C, complement; FCR, Fc receptor; G-CSF, granulocyte-colony stimulating factor; GM-SCF, granulocyte monocyte-colony stimulating factor; FPR, formyl-peptide receptor.

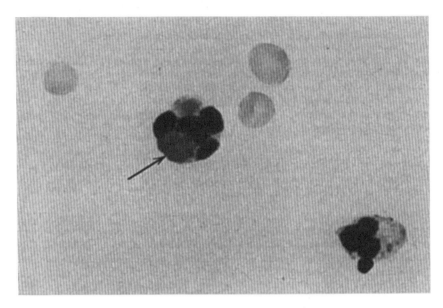

Fig. 2. Phagocytosis of autologous red cells was following treatment with periodic acid. May-Grunwald- Giemsa staining of guinea pig neutrophils (×1, 250). (From Bona C et al. Nature [London] 1967; 213:824–825.)

By virtue of the broad specificity of hydrolyses contained in lysosomes, the phagocytized or pinocytized materials are completely degraded and, therefore, the neutrophils are unable to present antigen to T cells, which suggests that their major function is in innate immunity. Adaptive immunity via opsonins, antibodies specific for particulate antigen, enhances the function of neutrophil in the innate immune processes.

A major link between innate and adaptive immunity exists in the cytokine network. The cytokines produced by cells that mediate innate immunity display immunomodulatory properties on lymphocytes, and the cytokines that are secreted by lymphocytes modulate the function of cells involved in the innate immunity. In spite of the fact that the neutrophils are terminally differentiated, short-lived cells, they produce some cytokines or chemokines subsequent to exposure to antigen, such as LPS, which binds to Toll receptors, or C5a, which binds to complement receptors. Thus, LPS induces the synthesis of the cytokines, such as IL-1β, TNF-α, TGF-β, or IL-8 and MIP-1 chemokines *(53)*.

4.1.2. Eosinophils

Eosinophils constitute 3–5% of total WBCs. Structurally, they are cells of 10–15 µm in diameter, with bilobated nuclei and cytoplasm that is full of granules that stain bright red with eosin. The granules contain unique crystalloid

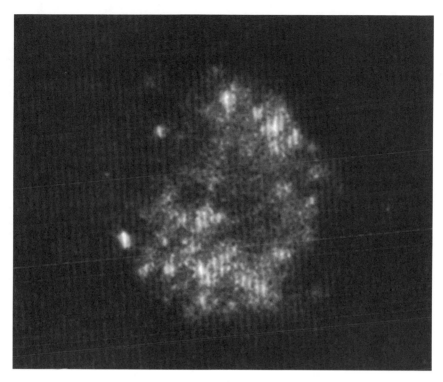

Fig. 3. Pinocytosis of fluorescein-labeled *Salmonella typiymurium* endotoxin by guinea pig neutrophil. The pinocytosis was observed in fluorescent microscopy 45 min after incubation of cells with labeled endotoxin.

core structures (Charcot–Leyden) that are composed of several basic proteins (Fig. 5).

In contrast to neutrophil granules, eosinophil granules contain fewer hydrolytic enzymes (arylsulfatses, acid phosphatase, ribonuclease, cathepsins, and lysophospholipases) but are richer in major basic proteins, which are toxic for eukaryotic cells, and cationic proteins, which are toxic for prokaryotic and eukaryotic cells.

The eosinophils express receptors for Fc fragments of IgG, IgA, IgE, receptors for complement (C1q, C5a), and growth factors (G-CSF and GM-CSF).

Eosinophils can internalize macromolecules and, in certain conditions, generate peptides from the processing of internalized macromolecules. Antigen-presenting property was shown by the ability of murine and human eosinophils to present peptides derived from ovalbumin (OVA) to activate OVA-specific T cells *(54)* and by the ability of human eosinophils to present peptides derived from foreign proteins *(55)*. The antigenic-presenting property is related to the

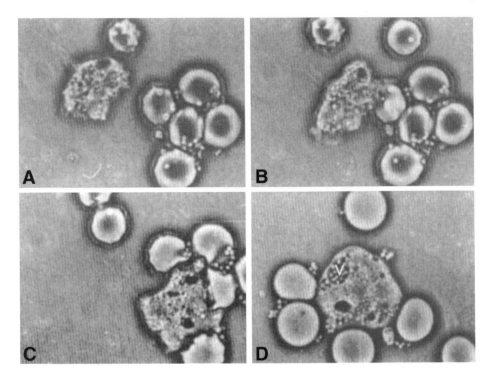

Fig. 4. Phenomenon of immunoadherence. Red blood cells coated with specific antibodies were incubated with complement and bacteria and then with guinea pig peritoneal cells. The figure represents four different steps analyzed by microcinematography. It is noteworthy that in the last figures, the majorities of bacteria were phagocytized and are present in vacuole (V) .

ability of eosinophils activated by GM-CSF to induce higher expression of class II molecules, which present the peptides to CD4 T cells *(55)*.

The major function of eosinophils in innate immunity is related to defense reaction against higher-ordered eukaryotic parasites such as helminths. They also play a role in allergic diseases. In both instances, the number of eosinophils in the blood is increased (eosinophilia).

4.1.3. Basophils

Basophils represent 1% of WBCs in humans but are found in all vertebrate—and some invertebrate—species. Frederick von Recklinghausen reported the first description of basophils in 1863, and, in 1879, Ehrlich described the same cells in various tissues and called them Mastzellen: the mast cells. These cells were named basophils because of strong metachromatic staining of granules

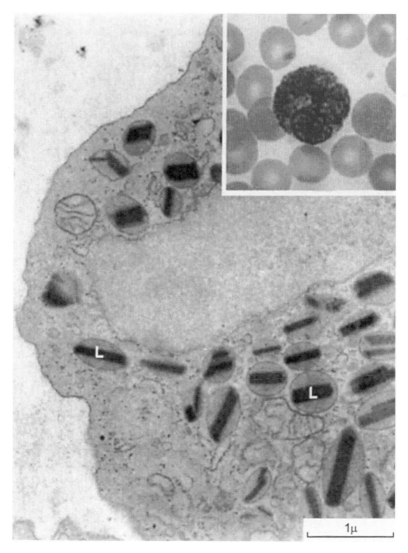

Fig. 5. Electron micrograph and light microscopy of an eosinophil. The cytoplasm of this guinea pig eosinophil contains many granules. The granules contain a unique crystalloid core structure (Charcot–Leyden) composed of several basic proteins (L).

with Toluidine blue, which is because their contents are rich in anionic substances (Fig. 6). The granules of basophils and mast cells contain proteoglycan, biogenic amines, leukotrines, and hydrolytic enzymes (Table 7). Several receptors and glycoproteins are associated with the membranes of basophils and mast cells (Table 8).

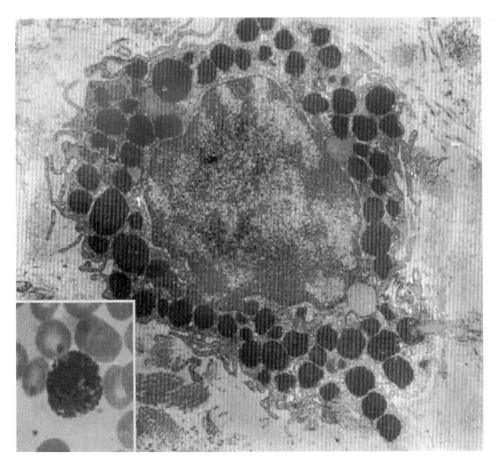

Fig. 6. Electron micrograph and light microscopy of a mastocyte. The cytoplasm is packed with large granules strongly metachromatically stained with Toluidine blue because their contents are rich in anionic substances. The granules of basophils and mast cells contain proteoglycan, biogenic amines, leukotrines, and hydrolytic enzymes.

The binding of ligands to some receptors caused degranulation of basophils, leading to the release of a broad variety of proteins and biogenic amines, which play an important role in innate immunity, inflammatory processes, and allergic diseases. Among these receptors, one may cite FcεR, which is capable of binding IgE-antigen complexes. The activation of basophils via the IgE receptor plays an important role in inflammation and adaptive immunity but not in innate immunity because IgE activation is totally dependent on Th2 cells. IgE-mediated degranulation leads to the release of histamine, heparin, β-glucuronidase, and eosinophilic chemotactic factor. All these factors are important mediators of acute inflammatory processes.

Table 7
Content of Granules and Protein Secreted by Mast Cells

Biogenic amines: histamine and serotonin
Peptidoglycans: chondroitin sulfate A, B, E, heparin
Proteases: tryptase chymase carboxypeptidase, cathepsin G,
    neutral protease (MMCP 1,2,3,4,5,6)
Hydrolases: β-glucuronidase, lysophospholipase, elastase,
    acid phosphatase,
Oxigenase: cyclo oxigenase-2
Bioactive proteins: endothelin, eosinophil chemotactic factor,
    leukotriene, major basic protein
Interleukins: IL-4, TNF-α, IL-Iβ , IL-13, IL-9

Toll receptors (TLR 2, 4, and 9), which are capable of binding to LPS and CpG, and complement receptors are also expressed on the surface of mast cells.

Like neutrophils, human and murine mast cells can phagocytize and kill gram-positive and gram-negative bacteria *(56–58)* through a combination of nonoxidative and oxidative killing system. The phagocytosis of bacteria is mediated by opsonizing complement components *(59)*. This was elegantly demonstrated by taking advantage of a mast cell-deficient murine strain W/Wv. This mouse strain bears a mutation at the W locus, which encodes the c-Kit receptor for stem cell factor (SCF), a growth factor required for the differentiation of myeloid progenitor in basophils *(60)*. These mice are less efficient in clearing the bacteria and succumb faster to bacterial infection when compared to wild mice *(61)*.

The mast cells produce several interleukins subsequent to activation resulting from the binding of ligands to Fc receptors such as IL-4, TNF α, IL-1, IL-3, IL-6, and GM-CSF, endothelin (ET-1) *(62)* and leukotrines (LTC4) *(63)*. The mast cells play an important role in innate immunity by recruiting neutrophils and eosinophils through chemotactic factors such as eosinophil chemotactic factor, leukotriene B4, and others. Thus, it was shown that neutrophil influx after peritoneal injection of *E. coli* is reduced after pretreatment with leukotriene inhibitor *(64)*. Furthermore, studies carried out in MC-deficient mice have shown that reduced killing ability of bacteria correlated directly with reduced neutrophil infiltration in the lung and increased mortality and morbidity in a model of acute septic peritonitis *(58)*.

The interaction of mast cells with lymphocytes is supported by observations showing that after the phagocytosis of live bacteria or bacterial products, the mast cells process antigen and are able to present peptides, which are associated with MHC class I molecules, to antigen-specific T-cell lines *(65,66)*.

Table 8
Receptors Associated With Mast Cell Membrane

Receptor	Ligand
CD117(c-kit)	SCF
Adenosin receptors (A2A, A2B, A3)	Adenosine
ETB	Endothelin-1
Interleukin receptors	
CD125	IL-5
CD118	IFN-α and -β
α-integrin family	
CD11a	ICAM-1.3
CD11b	ICAM-1
CD11c	Fibrinogen, iC3b
β-integrin family	
CD18	ICAM-1-3, fibrinogen
iC3b	
CD29	Collagen, laminin
Fibronectin	
Fc receptors	
CD23	Ig Fcε
CD64 (FcγRI), CD32 (FcγRII) , CD16 (FcγRIII)	Ig Fcγ
Growth factor receptors	
CD114	G-CSF
CD116	GM-CSF
LPS receptors	
CD14, TolR 2, TolR 4	
Complement receptors	
CD88	C5a
Chemokine receptors	
CCR3	CCL24, CCL11
CCR2	CCL13, CCL2
Cannabinoid receptors	
CB1	Endocannabinoid
CB2	Endocannabinoid
Other membrane-associated molecules	

CD65 (poly-*N*- acetyllactose amine), CD69 and CD165 (sialomucine), CD66 (C-type lectin)
CDw17 (lactosyl ceramide), CD33 (sialoadhesin), CD48 having as a CD2 ligand

Abbreviations: SCF, stem cell factor; ICAM, intercellular adhesion molecule.

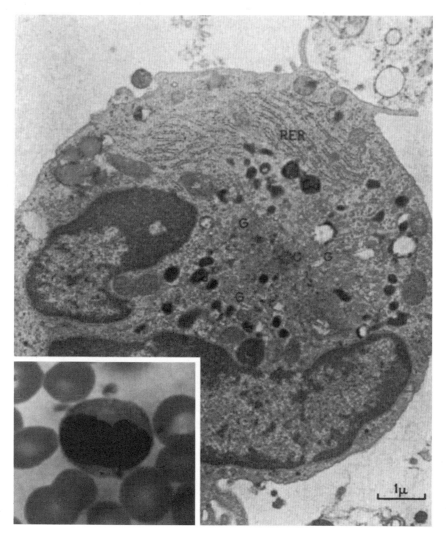

Fig. 7. Electron micrograph and light microscopy of a guinea pig lymph node and blood monocyte. The monocytes are spherical cells 10–40 μm in diameter with an oval or kidney-shaped nucleus with two prominent nucleoli. The cytoplasm is rich in rough endoplasmic reticulum (RER) developed Golgi apparatus (G), mitochondria, and lysosomes (Cd). A centriole can also be observed (C).

4.1.4. Monocyte-Macrophages

The blood monocytes are spherical cells of 10–40 μm in diameter with oval or kidney-shaped nuclei with two prominent nucleoli. The cytoplasm is rich in rough endoplasmic reticulum (ER)-developed Golgi apparata, mitochondria, and lysosomes (Fig. 7). Blood monocytes migrate in various tissues and inter-

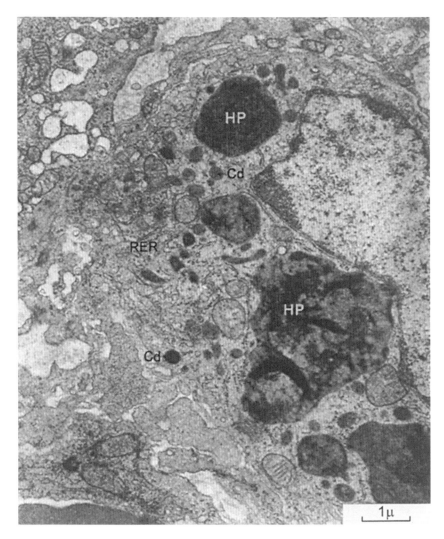

Fig. 8. Electron micrograph of a guinea pig splenic macrophage. The cytoplasm contains large heterophagosomes (HPS); numerous lysosomes (Cd); mitochondria; and a well developed RER.

nal cavities such as the peritoneum, pleura, or pericardium. Fixed and differentiated monocytes in various tissues are most commonly called macrophages. Macrophages can be divided in normal and inflammatory macrophages. Normal macrophages include macrophages in connective tissues and skin (histiocytes), liver (Kupffer's cells), lung (free and fixed), spleen and lymph nodes, central nervous system ([CNS]; microglia), cartilage (chondroclasts), bones (osteoclasts), and serous cavities (peritoneal, pericardia, and pleura) (Table 8).

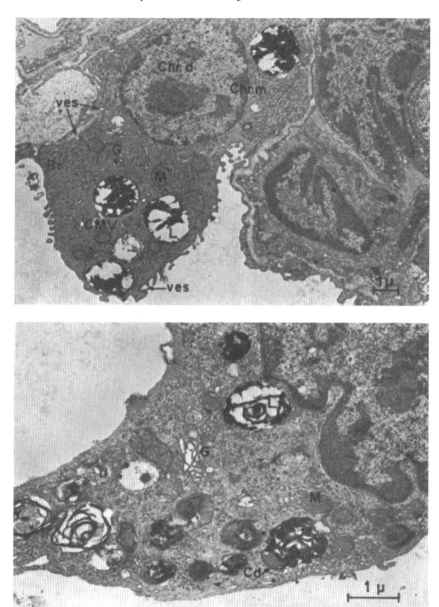

Fig. 9. Electron micrograph of guinea pig lung macrophages. In the nucleus, the diffuse chromatin (Chr d) is predominant and dense heterochromatine (Chr m) is located in close contact with the nuclear membrane. The cytoplasm contains a developed Golgi apparatus (G), numerous mitochondria (M), large empty vesicles (ves) and multivesicular bodies (CMV), and a few lysosomes (Cd).

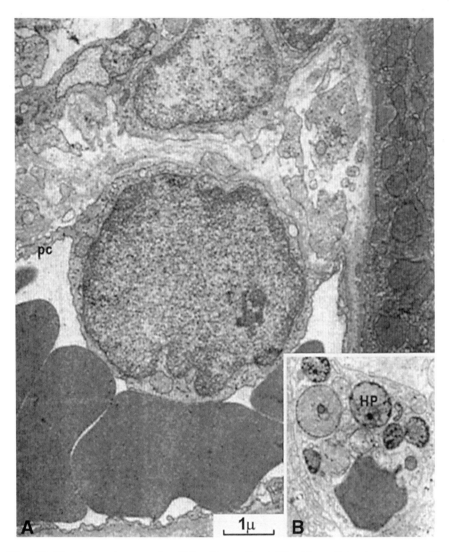

Fig. 10. Electron micrograph of Kupffer cells. A Kupffer cell is characterized by a large nucleus with cytoplasm prolongation (pc). The left square shows an abundance of heterophagosomes.

Despite the fact that macrophages undergo some morphological changes after fixation in tissues, they share basic structural features with blood monocytes (Figs. 8–10). However, the macrophages isolated from different tissue display a diversity of phenotypes and functions. The heterogeneity of fixed macrophage population may arise in part on signal received from immediate microenvironment and from unique condition within specific tissues.

Tissue macrophages may also differ in the expression of antigen or other molecules that are associated with their membranes. For example, human lung macrophages express an antigen that is not found at the surface of alveolar or peritoneal macrophages. In contrast to peritoneal macrophages, which express poor-class II MHC molecules, human alveolar macrophages express high levels of class II molecules.

Thus, functional heterogeneity of macrophage population depends on tissue environmental factors, which contribute in different ways to the maturation of blood monocytes into macrophages.

The lysosomes of monocyte-macrophages are rich in hydrolyses that are bable to degrade and process phagocytized particulate antigen or pinocytized macromolecules. In addition, the macrophages synthesize and secrete peptide hormones (erythropoietin, adrenocorticotropic hormone, β-endorphin, thymosin), some complement components, coagulation factors, arachidonic acid metabolites (prostaglandin, leukotriens, thromboxanes), and various interleukins (IL-1, IL-6, TNF-α, TGF-β, interferons) and growth factors (fibroblast and platelet-derived growth factors and colony-stimulating factors) (reviewed in ref. *67*). These broad varieties of bioactive substances produced by macrophages suggests that beside their major role in innate immunity, they can interact with other cells by regulating their functions and contributing to the maintenance of macromolecular homeostasis.

The major role of macrophages in innate immunity consists in their ability to phagocytize and destroy bacteria and to inhibit the growth of obligatory intracellular bacteria when they are activated by interleukins, which are secreted by lymphocytes. The monocyte-macrophages are able to present peptides, which result from the processing of internalized microbes or self- and nonself-macromolecules to both CD4 and CD8 T cells, because they express both class I and class II MHC molecules.

4.1.5. Dendritic Cells (Table 9)

Dendritic cells, discovered by Steinman and Cohn *(68)*, play an important role in innate and adaptive immunity. The dendritic cells are the most efficient antigen-presenting cells in initiation of specific immune responses, because the mature dendritic cells express class II and class I MHC molecules and costimulatory factors that are required for the activation of T cells *(69)*. The distinctive tissue distribution of dendritic cells has been outlined using a common set of criteria, especially the isolation of MHC II-rich, nonadherent, nonphagocytic cells. Large, stellate, MHC class II-rich cells are present in the blood and lymph *(70)* (Fig. 11). They are found in the T-cell area of peripheral lymphoid organs: spleen, lymph nodes, and Peyer's patches *(71)*. In various species, the dendritic cells also are found in peripheral tissues, including skin, airways, gut, and vagina *(72–76)*. Murine dendritic cells are characterized by

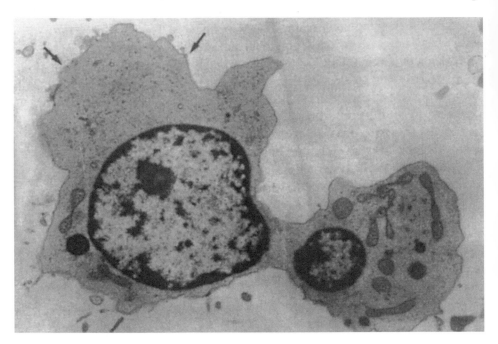

Fig. 11. Electron micrograph of a dendritic cell. In the nucleus, the diffuse chromatin is predominant and a nucleoli could be identified The cytoplasm is rich in mitochondria and smooth endoplasmic reticulum and contains a few lysosomes. (From Knight SC Int Rev Immunol 1990;6:166.)

the expression of some cytodifferentiation antigen, such as CD11c; CD11b; 33D1; CD8α; high expression of MHC class II molecules (reviewed in ref. *77*); endocytic receptors, such as DEC-205 *(78)* or mannose/fucose receptors *(79)*; costimulatory molecules (CD40, CD86, CD89); receptors for interleukins, such as IL-3R *(80)*; and receptors for chemokines *(77)*. Whereas the immature dendritic cells express CCR1-CCR5 chemokine receptors, the mature dendritic cells express only CCR7 chemokine receptor.

The role of dendritic cells in innate immunity is illustrated by the fact that they express almost all Toll receptors involved in the recognition of PAMPs, which transduce signals leading to activation of NF-κB through MyD88-dependent or -independent pathways (reviewed in ref. *81*).

Dendritic cells are a heterogeneous cell population composed of several subsets of lymphoid or myeloid origin *(82)*. Plasmacytoid dendritic cells of lymphoid origin are localized in the thymic cortex and T-cell zone cells of lymphoid organs. They are able to take up and process antigen and to prime both CD4 and CD8 T cells. After maturation, they secrete IL-12 and type I IFN *(83)*. In mouse, plasmacytoid dendritic cells express CD8α, CD4, CD11a,

Table 9
Tissue Localization of Monocyte-Derived Macrophages

Name	Organ location
Microglia	Brain
Kupffer cell	Liver
Chondroclast	Growing cartilage
Osteoclast	Bone
Histiocyte	Connective tissue
Mesangial cell	Kidney
Alveolar macrophage	Lung
Macrophage	Peripheral lymphoid organs, peritoneal, pleural, pericardic cavities, placenta, milk

Adapted from ref. *79.*

CD11c, CD40, CD43, B220 (CD45R), CD54 antigen, IL-3 R, and class II MHC molecules. In humans, plasmacytoid dendritic cells express CD45RA, CD123 BDCA-2, and BDCA-4.

Interstitial, CD8α- dendritic cells of myeloid origin are localized in marginal zone of spleen, subcapsular sinuses of lymph nodes, and the subepithelial dome of Peyer's patches. They are able to take up and process antigen and to prime naive T cells (reviewed in refs. *84,85*).

Langerhans cells (LCs) are also derived from myeloid lineage dendritic cells *(86)*. They express distinctive markers such as Birbeck granules, langerin, and E-cadherin *(77)*. They are localized in the skin and epithelia. After antigen stimulation and maturation, the LCs migrate to T-cell zones of peripheral lymphoid organs. They are able to capture and process antigen *(86,87)*. We have shown that they are transfected in vivo after subcutaneous administration of naked DNA. Transfected LCs migrate to regional lymph nodes and are able to present peptides to and stimulate both CD4 and CD8 T cells *(88,89)*. Our data and those reported by others *(90,91)* strongly suggest that transfection and activation of dendritic cells represent a key element in the immune responses that are induced by DNA vaccination. The phenotypic characteristics of dendritic cell are illustrated in Table 10.

In the blood and various tissues, the dendritic cells are immature. Following the ingestion of antigen by pinocytosis or phagocytosis, immature dendritic cells undergo maturation both in vivo and in vitro *(92,93)*. The maturation leads to reduced uptake capabilities, increased antigen processing, and enhanced expression of class II and costimulatory molecules. Mature dendritic cells are more immunogenic than immature dendritic cells.

Table 10
Phenotypic Characteristics of Mature Dendritic Cells Subsets

A. Murine dendritic cells

Myeloid-derived dendritic cells		Lymphoid-derived dendritic cells
Interstitial	Langerhans dendritic cells	Plasmoid dendritic cells
CD11c	CD11c	CD11c
CD11b	CD11b	CD11b±
MHC class II	MHC class II	MHC class II
CD4	CD4	CD8 α
CD13		
CD33		
CD123		
CD86	CD86	CD86
CD40	CD40	CD40
DEC205	DEC205	
	Birbeck granule	
	Langerin	

B. Human dendritic cells

Interstitial	Langerhans dendritic cells	Plasmoid dendritic cells	
CD11c	CD11c	CD11c	
CD11b	CD11b		
CD1a	CD1a		
MHC class II	MHC class II	MHC class II	
CD4	CD4	CD4	
CD13	CD13		
CD33	CD33		
CD86	CD86		
CD40	CD40		
DC-LAMP	DC-LAMP		
TLR 1,2, 4,5, 8,		TLR 7,9	
	Birbeck granule		
	Langerin		
		CD62L	
		CD123	
Follicular dendritic cells			
CD11b	CD14	CD54	CD32
CD23	CD19	CD73	VCAM-1
CD64	CD21	CD45	
CD19	CD29	CD23	
CD21	CD40	CD74	

Abbreviations: TLR, toll receptor; DC, dendritic cells; VCAM-1, vascular cell adhesion molecule-1.

During maturation, the level of cysatin C, which is an inhibitor of cathepsins, is downregulated. This allows the processing of the invariant chain in endosomes, favoring the generation of MHC-peptide complexes and their movement to the cell surface where they can be recognized by T cells *(94)*. Upon maturation, myeloid dendritic cells produce several cytokines, such as IL-10, IL-12, IL-15, IL-23, and IFN-γ. The LCs produce IL-12, and lymphoid-derived plasmoid dendritic cells produce IL-12, IFN-γ, and IFN-α *(95–97)*. A hallmark of the dendritic cell maturation process is the upregulation of the CCR7 receptor for CCL19 and CCL21 chemokines that are produced in the T-cell area of lymphoid organs *(98)*. These chemokines favor the migration of immature dendritic cells to lymphoid organs. The dendritic cells also produce chemokines. Whereas myeloid-derived dendritic cells produce CCL17 and CCL22, the plasmoid dendritic cells produce CCL3 chemokine *(99)*.

Recent studies have underlined the role of dendritic cells in innate immunity by their ability to activate the NK cells *(100,101)*, which supports the concept that dendritic cells can play an important role in the immune surveillance of malignancies and antimicrobial defense reactions *(102)*.

Follicular dendritic cells are localized in primary follicles and the light zone of germinal centers induced by antigen stimulation. They bind and retain immunocomplexes and activate resting B cells to become effective antigen-presenting cells *(103)*, Follicular dendritic cells promote the proliferation and maturation of B cells and prevent B cells from undergoing apoptosis *(104)*. In contrast to macrophages and dendritic cells, the follicular dendritic cells do not internalize and process antigen.

4.1.6. NK Cells

NK cells constitute 10–15% of peripheral blood lymphocytes. Their morphological structure resembles the circulating resting lymphocyte except for the richness in granules, which exhibit different staining patterns compared to the granules of polymorphonuclear cells (Fig.12). In contrast to lymphocytes, the NK cells do not express TCR, CD3, CD4, or CD8, which are characteristic of T lymphocytes. They express CD2, CD56, CD 57, CD58, CD11a cytodifferentiation antigen, and CD16, which is the receptor for Fcγ fragment of IgG. A subset of NK cells expresses a receptor for a Fcμ fragment *(105)*. The NK cells can kill virus-infected or tumor cells.

The NK cell population is heterogeneous: one subset, which represents the majority of NK cells (90%), expresses a low CD56 level and a high amount of CD16; the second subset expresses a low amount of CD56 and lacks CD16 *(106)*. This suggests that the first subset mediates ADCMC lysis of target cells, whereas the second subset mediates spontaneous cytotoxic reaction. CD16, which is FcγRIII, plays a major role in ADCMC because it binds to an Fcγ fragment of antibody that is specific for an antigen expressed by target cells; this brings NK

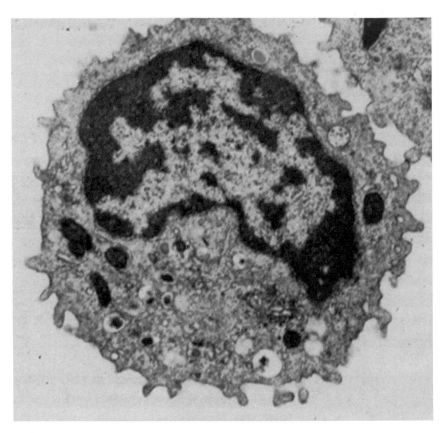

Fig. 12. Electron micrograph of a human NK cell. In the nucleus, the dense chromatin is predominant. The cytoplasm contains numerous vacuoles, dense particles, and mitochondria. (Courtesy of Dr. A. Sulica Laboratory of Immunology, Romanian Academy, Bucharest.)

and target cells in close contact and leads to exocytosis of granules and the release of perforin, which mediates the killing of the target cell.

The NK cells express nonclonal receptors such as CD94/NKG2, which binds to nonclassical HLA-E, and KIR receptor. The KIR receptor represents a family of inhibitory receptors that recognizes class I MHC molecules (HLA-A, B, and C). These receptors recognize different allotypic forms of HLA-A, B, and C (reviewed in ref. *41*).

The NK cells produce various cytokines such as IL-2, IL-15, IFN-γ, IL-12, IL-10, and TNF-α, and lymphotoxin. The lymphotoxin may play an important role in apoptosis and killing of tumor cells (reviewed in ref. *106*).

NK cells play a role in innate immunity—in particular, in the earliest phases of viral infections and in elimination of tumor cells.

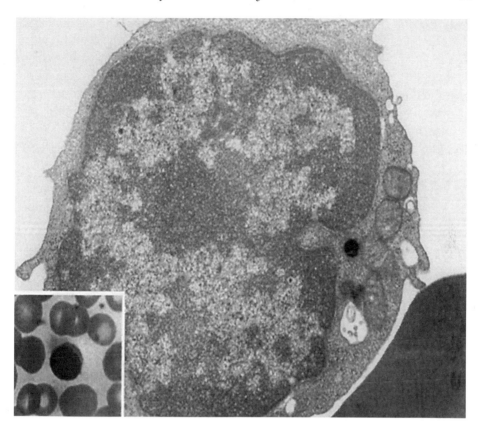

Fig. 13. Electron micrograph and light microcroscopy of a guinea pig lymphocyte. The lymphocytes are small and round cells of 7–9 μm in diameter, with a large nucleus dominated by heterochromatin, a thin rim of cytoplasm containing a few lysosomes, and mitochondria.

4.2. Lymphocytes: Effector Cells of Adaptive Immunity

Lymphocytes are the primary immune cells that mediate adaptive immunity. Lymphocytes are of two main types: B lymphocytes, which derive from the bursa of Fabricius in birds and from bone marrow in mammals, and T lymphocytes, which derive from the thymus. Morphologically, there are no differences between the two subsets. The lymphocytes are small and round cells approx 7–9 μm in diameter, with large nuclei dominated by heterochromatin, thin rims of cytoplasm containing a few lysosomes, and mitochondria (Fig. 13). The major difference between the two populations consists of the structure and function of the antigen-specific receptor. The cognitive B-cell receptor (BCR) is the immunoglobulin (i.e., IgM on young B cells; IgM and IgD on mature, resting B lymphocytes; and IgG, IgA ,or IgE on activated and differentiated B cells).

In Fig. 14, the presence of the IgG receptor is visualized subsequent to incubation of a rabbit lymphocyte with ^{125}I-labeled anti-rabbit IgG antibody.

The lymphocytes that derive from a given clone bear a structurally identical Ig receptor, which is able to bind the antigen. Figure 15 illustrates an autoradiograph that is showing the binding of biosynthetically ^{14}C-labeled LPS to the Ig receptor. Through an Ig receptor, the B cells can bind to an epitope that is present on the surface of native antigen as well as on peptide epitopes derived from the degradation of antigen.

B cells display two major functions: the production of antibodies and the presentation of peptides to T cells.

The synthesis and secretion of antibodies are induced by the activation of B cells subsequent to binding of the antigen to the BCR and their subsequent differentiation into plasma cells. Figure 16 illustrates main cytological features of plasma cells, which are oval cells 30 μm in diameter with strong basophilic cytoplasm that is filled with highly developed ER.

A B-cell subpopulation is divided into two subsets. The B-1 subset expresses CD5 antigen and produces mainly IgM antibodies that are specific for self-antigen *(107)* or displays multispecific binding properties to self- and nonself-antigen *(108)*. The B-2, CD5$^-$ B subset represents the majority of B cells and produces antibodies against foreign antigen and pathogenic autoantibodies *(109)*.

The second important function of B cells is the ability to internalize macromolecules through fluid pinocytosis to process the antigen and to present the peptides associated with MHC molecules to T cells. Figure 16 illustrates the pinocytosis of horseradish peroxidase by an activated B cell.

Third, the stimulated B cells are able to synthesize and secrete cytokines and chemokines. They bear receptors for cytokines and chemokines.

The T-cell population is divided into three major subsets that are based on the specific expression of CD antigen CD4, CD8, and NK T cells and into two subsets that are based on the genes that encode the TCR, such as α/β T cells and γ/δ T cells.

In contrast to B cells, which recognize the antigenic determinants on the surface of native antigen, through the TCR, the T cells recognize only peptides that are derived from the processing of antigen by antigen-presenting cells. CD4 T cells recognize peptides in association with class II or CD1 MHC molecules; the CD8 T cells recognize peptides in association with class I MHC molecules; and the NK T cells recognize peptides in association with CD1 molecules.

The CD4 subset is composed of discrete subsets, which can be distinguished by their functions, such as synthesis of cytokines, mediation of Ig class switching, regulatory properties, and expression of different transcription factors. These subsets do not express specific CD antigen. These discrete subsets in mice are called Th1, Th2, Th3, and the regulatory cells Tr1, CD4$^+$ CD25^{high}.

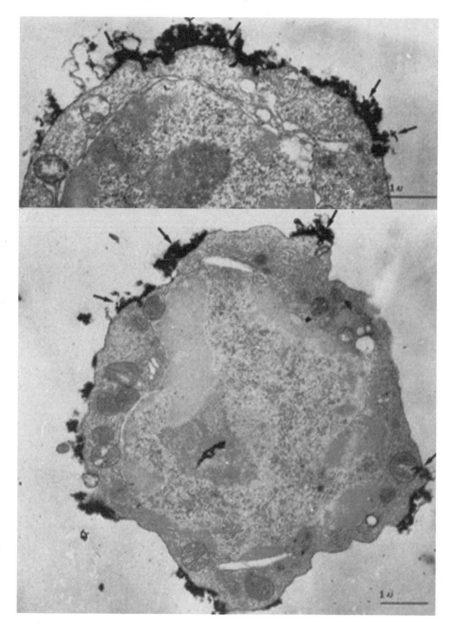

Fig. 14. Electron micrograph of a rabbit lymphocyte incubated with ^{125}I-labeled goat antirabbit IgG. The surface of lymphocytes shows a discontinuous strong peroxidase reaction, indicating the binding of labeled antibody to surface IgG of lymphocytes. (From Bona C., et al. Eur J Immunol 1972;2:434–439.)

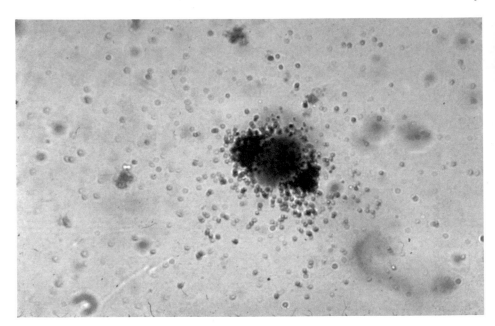

Fig. 15. Autoradiograph of murine splenic lymphocytes incubated with [14]C-*Salmonella entertidis* lipopolysaccharide (LPS). Splenic lymphocyte from a mouse immunized with *Salmonella enteritidis* LPS. Cells were incubated with ^{14}C-labeled LPS, fixed; and then coated with photographic emulsion. Radioactive emission of β-ray caused deposition of silver grains at the level of binding of LPS by lymphocytes receptors.

CD4 T cells mediate cellular immune responses such as delayed type hypersensitivity and cytotoxic reactions. CD4 T cells collaborate with B cells in the humoral responses by virtue of providing the second signal required for the activation of B cells.

NK T cells are characterized by an NK marker, such as NK1.1 in mice. Sixty percent of NK T cells express CD4, and 40% lack CD4 and CD8 markers (double-negative). The TCR is encoded by an invariant *Vα14-Jα28* gene and 55% by Vβ8,2, 14% Vβ7, and 7% Vβ2 *(110)*. They recognize lipids and glycolipids in association with nonpolymorphic class I-like, CD1, MHC molecules *(111,112)*.

The T cells expressing TCR-γ/δ are present in the female reproductive tract, intestinal epithelium, lung, and bladder *(113)*.

In humans, a subset expressing a TCR that is encoded by *Vγ9 /Vδ2* genes appears to be important because they can be stimulated by nonpeptidic phosphoantigen and do not require the presentation by polymorphic and nonpolymorphic MHC molecules. These subsets of T cells play a role in the

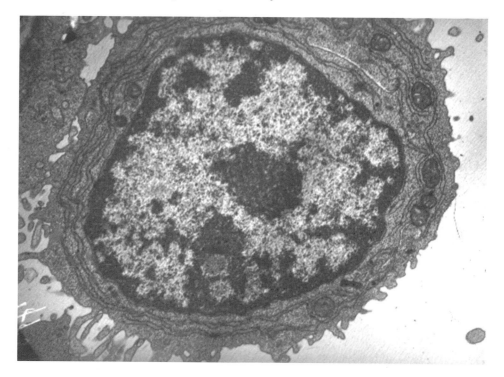

Fig. 16. Electron micrograph of a guinea pig plasma cell. The cytoplasm is filled with rough endoplasmic reticulum and few mitochondria.

regulation, initiation, and progression of some infectious diseases. For example, their number is increased in infection with *Mycobacterium tuberculosis*, and they may also inhibit the replication of *Plasmodium falciparum* merozoites and may lyse cells infected with HIV *(114)*.

The T cells produce various cytokines that exhibit immunomodulatory properties and receptors for cytokines and chemokines (reviewed in ref. *115*). T and B cells express various CD antigen; some are expressed specifically on a given subset, whereas others are shared by various subsets or with cells that mediate innate immune defense reactions (Table 11).

5. THE ORGANS OF THE IMMUNE SYSTEM

The lymphoid organs are divided into two categories: central and peripheral lymphoid organs. The central lymphoid organs are represented by bone marrow that contains the stem cells; these stem cells develop the precursors of cells that mediate both innate and adaptive immunity—a process called hematopoiesis. Hematopoiesis continues throughout a lifetime. In birds, the B lymphocytes originate from the bursa of Fabricius.

T lymphocytes are derived from thymus, which represents the second central lymphoid organ.

The mature lymphocytes leave bone marrow/bursa of Fabricius or thymus and are distributed through lymph and blood circulatory systems to peripheral organs.

The peripheral organs are the lymph nodes, the spleen, lymphoid tissue associated with upper respiratory tract (bronchial-associated lymphoid tissue [BALT]), lymphoid tissue associated with gastrointestinal tract (gut-associated lymphoid tissue [GALT]), and lymphoid tissue associated with skin (skin-associated lymphoid tissue [SALT]).

Bone marrow is the main organ of hematopoiesis throughout life. It is made up of a fine meshwork of reticular fibers, which contains stromal cells, reticular cells, fibroblasts, and adipocytes, and the hematopoietic stem cells (HSCs), which are the progenitor of erythroid, thrombocytic, myeloid, and lymphoid lineages. Vessels irrigating the bone marrow enter into bones in the subendostal arteriovenous complex, which empties into the medullary sinusoids. Stromal cells and cells differentiated from the progeny of various lineages are in close contact with the intersinusoidal spaces.

The thymus is the main organ that produces T cells. It is made of two symmetrical lobes located in the superior mediastinum. The thymus has no afferent lymphatic supply, and the blood reaches the organs from arteries branched from the subclavicular artery; these arteries enter into the medulla and septa. The parenchyma of each lobe is divided into lobules by septa. The peripheral zone of lobule that contains the epithelial cells and the majority of lymphocytes is called the cortex. The central zone that contains epithelial cells, dendritic cells, myoid cells, Hassal' corpuscules, and small lymphocytes is called the medulla (Fig. 17).

After maturation, the lymphocytes, which are produced into bone marrow and thymus, enter into circulation and into peripheral lymphoid organs (lymph nodes, spleen, BALT, GALT, and SALT).

The lymph nodes are surrounded by a capsule and are divided into two distinct zones: the cortical zone, which contains packed lymphocytes in follicles, and a less cellular-dense zone called the medulla. Primary follicles consist of a meshwork of follicular dendritic cell-holding B lymphocytes, surrounded by zones containing T cells (Fig. 18). After antigen stimulation, the structure of primary follicles changes, and the central zone contains germinal centers organized in several compartments; these are the follicular mantle, apical light zone, basal light zone, and dark zone (Fig. 19). The dark zone contains mainly rapidly dividing B cells called centroblasts that lack surface Ig and maturate into centrocytes and migrate into the basal light zone, where they differentiate into plasma or memory cells. These cells migrate to the apical light zone. The germinal centers appear 3–7 d after immunization and are extinct after 4 wk.

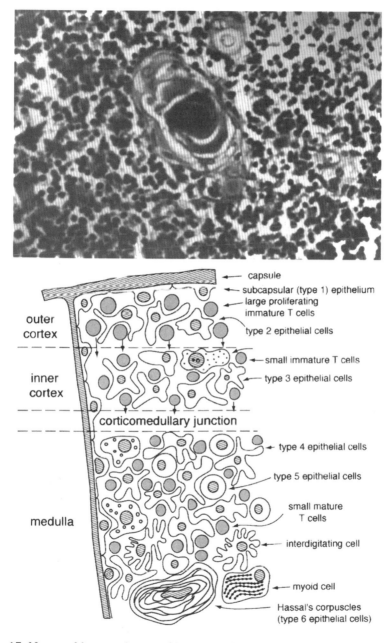

Fig. 17. Neonatal human thymus. Upper panel represents a micrograph showing the thymic cortex packed with lymphocytes and in the center, a Hassal's corpuscle composed of aggregated epithelial cells some are keratinized). The bottom of the figure is a diagram of thymic lobule. (This figure is a composite of two figures from Bona C, Bonilla F. Textbook of Immunology. Harwood Academic Publ., USA 1990, pp.30, 31.)

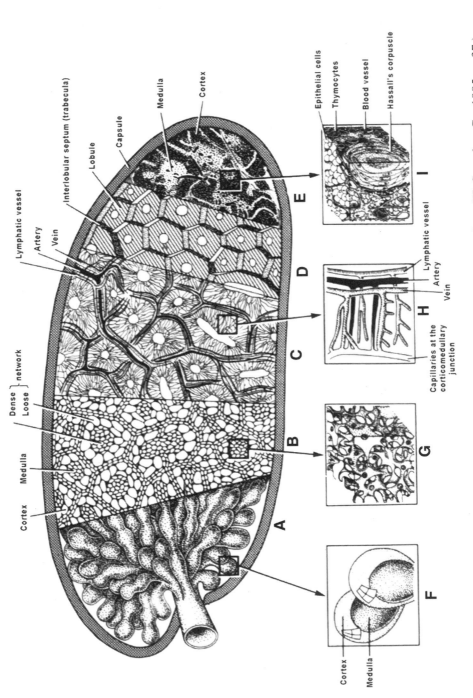

Fig. 18. Diagrammatic cross-section of a lymph node. (From Bellani JA. Immunology III. Saunders Co. 1985, p. 37.)

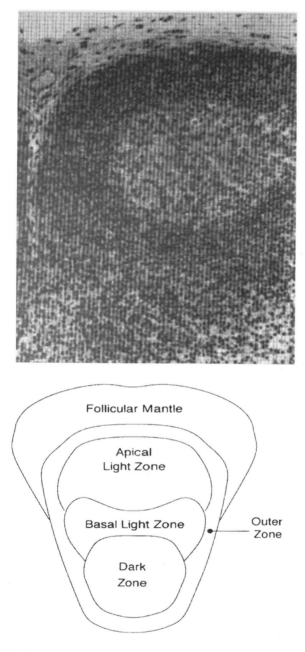

Fig. 19. Germinal center at the periphery of the lymph node cortex and diagram of the architecture of a germinal center. (Composite figure from Bona C, Bonilla F. Text book of Immunology. Harwood Academic Publ USA 1990, pp. 36, 38.)

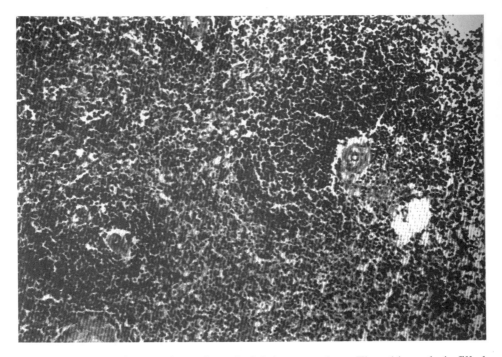

Fig. 20. Light microscopic section of adult human spleen. The white pulp is filled up with small lymphocytes. The periarteriolar sheats appear as islands in a sea of red pulp containing sinusoids filled with erythrocytes. (From Bona C, Bonilla F. Textbook of Immunology. Harwood Academic Publ USA 1990, p. 34.)

The spleen is another important peripheral lymphoid organ, which in some species has hematopoietic capacity during life. Splenic parenchyma is surrounded by a connective tissue capsule. It is irrigated by a single splenic artery, which enters in the hillum, and is then divided into branches. Cuffs of lymphocytes, called periarteriolar lymphoid sheets (PALS), surround small arteries. Parenchyma consists of two distinct tissues: red and white pulp. The red pulp is rich in macrophages that exhibit a high ability to clear aged cells, microbes, viruses, and macromolecules. The white pulp consists of lymphoid follicles that contain mainly B cells and dendritic cells. The PALS contain mainly T cells. The white pulp surrounding PALS is called the marginal zone, an area where the arterioles open in a loose matrix composed of reticular cells and fibroblasts (Fig. 20).

GALT is composed of the tonsils, appendix, Peyer's patches, and lymphoid tissue contained in lamina propria.

BALT is composed of lymphoid tissue associated with both the upper and lower respiratory tract.

6. RELATIONSHIP BETWEEN INNATE AND ADAPTIVE IMMUNITY

The response of innate immunity against microbes is prompt but incomplete, because it is less discriminative. However, innate immunity instructs the adaptive immunity, which develops slower but is mediated by more efficient and specific effectors of humoral and cellular immune responses. The germline genes that encode adaptive immunity are subject to Darwinian antigen-selective pressure, and the repertoire diversifies during the life through somatic variation processes such as recombination of various gene segments, somatic mutations, gene conversion, and N-addition, conferring fine specificity of BCRs and TCRs.

The crosstalk between the cells that mediate innate and adaptive immunity takes place at the level of immune synapses and through the cytokine network. The cytokines produced by cells that mediate innate immunity can influence the magnitude of adaptive immune responses, and the cytokines secreted by lymphocytes may enhance innate immune defense reactions.

6.1. Antigen Presentation

In contrast to B cells, which recognize the epitopes on the surface of native antigen via BCR, T cells can recognize fragmented antigen after processing. The antigen internalized within antigen-presenting cells (APCs) is degraded, and the resulting peptides are bound to MHC molecules that are presented to T cells.

Antigen presentation takes place in macrophages and dendritic cells, which are effectors of innate immunity, as well as in B cells. The processing of phagocytized particulate antigen or pinocytized macromolecules generate peptides that are presented to CD4 T cells in association with MHC class II molecules. The peptides recognized by CD4 T cells are generated via the exogenous pathway.

The CD8 T cells recognize peptides derived from endogenous proteins, such as viral proteins that result from viral replication, or from proteins that leak from phagosomes containing microbes, fungi, or parasites. These peptides are generated via the endogenous pathway.

The exogenous pathway leading to the generation of peptide class II complex consists of three major events. The first event takes place in endosomes after the internalization of antigen. The peptides are generated within low-density endosomes after fusion with dense lysosomes, leading to the activation of lysosomal hydrolases in acid pH medium.

The second event takes place in the ER, where class II molecules and invariant (Ii) chains are synthesized. The nascent class II molecules bind Ii chains, and the formation of heterodimers is facilitated by chaperone molecules present in ER. Class II–Ii heterodimers are then translocated via the Golgi secretory pathway into endosomes where the Ii chain is hydrolysed.

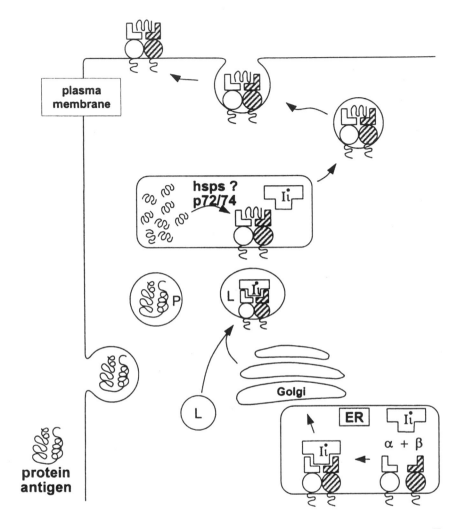

Fig. 21. A model for antigen processing and presentation by class II+ APCs. (From Bona C, Bonilla F. Textbook of Immunology. Harwood Academic Publ USA 1990, p. 241.)

The third event consists of sorting the peptides by empty class II molecules. The formation of peptide class II complex is then translocated to the membrane, where it can be recognized by CD4 T cells. (Figure 21 illustrates the major events of exogenous pathway.)

Of all APCs, the dendritic cells are the most efficient. This was demonstrated by studying the number of APCs required for the presentation of an influenza virus hemagglutinin-derived peptide to CD4 T cells. In this experiment, a viral epitope recognized by CD4 T cells was expressed in a chimeric Ig molecule by replacing the CDR3 segment of *VH* gene with a viral peptide. Various APCs were pulsed with the same amount of chimeric Ig molecule, and then various numbers of APCs were incubated with a fixed number of peptide-specific T-cell hybridoma cells. The maximal activation of the T-cell hybridoma was obtained with 500 dendritic cells, 8000 B cells, and 10^6 spleen cells *(116)*. These results clearly demonstrated that there is a hierarchy among APCs with regard to the efficiency of processing and presentation of peptides to T cells.

The endogenous pathway begins with the processing of proteins by the proteosomes. The peptides released from proteosomes are translocated to the ER by protein-specific antigen peptide (TAP), which belong to the ATP-binding casette family of protein transporters. In the ER, newly synthesized heavy chains of class I molecules interact with calnexin and BIP proteins, which facilitates the formation of heterodimer by binding β2-microglobulin to the heavy chains. After the heterodimer is formed, calnexin is released and the class I molecule forms a complex with calreticulin. The calreticulin-class I complex binds to the TAP-peptide complex, a process allowing for the release of the peptide from TAP and its bond to empty class I molecules. The complex is then translocated via the *trans*-Golgi to the membrane, where it is recognized by CD8 T cells. (Figure 22 illustrates the major events of endogenous pathway.)

6.2. Immune Synapses

Cell–cell interaction between the cells that mediate innate and adaptive immunity requires the formation of highly organized patterns of protein receptors and ligands, clustering of the cytoskeleton, and submicroscopic rafts at the level of the intercellular junction. These events take place at the level of the immune synapse (IS), defined as intercellular contact between at least one type of cell of the immune system *(117)*. The IS plays an important role in the recognition and activation of lymphocytes, favoring the binding of the antigen receptor to antigen, the interaction of the receptor proteins with their corresponding ligands, and, in certain cases, the transfer of antigen from one cell to another. The IS is a clearly organized transient structure of protein and lipid complexes that occurs at the level of the junction of membrane of two cells causing the segregation of proteins and lipids in micrometer-scale domains *(117)*. The molecular interactions in the IS between receptors and ligands into apposed cell membranes integrate innate and adaptive immunity processes.

Underitz *(118)* first described IS between bone marrow cells. Later, Mosier *(119)* observed the formation of intercellular contact between immune cells from mice immunized with heterologous RBC 24 h after culture in a Mishel–Dutton system. After 48 h of culture, the B cells in the lymphocyte synapses

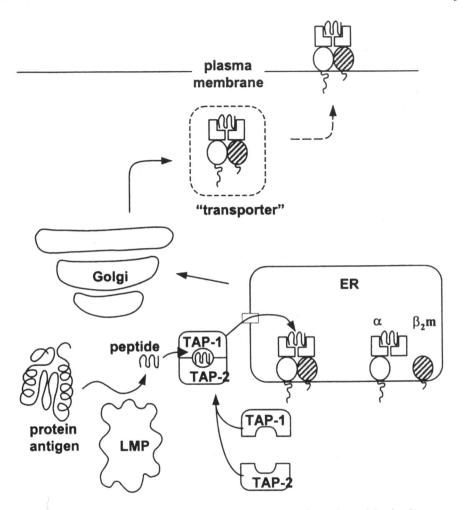

Fig. 22. A model of antigen processing and presentation of peptides in the context of class I molecules to CD8 T cells. (From Bona C, Bonilla F. Textbook of Immunology Harwood. Academic Publ USA 1990, p. 238.)

produced anti-RBC antibodies as assessed by PFC assay. Cline *(120)* described the requirement of IS for the proliferation of T cells incubated with macrophages pulsed with a foreign antigen, the tuberculin.

Figure 23 illustrates spontaneous formation of IS after incubation of guinea pig syngeneic macrophages with thymocytes. The T cells tightly adhered to a macrophage. Lipsky and Rosentahl *(121)* showed that the formation of IS required living and metabolically active macrophages.

The cellular and molecular events in the formation of IS were studied in IS formed between B and T cells, between dendritic cells and naïve or antigen-

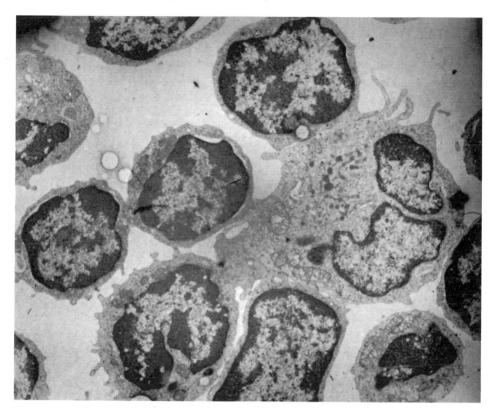

Fig. 23. Electron micrograph showing synapse formation between a macrophage and lymphocytes in a guinea pig lymph node. (From Lipski PE, Rosenthal AS. J Exp Med 1973;138:900–910.)

specific T cells, between B cells and cells expressing FcR, and between NK cells and target cells.

Wulfing et al. *(122)* showed the formation of ISs between antigen-specific T and B cells bearing the appropriate MHC-peptide complex. They observed that the formation of a tight junction between cells leads to an increased elevation of intracellular calcium accumulation, which is a sign of the activation of T cells that precedes the clustering of ICAM-1 molecules at the levels of junction. ICAM-1 is the ligand of the LAF-1 receptor on T cells that is also clustered at the level of the cellular junction. Further studies showed that ISs are composed of supramolecular activation clusters (SMACs), which are comprised of a central core containing TCR and MHC-peptide complex; CD28, CD80, and CD86 costimulatory molecules (cSMACs); and a peripheral layer composed of ICAM-1 and LFA-1 (pSMAC). The ability of proteins of apposed membranes to form IS depends on their size, elasticity, tethering of the mem-

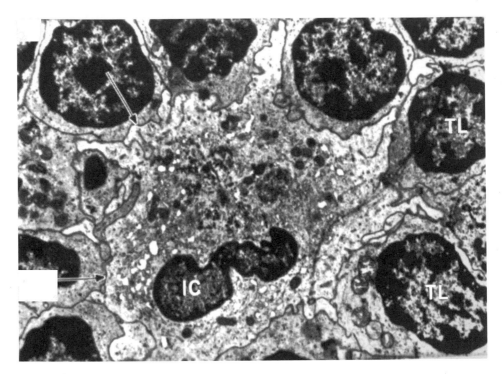

Fig. 24. Electron micrograph showing clustering of dendritic cells with T cells (TL). (Courtesy of Dr. R. Steinman, Rockefeller University, New York.)

brane, and local separation between membranes *(123)*. It interesting to note that in B–T cell-ISS, except for the clustering of ICAM-1 and MHC molecules, no reorganization of cytoskeleton was observed.

IS formation between dendritic cells and T cells was also observed. Austyn et al. *(124)* demonstrated that the clustering of dendritic cells with T cells precedes and is essential for the activation of T cells. Inaba et al. *(125)* showed that clustering of dendritic cells with T cells can be antigen-independent or antigen-dependent.

Figure 24 illustrates the ultrastructural aspect of a dendritic cell and T-cell immunosynapse.

The spontaneous formation of IS between dendritic cells and naïve T cells may explain the ability of dendritic cells to stimulate naïve T cells *(125)*. Revy et al. *(126)* showed that the formation of IS between dendritic cells and naïve T cells may take place in the absence of antigen or MHC molecules. The incubation of T cells with dendritic cells is associated with an intense T-cell membrane ruffling observed minutes after incubation of cells and by an accumulation of calcium 10 min after interaction. This was followed by the rotation of the T-cell microtubule organizer center toward synapses, suggesting that polarization and the clustering of this organelle is essential in the initiation of IS formation. The IS formation leads to a local increase of tyrosine phosphatase and PKC-π serine-threonine kinase. In contrast to clustering of molecules comprised of cSMAC and pSMAC at the level of the synapse, the exclusion of CD43 was constantly observed. This suggests that the CD43 functions as a repulsive molecule in IS formation.

Al-Alvar et al. *(127)* showed that the IS formation between dendritic cells and naïve T cells is dependent on profound reorganization of the T-cell skeleton, which is characterized by the accumulation of filamentous actin (F-actin) and fascin at the level of the junction. The role of the actin cytoskeleton reorganization is supported by observations demonstrating the inhibition of IS formation by cytochalasin D, a potent inhibitor of F-actin formation, by jasplakinolide, which prevents actin rearrangement by stabilizing F-actin, and by latrunculin A, which inhibits actin cytoskeleton rearrangement.

An insight into the quantitative aspects of clustering of molecules was studied in vitro by incubating T cells with phospholipid bilayers embedded with various molecule involved in synapses *(128)*.

In this system, it was shown that the interaction of T cells with the bilayer requires only 2–5 min and lasted at least 1 h. At the level of synapses, 0.7 molecules/μm^2 of class II, ICAM-1 to an average density of 100 molecules/μm^2, and CD80 at a density of 35 molecules/μm^2 were accumulated in the synapse.

In this system, Bromley and Dustin *(128)* also studied the effect of chemokines on IS formation. They showed that the addition of CXCL12 and CCL21 to ICAM-1 bilayer significantly increased the adhesion of T cells. The chemokine-stimulated adhesion is dependent on G-protein signaling. Indeed, the pretreatment of T cells with pertussis toxin inhibited the chemokine-induced adhesion to bilayers containing ICAM-1. This result suggests that chemokines may enhance LFA-1–ICAM-1 interaction that mediates adhesion in IS.

The occurrence of IS between B cells and myeloid-derived cells was also described. B cell synapses favor efficient recognition of antigen borne by microbes, viruses, or microbial toxins bound to various receptors. Macrophages and dendritic cells bear a class of receptors that mediate innate immunity and are specialized to interact and internalize microbes. Although some of the microbial antigen are processed within lysosomal compartment, others are not. We have shown that the LPS internalized into endosomes of guinea pig macrophages and neutrophils is not degraded because the lysosomal fraction prepared from these cells was able to induce the Schwartzman phenomenon in rabbits *(5)*.

We also described the formation of IS between B cells and macrophages in which the B cells were wrapped by several macrophages. Furthermore, in this

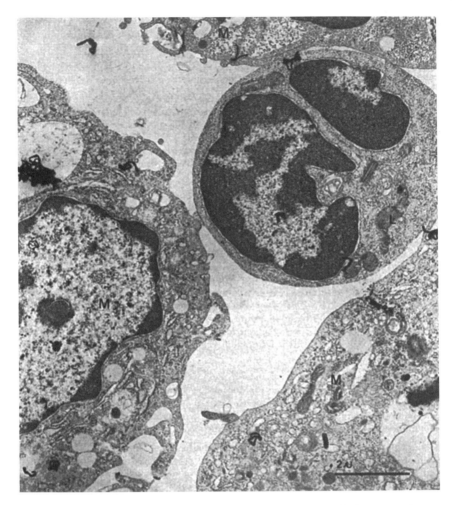

Fig. 25. Electron micrograph showing the transfer of LPS from macrophages to a lymphocyte. Guinea pig macrophages were pulsed with ^{14}C-LPS and then incubated for 1 h with lymph node lymphocytes. The cells were centrifuged, fixed, and then coated with photographic emulsion. Radioactive emission of β-rays caused deposition of silver grains. Silver grains are observed in the phagosomes of macrophages and at membranes of contact between a lymphocyte, which adhere to two macrophages.

study we demonstrated that the macrophages transfer the antigen associated with their membrane to B cells. In this experiment, guinea pig macrophages were pulsed with ^{14}C biosynthetically labeled LPS and then incubated with B cells. The cells were centrifuged and the pellet was processed for electron microscopic autoradiography *(129)*. Figure 25 shows the presence of silver grains (i.e., labeled LPS) on the surface of macrophages and in B cells that express surface Ig as assessed by the staining with peroxidase-labeled anti-Ig antibodies. Batista et al. *(130)* showed that the interaction of B cells with antigen–antibody complex that was immobilized via FcR at the surface myeloid cells leads to the formation of IS. In this experiment, HEL-specific B cells were incubated with myeloid cells loaded with HEL that was aggregated by anti-HEL antibodies. A kinetics study showed that most of the B cells adhered to the target cells after 10 min. The formation of the synapse was associated with macromolecular reorganization of the B-cell membrane that was characterized by the polarization of the Ig receptor, the concentration of GMP gangliosides and phosphotyrosine-containing proteins, and the depletion of CD22 from the center of the synapse. As in the case of dendritic cell–T cell ISs, in B–T cell ISS, the CD45 was excluded. The transfer of the antigen in IS was demonstrated in an elegant experiment in which B cells were incubated with fibroblasts that were transfected with a construct that expressed a chimeric gene, encoding a membrane form of HEL linked to a GFP reporter. In this experiment, it was shown that HEL-specific B cells aggregated rapidly (10 min) with the target cells, and by 20 min after the formation of IS, green fluorescent material was observed within B cells. The transfer of the antigen at the level of the synapse induced the activation of B cells, leading to upregulation of CD86 costimulatory molecule *(130)*.

ISs between follicular dendritic cells and B cells were described in the lymph node germinal centers. In an electron microscope study, Nossal et al. *(131)* demonstrated the persistence of radiolabeled antigen at the surface of follicular dendritic cells at the junction with B cells. The immunogenicity of antigen associated with follicular dendritic cell membrane was long-lasting. They also proposed that the presentation of antigen by follicular dendritic cells plays an important role in the induction of primary and secondary immune responses and in the generation of memory cells. Other studies showed that follicular dendritic cells capture immune complexes containing antigen, antibody, and complement component via the FcR. These complexes, which are bedlike structures called iccosomes are identified on the surfaces of follicular dendritic cells, can be captured by the centrocytes in the germinal centers. The centrocytes may process the antigen, and the peptides derived from the processing are presented to T cells, which contribute to affinity maturation of the immune responses *(132)*.

The ISs were also observed between target cells and NK cells, which play an important role in innate immunity *(133)*.

6.3. Crosstalk Between Cells That Mediate Innate and Adaptive Immunity Through the Cytokine Network

Beside the crosstalk through direct cell-to-cell contact at the level of ISs, the cells mediating innate and adaptive immunity can speak to each another via cytokines. The cytokines evolved along with the immune system. Some cytokines

Table 11
**Cytodifferentation Antigens, Receptors and Enzymes Associated
With the Membrane of Lymphocytes**

Cytodifferentation antigens	Ligand	Lymphocytes B	T	Effect
CD1	Lipid glycolipid	+	+	Antigen presentation
CD 2	LAF-3, CD48, CD59	+[a]	+	
CD 4	MHC Class II		+[b]	Coreceptor
CD 5	CD72, C-type lectin	+**	+	
CD 8	MHC Class I	+[b]		Coreceptor
CD19		+		Signal transduction
CD 20		+		
CD21			+	Signal transduction
CD24-HSA	CD62P	+	+	Endotelial cell activation
B220 (mouse)		+		
CD28	CD 86	+		
CD45Ro		+		Signal transduction
CD48	CD 2	+	+	
CD58	CD 2		+	
CD59	CD 2		+	
CD 70	CD27	+		
CD75 (syaloglicprotein)	CD22	+		
Cd77 (glycoshinolipid)	CD1	+		
CD90 (Thy1-mouse)		+		

Molecules associated with lymphocyte's antigen receptor

CD 3 (TCR)	+			Signaling
CD 79 (BCR)	+			Signaling
CD179 (pre-B BCR)	+[b]			?

Costimulatory molecules

CD 6	CD166, Alcam	+		Costimulation
CD28	CD80,CD86	+		Signaling
CD54 (ICAM-1)	LAF-1	+		Adhesion,signaling
CD80	CD28,CD152	+		Signaling
CD86	CD28,CD156	+		Signaling
CD162	LAF-1	+		Signaling
CD178 (Fas ligand)	CD95	+		Apoptosis

(Continued)

Table 11 *(continued)*

Receptors

A. Fc receptors

Receptor	Ligand			
CD16 (FcRγII	IgGFc	+		
CD 64(FcγRI),	IgGFc	+		
CD 23(FcεR)	IgEFc	+	+	
CD 32(FCγRII)	IgGFc	+		

B. Complement receptors

Receptor	Ligand			
CD21	C3d	+		
CD35	C3b	+		
CD46	C3b,C4b	+		

C. Integrin receptors

Receptor	Ligand			Function
CD11a	CD54, CD102	+	+	Cell adhesion
CD11b	CD56, iC3b, fibronectin	+	+	Cell adhesion
CD11c	iC3b, fibronectin	+	+	Cell adhesion
CD18	CD11a.b.c	+	+	Cell adhesion
CD31	Vitronectin	+		Adhesion
CD49a	Laminin, collagen	+[a]		Adhesion
CD49b	Laminin collagen	+	+	Adhesion
CD49c	Fibronectin	+[a]		Adhesion
CD51	Vitronectin, fibronectin	+[a]		Adhesion
CD87	Vitronectin	+		Adhesion
CD104	Laminin	+[a]		Adhesion

D. Interleukin receptors

Receptor	Ligand			Function
CD25 (IL-4R)	IL-4	+[a]	+[a]	Activation
CD119 (IFNγ R)	IFNγ	+	+	Activation
CD120 (TNFR)	TNF, LT	+	+	Apoptosis
CD121 (IL-1R)	IL-1	+		Activation
CD122 (IL-2, IL-15R)	Il-2, IL-15	+	+[a]	Activation
CD123 (!L-3R)	IL-3	+[a]		Activation
CD124 (IL-4 R)	IL-4,IL13	+	+[a]	Activation
CD125 (IL-5 R)	IL-5	+		Activation, differentation
CD126 (IL-6R)	IL-6	+	+	Signaling
CD128 (IL-8R)	IL-8	+[b]	+[b]	Chemotaxis
CD10 (IL-10R)	IL-10	+[b]		Activation
CD212 (IL-12R)	IL-12	+[b]	+[b]	Activation
CD213 (IL-13R)	IL-13	+		Activation

E. Chemokine receptors

Receptor	Ligand			Function
CXCR5	BCA-1	+		Adhesion
CCR6	MIP 1-α	+		Adhesion
CXCR3	MIG, IP-10, I-Tac		+[a]	Adhesion
CXCR6	B6 inducible cytokine		+[a]	

Table 11 *(continued)*

XCR1	Lymphotactin, SCM-1B	+		Adhesion
CXCR1	Fractalkine	+[a]		
CCR2	MCP-1 MCP-5	+[a]		
CCR1	MIP-1α, MCP-4, LEK	+[a]		
CCR3	Eotaxin	+[a]		
CCR4	TARK	+[a]		
F. Other receptors				
CD22	Neuraminic acid	+	+	Adhesion
CD14	LPS	+		Activation differentation
CD36 (scavenger R)	Oxidized LDL	+		Scavenger
CD40	CD40 ligand	+		Activation
CD71	Transferin	+[a]	+[a]	Internalization
CD95	Fas ligand	+	+	Apoptosis
CD117	c-Kit	+	+	Signaling
G. Enzymes				
CD156	Metalproteinase	+	+	Enzymatic activity
CD143	Dipeptidylpeptidase	+	+	Enzymatic activity
CD73	Ecto-5' nucleotidase	+[b]	+[b]	Enzymatic activity

[a]Activated cells
[b]Subset

produced in vertebrates have homologs in invertebrates. Cytokine-like molecules similar to IL-1, IL-2, IL-6, TNF-α, PDGF, and TGF-β1 were described in mollusca; insecta, IL-1, TNF-α, and PDGF were described in nematoda; and IL-1 and TNF-α were described in tunicata (reviewed in ref. *134*).

The cytokines are produced by the cells of the immune system but can be synthesized by other cell types. The effect of cytokines is pleiomorphic, because the receptor for a particular cytokine may be expressed in various cell types. The cytokines display a broad range of properties that influence cell division, differentiation, metabolism, and the expression of immune functions. Immunomodulatory properties of some cytokines are redundant because different cytokines can bind to the same receptor and others can bind to distinct receptors.

The cytokines produced by the immune cells represent a network of soluble molecules that links innate and adaptive immunity. In contrast to the idiotype network, which is clonally restricted by virtue of the specificity of lymphocyte receptors that are able to recognize a single idiotype, the cytokine network is not clonally restricted because of the pleiotropic properties of cytokines and the nonclonal distribution of the cytokine receptors.

Table 12
Cytokines Produced by Cells Mediating Innate Immunity Exhibiting Immunomodulatory Properties on Lymphocytes

Cytokine	Producer	Target	Effect
IL-1	Monocytes, macrophages	T cells	Activation
	Dendritic cells	Th1	Production of IL-1
IL-12	NK cell, monocytes, dendritic cells	Th1	Proliferation, synthesis of IFNγ
IL-18	Macrophages, dendritic cells	Th1	Synthesis of IFNγ
IL-3	Mast cells	B cells	Growth, differentiation
		γ/δ T cells	induces transcription of TCR-γ
IL-4	Mast cells, NKT cells, Platelets	B cells	Activation, class switching
		Th2	Proliferation, cytokine production
		CTL	Proliferation
IL-13	Mast cells, activated dendritic cells	B cell	Activation, class switching
IL-6	Macrophages, astrocytes	B cell	Growth, endothelial cell differentiation
IL-8	Monocytes, macrophages	Chemokine activity	Activated neutrophils
IL-15	Monocytes, macrophages	Th1, DC, CTL	Differentiation
IFNFγ	Macrophages, NK cells	Th1	Differentiation
IFN-α and -β	Monocytes, macrophages	B cells	Antibody production
		T cell	Survival, CTL activation

Abbreviations: DC, dendritic cells; NK, natural killer cell; CTL, cytolytic T cells; Th, T helper.

Table 12 illustrates the effects of cytokines produced by cells that mediate innate immunity on lymphocytes.

2

Ontogeny and the Development of Cells Mediating Innate and Adaptive Immunity

1. ORIGIN OF IMMUNE CELL PROGENITORS DURING EMBRYOGENESIS

All white blood cells (WBCs) are derived from a common precursor: the hematopoietic stem cell (HSC). This paradigm emerged from an elegant experiment demonstrating the repopulating of all mature WBCs in lethally irradiated adult animals subsequent to infusion of a single HSC *(135)*. This experiment demonstrated that HSCs exhibit two exquisite properties: self renewing capacity throughout life and multipotential differentiation ability.

In all vertebrates, HSCs have two origins: extraembryonic (in the yolk sac) and intraembryonic (within the embryo itself). In lower vertebrates, the yolk sac appears to be the earliest hematopoietic organ in fish such as elasmobranches *(136)*, teleocasts such as angelfish *(137)*, and reptiles *(138)*. In rainbow trout, the HSCs produced in the yolk sac during the short larval period migrate to the intermediate cellular mass (ICM), which forms from the paraaxial mesoderm during early gastrulation. Oellacher considered that the ICM represents the site of blood cell formation in most low vertebrates *(136)*.

Studies of hematopoiesis in mouse embryos suggest that hematopoiesis begins in the mesodermal compartment of the yolk sac at d 7.5 of gestation. Extraembryonic hematopoiesis in the yolk sac is defined as primitive hematopoiesis. At d 7.5 of gestation, only primitive erythropoiesis was observed, which consisted of the generation of erythrocytes with extruded nuclei and the expression of the fetal hemoglobin gene *(139)*. Cumano et al. found only myeloid precursors within the mouse yolk sac at d 8.5 of gestation *(140)*, whereas others reported the presence of B- and T-cell precursors in the yolk sac excised on d 8.5 of gestation (before that the yolk sac and embryo became connected through circulation) *(141,142)*.

Moore and Metcalf assumed that in higher vertebrates, the blood island in the yolk sac is the first hematopoietic tissue and the early site of HSC generation *(143)*. By d 12 of gestation, the HSCs migrate to the fetal liver and later to the bone marrow and spleen. The shift of primitive hematopoiesis from the

From: *Contemporary Immunology: Neonatal Immunity*
By: Constantin Bona © Humana Press Inc., Totowa, NJ

yolk sac to the fetal liver and then to bone marrow leads to adult-type definitive hematopoiesis.

The contribution of yolk sac hematopoiesis to definitive hematopoiesis is supported by experiments that show that the HSCs present at d 9 and 10 of gestation can repopulate hematopoiesis in conditioned newborns instead of irradiated adult mice *(144)*.

However, experiments carried out in chickens have challenged the paradigm that HSCs derive solely from the yolk sac. In these experiments, cells from quail embryos were grafted into chicken yolk sacs *in ovo* before vascularization. The hematopoiesis in this system emerged from the embryo (quail and chicken cells can be easily distinguished by size of their nucleoli) *(145)*. This *in ovo* adoptive transfer experiment showed that all cells in the thymus, spleen, and bursa of Fabricius derived from quail cells *(146)*. Histological studies showed hematopoietic foci located within the dorsal mesentery of the embryo *(147)*. In vitro experiments demonstrated that HSCs isolated from the aortic wall of the chicken embryo are able to generate erythroid and myeloid colonies *(148)*. Aortic hematopoietic clusters observed in chicken embryos were identified later in many lower and higher vertebrate species.

In lower vertebrates, HSCs derived from the embryonic mesoderm occur in distinct tissues and different locations in different species. In the Antarctic teleost pronephritic kidney, HSC progenitors were observed at 1 h posthatch, whereas in the splenic analog, they were not observed until 4 wk posthatch *(149)*. In some teleocast such as zebrafish, HSCs also were identified within the ICM *(150)*. Markers of higher vertebrate HSCs such as SCL, GATA1, c-Myb, and Flo-1 were identified in zebrafish HSCs *(151)*. In rainbow trout, the ICM progressively increases up to 12 d postfertilization and disappears by d 15 *(152)*.

In the first blood islands of early larval-stage amphibian Xenopus and Rana embryos, HSCs appear at the early neural stage in the developing dorsal aorta, postcardial veins and pronephros *(153)*, the intraembryonic mesodermic region called DLP, and VP1, which represent the sites of primitive hematopoiesis. In the late larval stage, the HSCs migrate and seed lymphoid organs during metamorphosis. At this stage, HSCs express markers characteristic of higher vertebrate HSCs—CD45, SCL, and GATA-1 *(151)*.

In the mouse embryo, hematopoiesis occurs in the aorta, gonad, and mesonephros region (AGM) and its analog, the tissues derived from the para-aortic splachnopleura (p-Sp) such as the dorsal aorta, umbilical, and omphalomesenteric arteries; the hind gut; and the septum transversum. At d 10.5 of gestation, the AGM region contains about 100 HSC precursors that exhibit long-term repopulating capacity, as assessed in transfer experiments in lethally irradiated adult mice *(154)*. Cumano et al. *(140)* showed the presence of HSCs in cultures of p-Sp harvested from mouse embryos at d 9.5 of gestation and in cultures of

AGM excised from 10.5-d-old embryos. Lymphoid precursors indicative of definitive hematopoiesis also were found in cultures of p-SP from mouse embryos *(155,156)*. By d 12, the number of precursors in this region decreased, suggesting that the AGM region is not the site of hematopoiesis throughout the entire embryonic period *(156)*. Cultures of the AGM region excised from 11.5-d-old embryos in the presence of stem cell growth factor (SGF), interleukin (IL)-3, IL-6, and erythropoietin showed an increase in the total number of colony-forming units (CFUs).The addition of oncostatin M to the culture medium increased the number of mixed colony-forming cells (granulocytes, erythrocytes, macrophages, and megakaryocytes), suggesting that oncostatin M is a key element in the generation of multipotential HSC in the AGM. These multipotential HSCs may differentiate as assessed by fluorescence-activated cell-sorter (FACS) analysis of the expression of various markers for different lineages. A major fraction of cells (50–70%) expressed Mac-1 Gr-1 Th1.2, B220, Tar119, and c-Kit. This phenotypic analysis strongly suggests the differentiation of HSCs into myeloid and lymphoid common progenitors *(156)*. It is interesting to note that oncostatin M stimulated not only the expansion of HSCs but also the formation of endothelial cell clusters *(157)*.

In humans, the HSC progenitors that produce only myeloid and natural killer (NK) cells, but not lymphoid progenitors, are detected in the yolk sac as early as d 19 of the development of the embryo, 2 d before the onset of blood circulation. The origin of these HSC progenitors has not been well-defined but could be endothelial cells *(158)*.

Th extraembryonic (yolk sac) and intraembryonic origins of HSC precursors were studied by in vitro culture of the yolk sac and p-Sp and dorsal aorta excised from embryos ranging from 19 to 48 d of age. The tissues were seeded onto the MS-5 stromal cell line, and the presence of HSC precursors was analyzed after 7 d of culture. The $CD45^+CD56^+$ $CD94^+$ NK and $CD45^+$ $CD15^+$ myeloid cell progenitors were detected in the yolk sac and p-Sp cultures from 19-d-old embryos. Although the yolk sac cultures contained no lymphoid precursors, $CD45^+$ $CD19^+$ B-cell precursors were detected in cultures of p-Sp from 24- to 25-d-old embryos, and $CD4^+$ T-cell precursors were detected in p-Sp cultures from 26- to 27-d-old embryos *(158)*.

These results clearly demonstrate that in human embryos, the precursors of NK and myeloid cells derived from the yolk sac and p-Sp, whereas the precursors of lymphoid cells were of intraembryonic origin.

Studies of the generation of HSC progenitors strongly suggest that HSCs derive from mesodermal multipotential hematoblasts immediately after gastrulation in both lower and higher vertebrate species.

More recent studies suggest that the hematoblast, which is the progenitor of hematopoietic cells, and the angioblast, which is the progenitor of endothelial cells, are derived from a common progenitor called the hematoangioblast *(157,159,160)*.

Flk1, the fms-like receptor tyrosine kinase, which is expressed on a subset of mesodermal cells *(161)*, and CD105, which is a receptor for several members of the transforming growth factor (TGF)-β superfamily *(162)*, are markers of the bipotential hematoangioblast, the progenitor of both hematopoietic and endothelial cell lineages. Mice exhibiting targeted mutations in Flk-1 die *in utero* at day 8.5 of embryonic life with defects in blood island and vasculature formation *(161)*. In vitro cultures of Flk-1$^+$ cells from 8.5-d-old embryos give rise to cells expressing CD144 (cadherin), which is a marker of endothelial cells, and HSCs expressing CD45 and CD24 (heat stable antigen) *(163)*.

Angiopoietin-1 via binding to Tie-1 and Tie-2 receptors probably represents the growth factor that is required for the differentiation of the hemoangioblast into the angioblast and then into endothelial cells *(164)*. GATA-2 transcription factors are required for progression of the hemoangioblast to the hematoblast stage and then to the HSC *(165)*.

The differentiation of HSCs into mature cells that mediate innate and adaptive immunity is a multistep process with branching points for the various lineages *(166)*. This multistep process leads to the differentiation of pluripotential HSCs into lineage progenitors. Sometimes these progenitors display bipotential differentiation capacity, representing genuine branch points in differentiation processes. It is probable that different transcription factors are involved in the differentiation of cell types at branching points *(167)*. Whereas the multipotentiality and self-renewal capacity of HSCs ensure the continuous generation of white and red blood cells throughout life, the differentiation of progenitors of each lineage into mature cells leads to the death of cells. This is because of the short half-life of terminally differentiated cells. Memory lymphocytes may represent an exception.

Each step of the differentiation of a given lineage does not express a specific phenotype. However, each step requires different growth factors and cytokines, as well as activation of different transcription factors and different signaling pathways. This is probably related to the activation and inhibition of the expression of different genes in each step of the differentiation process.

2. ONTOGENY OF CELLS THAT MEDIATE INNATE IMMUNITY

Myelopoiesis is the process of the development of HSCs toward granulocyte and monocyte lineages. From the yolk sac and AGM region, the multipotential HSCs migrate to the fetal liver, which becomes the predominant hematopoietic organ during embryogenesis. Adult myelopoiesis takes place in the bone marrow *(168,169)*. In the bone marrow, the common myeloid precursor gives rise to polymorphonuclear cells. The development of mature neutrophils, eosinophils, and mast cells is a highly regulated process during which multipotential HSCs differentiate into different lineages. The differentiation program is guided by multiple microenvironmental factors such as stromal cells, and extracellular matrix components. Growth factors and cytokines lead to the activation of transcription factors and genes that are specifically expressed in certain steps of the differentiation process.

2.1. Neutrophil Development

In mice, HCSs in the fetal liver give rise to granulocyte-monocyte (GM) progenitors that are characterized by the phenotype $CD34^+$, Kit^+, Lin^-, and $IL-7R^-$. This cell population can be subdivided into Sca^+ and Sca^-. In vitro cultures of these cells in the presence of steel factor (SLF), granulocyte-macrophage colony-stimulating factor (GM-CSF), thrombopoietin, erythropoietin, IL-3, IL-6, and IL-7 give rise to mixed CFUs. The myelomonocytic progenitors in mixed CFU cultures begin to express Fcγ R II and III. Injection of these $CD34^+$ $FcγR^+$ cells into lethally irradiated recipients gives rise to $GR-1^+$ $Mac-1^+$ myelomonocytic cells. No B- or T-cell progenitors were detected in the cultures of $CD34^+$ $FcγR^+$ fetal cells *(170)*. These observations suggest that the differentiation potential of fetal liver granulocyte-monocyte colony-forming units (GM-CFUs) are entirely restricted to the myeloid lineage.

Similarly, in human fetal livers, the HSCs give rise to GM progenitors, which are characterized by expression of CD34 and Fcγ R II and III. CD34 is a sialo-mucin associated with the membrane of hematopoietic cells that interacts with CD62 ligand, which is a C-type lectin.

The differentiation of granulocyte progenitors is regulated by various cytokines, such as IL-3, GM-CSF, and, in particular, G-CSF, which is the major growth factor required for granulocyte production. The action of G-CSF is mediated through interaction with the G-CSF receptor. The critical role of G-CSF in neutrophil generation was demonstrated by the reduction of granulocyte precursors in G-CSF knockout mice *(171)*. The direct role of G-CSF-R in granulopoiesis comes from studies of patients with severe congenital neutropenia who exhibited a truncated cytoplasmic domain of the G-CSF-R *(172,173)*. In myeloid cells, the membrane proximal domain is essential for the transduction and differentiation signals in neutrophil progenitors. Binding of G-CSF to G-CSF-R results in rapid phosphorylation of four tyrosine residues that are involved in the recruitment of STAT3 and formation of Shc/Grb2/p140 and Grb/p90 complexes. In turn, the subsequent activation of the Syk kinases and PI3K activates Akt, which is an important factor involved in cell growth *(174)*.

The migration of granulocyte progenitors to bone morrow leads to their differentiation into mature neutrophils. The differentiation process is characterized by cytological changes, activation of early myeloid genes, and some specific transcription factors.

Neutrophil maturation proceeds from differentiation of myeloid progenitors into myeloblasts and then to promyelocytes, metamyelocytes, and, finally, neutrophils. Each cytological step of differentiation is associated with the activation of specific genes.

Early myeloid gene activation is responsible for the expression of the G-CSF-R and surface markers such as CD33 (sialo-mucin) and CD13 (metalloproteinase). Other early myeloid genes activated in the process of maturation of neutrophils include mim-1, myeloperoxidase, neutrophil elastase, myeloblastin, and lysozyme. The myelocyte stage is characterized by the expression of genes that encode for proteins contained in secondary granules such as lactoferrin and gelatinase (174,175). Activation of these genes and the progression of different precursors toward neutrophil maturation are regulated by different transcription factors.

Several transcription factors are expressed and activated in HSCs:

a. c-Myb is a transcription factor that recognizes a sequence known as the Myb response element. c-Myb contains an N-terminal DNA-binding domain, a central transactivating domain, and a C-terminal region that contains an evolutionary ESVES-conserved negative regulatory domain. Its role in hematopoiesis is clearly demonstrated in studies carried out using knockout mice that lack myeloid, lymphoid, and erythroid precursors (176).

b. Core binding factor (CBF) is a heterodimeric protein that contains three CBFα subunits that are bound to a CBFβ subunit. CBF is expressed in multipotential bone marrow HSCs. Animals bearing targeted mutated genes that encode both subunits lack all lineages of definitive hematopoiesis (177).

c. SCL is a helix–loop–helix transcription factor that is considered a key element of the regulation of hematopoiesis required for generation of multipotent HSCs (178).

d. GATA-2 is a transcription factor found only in hematopoietic cells. It mediates the differentiation of HSCs toward granulocyte differentiation by regulating C/EBPα levels (179).

   Different transcription factors are required for the differentiation of granulocyte progenitors and activation of various genes during the process of maturation. Thus, c-Myb is involved not only in the growth of HSCs but also in the activation of the CD13 promoter and the activation of the myeloperoxidase gene in response to G-CSF in early myeloid cells (180).

e. Homeobox proteins possess a specific helix–turn–helix DNA-binding domain and comprise a multiple-member family. HoxB4, which is one member of the Homeobox family, is expressed in the earliest HSCs. Hox A9 and Hox A10 are highly expressed in human CD34+ cells; however, their expression is downregulated during hematopoiesis (181).

Other transcription factors specifically regulate the expression of various genes in earlier phases of myelogenesis:

a. C/EBP is a member of a large leucine zipper 4 family. C/EBP is composed of six factors that bind to a similar consensus DNA sequence. Among them, C/EBPα is

detected in human CD33$^+$ CD34$^+$ myeloid progenitors, and its expression increases during the development of myeloid progenitors and their maturation into neutrophils *(181)*. Mice with a disrupted *C/EBPαα* gene show an early block in granulocyte differentiation. Cell lines from these mice express c-Kit but do not express Gr-1, CD34, or G-CSF-R markers. Transfection of fetal liver C/EBPα-/- cells with G-CSF or IL-6 restores the ability of these cells to generate neutrophils *(182)*.
C/EBPα plays a role in the activation of early myeloid genes. This was effectively demonstrated using the human U937 monocytoid line, which, after transfection with *C/EBPα* gene, expressed transcripts of *G-CSF-R, lactoferrin*, and *neutrophil collagenase* genes *(182)*. The expression of mim-1 also is regulated by this transcription factor *(174)*.

b. PU.1 is a member of the ETS transcription factor family that contains a conserved DNA-binding domain located in the C-terminal. PU.1 is phosphorylated on multiple serine residues by ERK1 and JNK1 kinases. PU.1 is expressed at high levels in murine myeloid progenitors and increases during granulocyte differentiation of CD34$^+$ cells in bone marrow *(181)*.
The role of this transcription factor in the maturation of neutrophils is supported by results derived from knockout mice that showed that fetal liver cells exhibit a complete defect in generating G-CFU and lack the expression of CD11b, CD18, and Gr-1 markers. PU.1 regulates the expression of *myeloperoxidase, elastase, lysozyme*, and *c-fes* genes during early phases of neutrophil development.

c. Myeloid zinc finger 1 is preferentially expressed in myeloid progenitors, and reduction of its expression prevents the formation of G-CFU *(183)*. This factor activates the CD34 promoter *(184)*.

d. Notch signaling via RBP-J Jak 3 promotes myeloid differentiation characterized by an increased number of neutrophils that express Fcγ R II and III and Gr-1 marker *(185)*.

In summary, these findings show that the differentiation of myelocyte progenitors into neutrophils is a multistep process in which different genes that encode receptors and specific markers are expressed subsequent to the activation of specific transcription factors.

2.2. Eosinophil Development

HSCs in the fetal liver and later in the bone marrow differentiate into common myeloblast progenitors (CMPs). In bone marrow, CMPs that express GM-CSF-R and G-CSF-R differentiate into monocyte and neutrophil progenitors as well as into CD34$^+$ eosinophil and/or eosinophil-basophil progenitors. In humans, eosinophil progenitors also are found in the cord blood. The events associated with the branching of CMP to the eosinophil lineage are not completely understood because, to date, no eosinophil growth factor or corresponding receptor has been discovered. Therefore, it is thought that some cytokines and transcription factors play a role in the maturation of eosinophil progenitors. Eosinophils that express Fcε R1 can differentiate in vitro from cord blood CD45$^+$ CMP in cultures supplemented with IL-3, GM-CSF, and IL-5 *(186)*.

These cells express proteins contained in eosinophilic granules such as Charcot–Lyeden crystal (16–18%), eosinophil peroxidase (7–8%), and eosinophil-derived neurotoxin (2–4%) *(187)*. Lundahl et al. *(188)* showed that the differentiation of CD45$^+$ CMP into eosinophils is associated with the upregulation of β7-*integrin* and *complement receptor* genes. The expression of EOS47, which is an early specific marker of eosinophil differentiation in the chicken hematopoietic system, is stimulated by GATA-1, c-Myb, Ets-1, and C/EBPα transcription factors. In transfection experiments, Nagny et al. *(189)* demonstrated that Ets-1 and C/EBPα proteins are physically associated with the EOS47 promoter. Overexpression of GATA-1 and GATA-2 in CMP promotes the differentiation and complete maturation of eosinophils, suggesting that these transcription factors play a crucial role in the maturation process of eosinophils *(190)*.

It is worth noting that an increased number of eosinophils were observed by addition of cysteinyl leukotrienes to cultures of bone marrow cells in the presence of GM-CSF, IL-3, and IL-4 *(191)*. However, the addition of IL-12 inhibited the differentiation of bone marrow cells cultured under the same conditions *(192)*.

Taken together, these findings suggest that some cytokines and the activation of some transcription factors direct the differentiation of eosinophil progenitors into mature eosinophils.

2.3. Development of Basophils and Mast Cells

Basophils and mast cells are derived from CD34$^+$ common myeloid progenitors. The differentiation of basophils from progenitors is independent of a defined lineage-specific growth factor. Therefore, one may argue that the differentiation of basophils and mast cells from progenitors results from a "default" pathway resulting from lack of a growth factor. This implies that other environmental factors, particularly cytokines, play an important role in the development of basophils and mast cells.

In vitro studies suggest that the basophils and mast cells represent different sublineages. Whereas basophils are derived from bone marrow CD34$^+$ HSC, the mast cells are derived from a progenitor that expresses CD34, c-Kit, and CD13 *(193)*. However, a recently prepared monoclonal antibody that is specific for CD203 binds to the progenitor of both basophilic and mast cells *(194)*. This information challenges the currently held concept that the basophil and mast cell are derived from different progenitors.

The basophils identified by a specific marker, namely, histamine decarboxylase, have been cultured in vitro subsequent to incubation of mixed, bipotential CFU progenitors (CFU eosinophil-basophil and CFU megakaryocyte-basophil) or unipotential precursors with different cytokines or growth factors *(193)*.

Several known cytokines allow the differentiation of bone marrow and human cord blood CD45$^+$ myeloid precursors into basophils:

a. IL-3 alone or together with stem cell factor or TGF-β induces the differentiation of basophils from CMP *(195)*. The IL-3 receptor CD123 is strongly expressed on basophils, and the SCF receptor CD117 is expressed on mast cells *(196)*. IL-3 functions as a basophilopoietin without evident effect on the maturation of mast cells.

b. IL-5 and eotaxin are involved in the differentiation of eosinophils and basophils from mixed CFU eosinophil-basophil progenitors *(193,197)*.

c. GM-CSF stimulates the production of histamine in monkey bone marrow cell cultures, suggesting that it may play a role in the differentiation of basophils *(193)*.

It is noteworthy that the presence of histamine decarboxylase, the synthesis of histamine, and the expression of Igϵ R are the most faithful markers used to identify the differentiation and the maturation of basophils and mast cells.

The subtle events involved in the differentiation of CMP into basophils and mast cells are not well understood. However, apparently the cytokine milieu, rather than specific growth factors, regulates the differentiation of common myeloid precursors into basophils and mast cells.

2.4. Development of the Monocyte-Macrophage System

The mononuclear phagocyte system, a major arm of innate immunity involved in the defense reaction against microbes and clearing of apoptotic cells, is evolutionarily conserved.

In both invertebrate and vertebrate species, the monocyte-macrophage lineage derives from the mesoderm. In insects, macrophages represent a subpopulation of blood cells called hemocytes. Like vertebrate macrophages, the hemocytes are derived from the mesoderm of the head or that associated with the aorta and heart *(198)*. In Drosophila, the hemocytes express CD36 and scavenger receptors, suggesting that they are the ancestors of vertebrate macrophages *(199)*.

In nematodes such as *Caenorhabitidis elegans*, which do not have blood cells, macrophage-like cells exhibit similar properties to fetal vertebrate macrophages and play a role in morphogenesis. Phagocytosis of apoptotic cells requires the expression of cc-7, which is homologous to murine ABC1 expressed in fetal macrophages *(200)*.

In lower vertebrates like Zebra fish, macrophages are derived from the yolk sac and, as in vertebrates, they are involved in the defense reactions against bacteria *(201)*.

In Xenopus larvae, macrophages are not derived from blood islands but from the mesoderm associated with the embryonic head located anterior to the heart *(153)*.

Study of the development of the monocyte system in mice suggests that, whereas fetal macrophages derive from the yolk sac *(202)*, the monocyte-macrophage lineage derives from the embryonic mesoderm.

Using colony-forming assays, Moore and Metcalf demonstrated that in mice, the precursors of macrophages are located in the yolk sac, which is the site of primitive hematopoiesis, on day 9 of gestation *(143)*. By d 10 of embryonic life, these precursors mature into macrophages, which leave the blood islands, enter the mesenchyme, and then migrate to various tissues via circulation. Fetal macrophages of yolk sac origin express F4/80 antigen *(203)* but are devoid of peroxidase activity, which is characteristic of adult macrophages *(204)*.

The monocyte-macrophage lineage derives from the embryonic hematoangioblast expressing Flk-1 and CD105 markers. The hemocytoblast differentiates into HSCs that migrate to the liver and give rise to common myeloblast progenitors (CMPs). Commitment of CMPs to monocyte progenitors coincides with granulocyte commitment because the bipotent GM-CFU that expresses the GM-CSF receptor can give rise to G-CFU as well as to M-CFU. In the fetal liver or later in the bone marrow, the M-CFU progenitor stimulated by G-CSF and other cytokines differentiates into monoblasts. In the bone marrow, the monoblast that expresses the M-CSF receptor (a product of c-fens protooncogene), lysozyme, and FcRγ II and III differentiate into promonocytes, which, in the blood stream, give rise to monocytes.

Mature blood monocytes express additional markers such as macrosialin, CD14, CD11b, and CD18 and possess strong phagocytic properties *(175)*.

Terminal differentiation of CMPs into monocytes is associated with the activation of Fes protein. This was demonstrated by studying the gain-of-function markers in the bipotential human U937 monocytoid line transfected with the C-fps/fes protooncogene. Transfected cells acquired macrophage cytological features and CD11b, CD11c, CD18, CD14, and M-CSFR marker expression characteristics for monocytes *(205)*. Maturation of monocytes also is associated with the ERK-MAP kinase pathway, as shown by increased phosphorylation of MEK1/2 and ERK1/2 in HL-60 cells treated with PMA *(206)*. Transcription factors regulate the expression of genes in various stages of the maturation of monocytes. Whereas some transcription factors are quite specific for the monocyte lineage, others activate genes in granulocyte progenitors. Egr-1, a member of the zinc-finger transcription family, is activated in various bipotential cell lines or bone marrow cells, which differentiate into macrophages after exposure to phorbol ester or cytokines *(181)*. Ectopic expression of Egr-1 in myeloid progenitor lines increases the expression of the M-CFU receptor *(207)*. The binding of C/EBP, PU.1, and c-Jun transcription factors to their corresponding DNA-binding motifs activates the promoter of the *GM-CSF receptor* gene and of the *lysozyme* gene that is expressed in monoblasts *(208,209)*.

It is noteworthy to point out that there are a few transcription factors that are specific for a given maturation step of the monocytic or granulocytic lineages. The majority of transcription factors are activated in CMP and in later phases

Table 13
Target Genes of Transcription Factors During Various Stages of the Development of Cells From Common Myeloid Precursors

Myeloid precursors	
Transcription factors	Target gene
C/EBP-α, PU.1	GM-CSF R
C/EBP-α, PU.1	G-CSF R
C/EBP-α, PU.1, c-Myb	M-CSF R
C/EBP-α, PU.1 c-MybL	Lysozyme
C/EBP-α, c-Myb	Min-1
C/EBP-α, PU.1, c-Myb, MZF-1	Myeloperoxidase
C/EBP-α, PU.1 CBF, c-Myb, SP-1	Neutrophil elastase
PU.1, SP-1	c-fes
C/EBP-α, PU. 1, c-Myb	Myeloblastin
C/EBP-α, PU.1, EPS	CD13
HoxA10	p21
C/EBP-α	p27
MZF-1	CD34

Mature cells		
	Neutrophils	
C/EBP-α, CDP, Sp-1, MZF-1		Lactoferrin
	Eosinophils	
GATA-1		Unknown
Ets-1, C/EBP-α		EOSA7 (birds)
	Monocytes	
PU.1, c-Jun		Macrosialin
Egr-1		Unknown
C/ EBP-α, Sp-1		CD14
PU.1, SP-1, GABP		CD18
PU.1, Sp-1		CD11b
ICSBP		IL-12
	Dendritic cells	
PU.1		CD11c

Adapted from refs. *162, 174, 175, 179, 181.*

of maturation. They can bind to the promoters of different genes. In addition, there is an extensive redundant effect of transcription factors on the activation of a single gene because DNA-binding motifs of different transcription factors can be present on the promoter of a single gene. Conversely, a single transcription factor might bind to the promoter of different genes. An example of redundancy of transcription factors is illustrated in Table 13.

Blood monocytes migrate to various tissues and mature into macrophages. In spite of the fact that tissue macrophages may display various cytological and distinct features, they express some common markers such as CD11b, IL-1β, FcγR, scavenger receptors, and CD11b, CD14, and CD18 markers.

An elegant demonstration of the capacity of mouse bone marrow monoblasts to differentiate into distinct types of macrophages was provided by Servet-Delpart et al. *(210)*. They showed that bone marrow immature monocytes expressing Flt3 ligand could differentiate in vitro into osteoclasts, microglia, or dendritic cells depending on culture conditions. For instance, bone marrow Flt3+ progenitors expressing CD11b after 6 d of culture in the presence of M-CSF and RANKL or tumor necrosis factor (TNF) give rise to osteoclasts. Similarly, the progenitors that express CD11b and F4/80 antigen cultured for 11 d in the presence of M-CSF and glial-conditioned medium differentiate into microglial macrophages.

There is recent evidence that blood monocytes in humans can differentiate into dendritic cells. In initial studies, it was shown that human blood monocytes cultured in the presence of GM-CSF and IL-4 differentiated into immature dendritic cells characterized by downregulation of the expression of CD14 and acquisition of CD1a antigen *(79)*. Upon in vitro stimulation of these cells with LPS, TNF-α, IL-1, and CD40L, they exhibit the phenotype of mature dendritic cells. Randolph et al. *(211)* showed that the differentiation of blood monocytes into dendritic cells can be achieved in the absence of cytokines subsequent to culturing the monocytes on an endothelial cell layer grown on a collagen matrix. Only the monocytes transmigrating across the endothelial layer into the collagen matrix acquire dendritic cell markers such as CD83, CD86, and dendritic cell-LAMP and lose CD14 and CD64 monocyte differentiation antigen.

The growth factors, cytokines, and cellular requirements of the differentiation of monocytes in various types of tissue macrophages are not completely elucidated and are the subject of intensive research. Recently, it was shown that the activation of caspases-3 and -9, which play a crucial role in apoptosis, are activated in blood monocytes during differentiation into macrophages, a process not associated with apoptosis *(212)*.

2.5. Development of Dendritic Cells

Dendritic cells were identified in the blood and in tissues such as peripheral lymphoid organs and thymus, skin and epithelia (Langerhans cells [LC]), and other tissues (e.g., interstitial dendritic cells).

It is difficult to identify lineage ontogeny of dendritic cells in the fetus because (a) there is not a specific dendritic cell-growth factor, and, consequently, there is not a receptor for a dendritic cell-specific growth factor that can be used as a cell marker; (b) the differentiation of common monocyte precursors, from which it is supposed that dendritic cells emanate, give rise to monocyte intermediates that can not be distinguished from dendritic cells; and (c) newly discovered markers of mature dendritic cells such as DEC10 in mice or dendritic cell-LAMP in humans are not expressed on the most primitive dendritic cell progenitor, which differentiates from CMP or CLP.

Major insights into dendritic cells have come from in vitro studies because new methods aimed at characterizing the progenitor of dendritic cells have been perfected. Senju et al. developed a new method to generate dendritic cells from 10-d-old embryo murine HSCs by culturing the HSCs on feeder cell layers of OP9 cells in the presence of GM-CSF *(213)*. Seven days after culture, the occurrence of irregularly shaped floating cells possessing strong phagocytic properties and expressing class II, CD11c, CD80, and CD86 antigen has been observed. Jackson et al. studied ex vivo differentiation of murine Sca1$^+$ Lin$^-$ HPCs into dendritic cells grown in the presence of GM-CSF alone or in various combinations with IL-4 and TNF-α *(214)*. Sca1+ HPC cultured for 9 d in the presence of a low dose of GM-CSF alone or in combination with IL-4 and/or TNF-α induced the differentiation of precursors into immature dendritic cells *(214)*. The cells generated in cultures exhibited the immature dendritic cell phenotype: CD11b^{bright}, CD11c^{mod}, CD86^{low}, class II^{low}, DEC 250^{low}, and CD4$^-$. The stimulation of these immature dendritic cells with LPS or CD40L resulted in dendritic cells exhibiting the mature phenotype CD40^{high}, secretion of IL-β and IL-12, and the ability to be strong stimulators in a mixed lymphocyte culture.

Studies of the differentiation of dendritic cells from bone marrow have advanced the hypothesis of a dual origin of dendritic cells from common myeloid and lymphoid progenitors. Several lines of experimental evidence support this concept. Inaba et al. showed that murine dendritic cells could be generated along with monocytes from cells within a single CFU after in vitro culture with GM-CSF but not with G-CSF or M-CSF *(215)*. dendritic cells generated in an ex vivo system expressed MHC class II molecules and were able to prime naïve T cells. In adoptive transfer experiments, it was shown that these dendritic cells homed to the T zone of lymphoid organs. Reid et al. demonstrated ex vivo differentiation of dendritic cells from human bone marrow bipotential CD34$^+$ cells and mixed CFU cultured with GM-CSF and TNF-α *(216)*. The dendritic cells recovered from the colony did not express CD14 but exhibited strong staining with anti-MHC class II, CD80, and CD86 monoclonal antibodies. Caux et al. showed that CD34$^+$ HSCs present in human cord blood could also differentiate into dendritic cells *(217)*.

The transcription factors NF-κB/Rel and PU.1 play an important role in the differentiation of dendritic cells of myeloid origin. Data indicating a reduced number of CD8α^- dendritic cells in mice with disrupted Rel or PU.1 genes strongly support this concept (reviewed in ref. *218*).

LCs are derived from blood dendritic cells. Strunk et al. demonstrated that CD34[+] progenitors expressing a skin homing receptor cultured in the presence of GM-CSF, IL-4, and TGF-β can differentiate into LCs expressing CD1a, langerin, E-cadherin, and Bierbeck granules *(219)*.

In human blood, Ito et al. identified another subset expressing CD1a and CD11c that can differentiate into LCs after culturing with GM-CSF, IL-4, and TGF-β *(86)*. The dendritic cells emanated from cultures also expressed markers characteristic of LCs such as langerin, E-cadherin, and Bierbeck granules. It is interesting to note that the development of dendritic cells from CMPs requires the activation of the Rel transcription factor. However, the LCs were present in Rel knockout mice. This observation raises interest regarding the myeloid origin of LCs *(220)*.

The concept of the lymphoid origin of a subset of dendritic cells arises from the observation that thymic, and some splenic, dendritic cells express markers of lymphoid cells such as CD8α, CD2, CD4, CD25, B220, and BP1 *(220–222)*. The concept of lymphoid origin is supported by adoptive transfer experiments of CD4[low] lymphoid precursors, which, after injection in lethally irradiate mice, gave rise to CD8α[+] cells exhibiting a plasmoid morphology *(223)*. In mice, the precursors of plasmacytoid CD8α[+] dendritic cells also are found in the bone marrow. These precursors can differentiate in ex vivo cultures supplemented with Flc-3 ligand as the sole growth factor *(224)*. Hochrein et al. showed that in vitro differentiated CD8α[+] dendritic cells have the capacity to produce type I IFN *(225)*. In humans, the equivalent of murine CD8α[+] plasmacytoid dendritic cells is characterized by the expression of IL-3R and CD68 (macrosialin); lack of expression of CD11b, CD11c, CD14, CD13, and CD33; and a high capacity to produce INF but not IL-12 *(226)*.

Human plasmacytoid dendritic cells can be generated in vitro from CD34[+] progenitors from fetal liver, cord blood, and bone marrow cultured with Flt-3 ligand alone or from CD34[+] CD38[–] fetal liver progenitors cultured for 7 d with murine stromal cells *(227)*. Liu et al. demonstrated that the thymus also contains plasmacytoid dendritic cells that develop from CD34[+] precursors *(228)*. Unlike interstitial dendritic cells of myeloid origin, the plasmacytoid dendritic cells do not require GM-CSF for their development.

In humans, CD34[+] HSCs that are able to generate dendritic cells are detected in the fetal liver until approx 20 wk after gestation after which they are found mainly in the bone marrow. After birth, 1–3% of cord blood cells express CD34 and, therefore, can be considered as multipotential HSCs. During the differentiation of CD34[+] CD45RA[–] progenitors into pre-dendritic cells, they gradually lose CD34 antigen and express CD4, CD45RA, IL-3R, and major histocompatibility complex (MHC) class II antigens *(228)*.

Immature dendritic cells differentiate into mature dendritic cells after stimulation by various agents. Thus, CpG and CD40 ligands induce the maturation of preplasmacytoid dendritic cells, which in turn are able to induce the differentiation of Th1 cells producing INF-γ. Stimulation with viruses induces the maturation of plasmacytoid dendritic cells that are able to activate regulatory T cells producing IFN-γ and IL-10. Stimulation with IL-3 induces the maturation of plasmacytoid dendritic cells that are able to induce the differentiation of Th2 cells producing IL-4, IL-5, and Il-10 *(228)*.

The prompt synthesis of IFNs by mature plasmacytoid dendritic cells after recognition of pathogens may represent a master function of these cells in innate immunity during development and throughout entire life. First, IFNs can activate other cells involved in the innate immune defense reactions, such as macrophages and NK cells. Second, IFNs may favor the initiation of the adaptive immune response by virtue of their pleiotropic effects on T and B cells, thereby triggering a whole spectrum of specific immune responses *(229)*.

More recently, the concept of different origins of the two subsets of dendritic cells was challenged by a report suggesting the presence in the bone marrow of a dendritic cell-progenitor that can differentiate into either CD8α⁻ or CD8α⁺ mature dendritic cells. These dendritic cell-progenitors are devoid of myeloid or lymphoid differentiation potential inducible by various growth factors *(230)*.

2.6. Development of NK Cells

NK cells are generated during fetal life from lymphoid common precursors that arise from the differentiation of HSCs. Mature NK cells originate from NK unipotential progenitors found in the fetal liver or from bipotential progenitors (NK and T cells) found in the fetal thymus. During adult life, NK progenitors are present within bone marrow.

Apparently, IL-15 secreted by stromal cells is the major growth factor directing the differentiation of NK precursors into mature NK cells. In the murine system, NK progenitors were identified in 14-d-old fetal livers. They express NK1.1 antigen, CD94 protein, and later Ly49E receptors that recognize Qa1^b nonclassical MHC antigen. A significant proportion of fetal NK cells binds the Qa1 tetramer *(231)*. The expression of Ly49E receptors significantly decreases after birth. Other members of the Ly49 receptor family such as Ly49A, C/1 D, G2, and H are almost indetectable during fetal life and in the first week after birth *(232)*.

Leclercq et al. demonstrated that in fetal thymus the NK cells arose from bipotential T/NK progenitors *(233)*. These bipotential progenitors differentiate into mature lytic NK cells upon in vitro culture with IL-15. A detailed kinetic and phenotypic analysis of clones derived from a 14-d-old fetal thymus showed that CD94 and NKG2 were expressed earlier than LY49E, which was acquired in a progressive and stochastic manner independent of the expression of CD94/NKG2 *(234)*.

In murine bone marrow, NK cells are derived from two different subsets of multipotential HSCs that express different phenotypes. The first subset, with both lymphoid and myeloid differentiating ability, expresses the phenotype Scal1$^+$, c-Kit$^+$, CD43^{high}, Ftl-3^{high}. In adoptive transfer experiments, it was shown that this cell subset gave rise to NK cells *(235)*. The second subset, which represents 1% of total bone marrow cells, displays a different phenotype: Scal2$^+$, c-Kit$^+$, CD44^{high}, HSA^{int}. This subset does not express Ly49, CD2, B220, Gr1, CD11b, NK1.1, CD4, CD8, and CD3 markers. These cells, when cultured for 5–6 d in medium containing IL-6, IL-7, SCF, and Ftl-3L and then for additional 4–5 d with IL-15, gave rise to NK1.1$^+$ cells displaying lytic activity *(235)*. These results suggest that the Scal 2$^+$ progenitors cultured in medium with a mixture of cytokines acquired the IL-15R and that IL-15 caused the terminal differentiation in mature NK cells that express the NK1.1 marker and later the Ly49 receptors. This observation suggests that the occurrence of lytic activity and the expression NK1.1 antigen precede the expression of the Ly49 receptor. In bone marrow culture, stromal cells are required for the induction of Ly49 *(236)*. In the absence of stromal cells, the progenitors dedifferentiate into NK1.1$^+$ cells that display cytotoxic abilities but lack Ly49 expression *(237)*.

In contrast to the expression of Ly49 during NK development, little is known about the expression of CD94/NKG2 during differentiation of NK from embryonic HSCs. NKG2 represents a family of genes. Whereas NKG2A associated with CD94 represents an inhibitor receptor complex, CD94/NKG2C and NKG2E are thought to be activating receptor complexes *(238)*. Lian et al. showed that there is a programmed order of the acquisition of CD94/NKG2 receptors during in vitro differentiation of embryonic HSCs into NK cells *(239)*. First, the CD94 transcript is detected in HSCs at the beginning of culture. A few days later, NKG2D transcript is detected, and at approx 8 d of culture, the transcripts of NKG2A and NKG2E are expressed. The NKG2C transcript was detected by RT-PCR at 10 d after culture. Thus, it appears that during the differentiation of NK cells, the inhibitory receptors that prevent autoagression and favor self-tolerance are expressed first, and the activating receptors are expressed later *(240)*.

In humans, CD56$^+$ NK cells develop from fetal livers, cord blood, and adult bone marrow CD45$^+$ HSCs cultured in vitro in the presence of IL-15. The differentiation of CD34$^+$, Ftl3$^+$, c-Kit$^+$ NK progenitors into CD34^{bright} IL-2R$^+$ IL-15 R$^+$ requires Ftl-3 and KL ligands that induce the expression of the IL-2 and

IL-15 receptors. These precursors in the presence of the stromal bone marrow environment or subsequent to stimulation by IL-2 and IL-15 give rise to mature NK cells characterized by the CD56$^+$, IL-2R$^+$, IL-15R$^+$ NKR$^+$ phenotype *(106)*. It is still not clear which factors are required for the expression of KIR receptor family.

Studies carried out both in mouse and human systems clearly demonstrated that the NK progenitors are derived from HSCs that differentiate into NK progenitors. Further, the maturation of NK precursors is dependent on cytokines, particularly IL-15 secreted by stromal cells.

Figure 26 illustrates the pathways of the differentiation of WBCs of myeloid origin.

3. ONTOGENY OF LYMPHOCYTES

Mature lymphocytes are derived from common lymphoid progenitors that arise from pluripotent HSCs, which differentiate from hematongioblasts of mesodermal origin. The commitment of HSCs to the lymphoid lineage is a stepwise process leading to irreversible differentiation into T and B lymphocytes. The commitment of HSCs to a given lineage follows a genetic program. However, the mechanisms underlying the accomplishment of the genetic program are unclear because they depend on a multitude of factors. Among these factors, one may cite (a) the cellular microenvironment, in which the expression of adhesion molecules and chemokines receptors might play a role; (b) the growth factors, which are required for the self-renewal of progenitors and their differentiation; and (c) cytokines, which may provide the activation signal or suppress the expression of genes at certain stages of the stepwise differentiation process. Because lymphopoiesis is a stepwise differentiation process, certain genes expressed in early phases can be silenced in more advanced stages of differentiation. Similarly, other genes can be activated in certain stages of irreversible commitment to a lineage. This may be related to activation and/or upregulation of certain transcription factors. The lineage commitment requires the stabilization of expression of transcription factors during the progressive differentiation genetic program of a lineage.

3.1. Development of B Cells

In the mouse, B cells are derived from HSCs of the yolk sac and the body of embryo. The HSCs migrate at d 12 to the fetal liver, which contains 1600–2000 antibody-forming precursors. These precursors migrate to bone marrow at d 15, which then becomes the major central organ in which the precursors mature. Such B cells exhibit cytodifferentiation antigen, including surface IgM and IgD, and the rearrangement of V genes that encode the specificity of the B-cell receptor (BCR). Early studies of bone marrow precursors of B cells showed

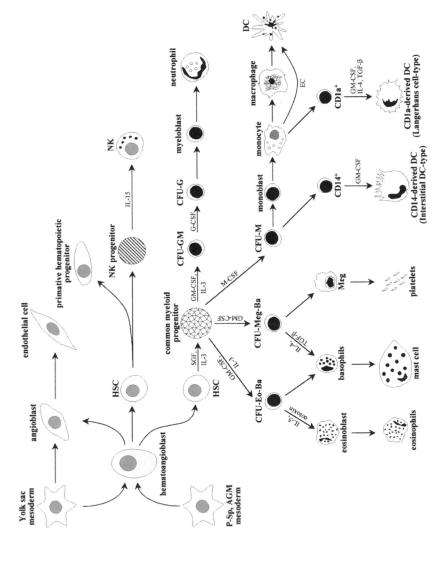

Fig. 26. Development of hematopoietic lineage during ontogeny, leading to generation of cells involved in innate immunity.

that some of them are devoid of the surface Ig receptor and express the μ heavy chain in the cytoplasm and that the V genes are not rearranged. This type of cell, called a pre-B cell, is considered to represent one element of the stepwise maturation process of B-cell progenitor development into mature B cells *(241)*.

Extensive studies led to the proposal of a unified model of B lymphopoiesis in which each step of differentiation process is characterized by the expression of various cell markers, Ig genes, and some specific transcription factors *(242)*.

The B-lymphocyte development model consists of several stages: pro-B cells derived from a stem cell lymphoid progenitor, pre B-1 cells represented by large cells that exhibit dividing capacity, leading to pre B-2 small cells, which differentiate into immature B cells and finally into mature B cells.

This model of B lymphopoiesis originates mainly from studies carried out in mice and humans and is consistent with the comparative phylogenetic studies of B-cell development in vertebrate species with species-specific differences related to the duration of pregnancy and the appearance of lymphoid organs during fetal life.

In lower vertebrate species, the tissues harboring early B-cell progenitors are still not well defined.

From a phylogenetic point of view, the elasmobranchs, which are cartilaginous fish such as sharks and skates, are the earliest species having a lymphoid system as defined by the presence of V genes that encode the BCR. During embryonic life, the kidney could be the initial site for the development of B-cell progenitors *(243)*. Later, when the embryo grows (5–10 cm long), renal lymphopoietic capacity declines and B-cell development switches to other tissues that may be considered to be an equivalent of bone marrow, i.e., Leyding organ, intestinal spinal valve, and spleen.

In the Aleutian skate (*Bathyreja aleutica*), cells expressing Ig were found in the embryonic spleen. Their number increases during embryonic development *(244)*. In another cartilaginous fish species, *Raja eglanteria*, the transcripts for IgM and IgX were found abundantly in 8-wk-old embryos in the spleen, Leyding organ, liver, gonad, and thymus *(245)*.

It is interesting to note that in these species, *in situ* chromosomal hybridization using Ig probes identified multiple IgX and IgM loci, suggesting that the V genes encoding Ig might be located on various chromosomes.

In teleosts, the kidney pronephros and mesonephros are the major sources of B cells. The presence of pre-B cells in the kidney is supported by the identification of non-rearranged multiple IgL transcripts in the pronephros of Atlantic cod and rainbow trout *(246)* and the high expression of Ikaros and RAG genes involved in the development and rearrangement of V genes in B cells *(247, 248)*. The differentiation of B-cell progenitors in the pronephros occurs later in ontogeny *(249,250)*. The origin of B-cell progenitors in the pronephros is unknown. Thompson et al. hypothesized that in zebrafish, the c-Myb$^+$ progenitors of the dorsal aorta move to the kidney *(251)*.

In Atlantic cod, the head of the kidney and the spleen appear as the first lymphoid organs at the time of hatching *(252)*. In catfish, the first B lymphocytes are observed in renal hematopoietic tissue and later in the spleen between d 7 and 14 after hatching *(253)*.

From these observations, several conclusions might be drawn: (a) In fish, pre-B cells and IgM- and IgX-bearing B cells are present during embryonic life; (b) the kidney appears to be the source of hematopoiesis and of B-cell progenitors; and (c) during embryonic development, the Leyding organ, liver, and gonad may be the site of B lymphopoiesis, which eventually may be considered the equivalent of bone marrow in higher vertebrates.

In amphibia, the larvae hatch 2 d after fertilization. The stem cells, lymphopoietic progenitors migrating from the lateral plate of the mesoderm, are detected in the liver and thymus during the first week of development. Larval B-cell development can be divided into two stages. The first stage starts at d 4 when RAG transcripts and B-cell precursors are detected, whereas by d 8, most IgM$^+$ B cells are pre-B cells lacking a rearranged light chain *(254)*.

The second phase extends from d 12 to 50, corresponding to the end of metamorphosis. Near the end of metamorphosis, the number of pre-B cells in the liver and spleen decline, and B lymphopoiesis switches to the bone marrow *(255)*.

Studies of the ontogeny of B cells in reptiles (e.g., Chalcides ocellatus lizard) indicate that the embryonic liver is the site for the differentiation of B cells *(256)* and that by d 40–41, 40–50% of spleen cells express cytoplasmic and surface Ig *(257)*.

In contrast to cold, lower vertebrate species, the avian species have a lymphoid organ called the bursa of Fabricius, which is the equivalent of bone marrow in mammalian species. The bursa of Fabricius has two major functions: (a) expansion of B-cell progenitors, and (b) the diversification of the antibody repertoire. The role of the bursa was elegantly demonstrated by Cooper et al. *(258)*, who showed that a bursectomy carried out on a 17-d-old embryo results in an agammaglobulinemic chicken. The bursa develops from the hindgut at day 4 of embryonic life from the endodermal bud surrounded by the mesoderm *(259)*. Using two monoclonal antibodies specific for stromal cells, Olah et al. showed that mesenchymal stromal cells migrate to the surface of the bursal epithelium around d 12 of embryonic life, preceding follicular formation *(260)*. Some of the stromal cells remain at the luminal surface and others migrate to the medulla. The stromal cells play an important role in the maturation of B-cell progenitors after interaction with HSCs.

The ontogeny of avian B cells can be divided into three phases. In the extrabursal stage, B-cell progenitors are derived from the intraembryonic mesenchyme *(261)*. This stage exists only during embryonic life and ceases after hatching. The most primitive B-cell progenitors are detectable in the yolk sac by d 5–6 and express only a D-J rearrangement characteristic for pre-B cells *(262)*. Complete VDJ rearrangement in the extrabursal progenitors is virtually complete by 15 d after incubation *(263)*. In birds, B-cell progenitors expressing Bu-1 antigen seem to be irreversibly committed to the B-lymphoid lineage prior to migration to the bursa *(264)*. The bursal stage is characterized by migration to and seeding of B-cell progenitors in the bursa, where the maturation of the precursors takes place after interaction with bursal stromal cells *(266)*. The postbursal stage begins during the late phase of embryonic life and continues at hatching when mature B cells (in the case of ducklings) migrate to the liver, bone marrow, and then lymph nodes and Harderian glands *(265)*. The colonization of peripheral organs takes place 10–17 d after hatching *(266)*.

Thus, the major differences between the ontogeny of avian B cells and those of the lower vertebrates and mammals consists of the generation of B cells from a single set of precursors during embryonic life and the maturation of B-cell progenitors in the bursa from which they colonize the peripheral lymphoid organs.

Murine mature B cells are divided into two subsets: (a) B-1 expressing CD5, which produces mainly IgM-polyreactive antibodies; and (b) the B-2 CD5⁻ subset, which produces antibodies specific for foreign antigen and pathogenic autoantibodies *(107,109)*. Both subsets are derived from common lymphoid HSCs.

In mice, pluripotential HSCs move from splanchnopleura to the fetal liver at d 12 of gestation. The fetal liver and the spleen represent the major sites of B lymphopoiesis during embryonic life, which continue until the first week after birth. The B cells arise from a common lymphoid precursor population that expresses $Sca1^{low}$ c-Kit^{low} and IL-$7R\alpha^+$ and is identified at day 14 in the fetal liver. These precursors are able to reconstitute all lymphoid lineages when injected into sublethally irradiated newborn mice. After culture on a stromal cell layer, in a medium supplemented with IL-7, they differentiate into immature CD19⁺ IgM⁺ B cells *(267)*.

The differentiation of B lymphocytes from multipotential progenitors is a stepwise process characterized by the expression of certain antigen and rearrangement of *V* genes. Pro-B cells that are characterized by the new phenotype B220⁺ c-Kit⁺, CD43⁻ TdT⁻ and the V pre-B receptor (encoded by the genes *VpreB1*, *VpreB2*, and λ5) arise from the progenitors committed to differentiation into the B lineage. The ligand for this receptor, as well as its function, is poorly defined. However, it plays an important role in furthering the differentiation process because *VpreB1*, *VpreB2*, and λ5 triple-deficient mice show impaired B-cell development *(268)*. Pro-B cells differentiate into pre-B-1 exhibiting the phenotype CD43[+], B220[+], c-Kit[+] VpreB[+] and the rearrangement of D and J segments of V genes. Both RAG1 and RAG2, which mediate the recombination of V germline gene segments, are expressed in pro-B cells. In contrast to fetal liver pre-B1 cells, the pre-B1 cells in bone marrow do not express TdT, which may explain why the fetal liver B cells lack N-addition in V genes *(269)*. The pre-B1 cells differentiate further into pre-B2, which are large dividing cells that exhibit complete VDJ gene rearrangement and express cytoplasmic μ-heavy chain. The RAG activity strongly decreases in pre-B1 cells in the next step, and pre-B2 small cells begin to rearrange the genes that encode k and λ-light chains, leading to the expression of surface IgM. In this stage, the RAG activity is again increased and the expression of CD43 antigen is lost. These cells differentiate into immature B cells, which are characterized by a B200[+], sIgM[+] phenotype. *(269)*.

Little is known about the fetal differentiation pathway of CD5[+] B1 cells. Clarke et al. proposed that the B1 phenotype results from the upregulation of CD5 on mature B2 cells during self-antigen-driven expansion *(270)*. The process of development of B2 cells is viewed as a transition from CD23[+] B200[high] IgM[low] IgD[high] CD5[−] to CD5[+] B220[low] IgM[+]. Hayakawa and Hardy consider that signaling via the B-cell receptor may play a role in the differentiation of the B1 subset *(271)*.

In rabbits, B-cell lymphopoiesis begins in the fetal liver and switches to the bone marrow late in fetal life and continues in the bone marrow throughout life. Pre-B cells are detected in the bone marrow beginning at d 14 of gestation in the fetal liver, reaching a peak at d 17–19, and disappearing at day 10 after birth. In fetal bone marrow, pre-B cells are detected at d 25. Pre-B2 small cells are detected in the fetal spleen at d 29 of gestation (data reviewed in ref. *272*). Previously, we showed that an extract from *Nocardia opaca* (NWSM) is a polyclonal stimulator of rabbit B cells just as LPS is a polyclonal stimulator of murine B cells *(273)*.

We found that B cells from fetal liver harvested at d 17–29 of gestation proliferate upon stimulation with NWSM and, at d 22, proliferate subsequent to stimulation with antiallotype antibodies. At birth (1-d-old pups), although the NWSM and antiallotype proliferative responses disappeared in fetal liver cells, a significant increase in NWSM and antiallotype responses was observed in spleen cells. Whereas B cells from the fetal liver harvested at d 17 of gestation lack the ability to synthesize Ig, Ig synthesis was observed at d 22 and gradually increased until d 29. In 1-d-old pups, whereas the liver cells were no longer able to synthesize Ig, the spleen cells from newborn rabbits exhibited the ability to spontaneously synthesize Ig, a process that was considerably enhanced after stimulation with NWSM *(274)*. Pre-B cells also were identified in rabbit fetal and postnatal omentum *(275)*. Apparently, at birth, the B cells are able to function in an immune response. This concept is supported by an experiment where the transfer of newborn lymphocytes into an adult rabbit was able to respond to a challenge with Shigella antigen *(276)*. In rabbits, the first peripheral organs colonized with B cells after birth are gut-associated lymphoid organs, such as the appendix, Peyer's patches, and sacculus rotundus, which is an organ found at ileal-cecal junction *(272)*.

In pigs, the first pre-B cells exhibiting VDJ rearrangement appear at d 29 of gestation in the yolk sac and at d 30 in the fetal liver, which, thereafter, is the major site of B-cell lymphopoiesis *(277)*.

B-cell development in the lamb is particularly interesting because the immune system matures rapidly during gestation, and the lamb can actually develop an antibody response after fetal immunization. Hematopoiesis occurs in the yolk sac at d 19–27 of the 145-d gestation period. The first B1 and B2 cells were detected in the spleen at approx d 81 and 48 of gestation, respectively *(278,279)*. The maximum proliferation of IgM$^+$ cells in the spleen was prominent between d 60 and 70. Little information exists concerning the origin of pre B cells during lamb gestation. If pre-B cells exist, they likely have a very short life because of the rapid differentiation into IgM$^+$ B cells. Similar to pigs, the gut-associated lymphoid system is the first organ colonized with B cells after birth *(279)*.

There is little information on nonhuman primate B-cell development. A recent study carried out on Rhesus monkey fetuses demonstrated that the first IgM$^+$ B cells were identified at d 65 of gestation (the term of gestation in Rhesus monkey is 165 d). The CD20$^+$ CD5$^+$ B cells expressing class II molecules appear in large numbers in the spleen, mesenteric lymph nodes, and small intestine at d 65 of gestation, and their number increases until birth. The most likely origin of CD5$^+$ B cells in monkeys is the omentum and fetal liver. By d 145, CD20$^+$ CD5$^-$ B2 cells become predominant in the B-cell follicles in various organs. They express not only surface IgM but also IgG and IgA *(280)*. These observations indicate that immune competence in monkeys may be achieved in the last trimester of fetal life, permitting the occurrence of an immune response soon after birth.

The human immune system, including B cells, is fully developed at birth. Throughout gestation, more than 90% of B cells in the fetal liver and spleen are CD5$^+$. The origin of the precursors of fetal CD5$^+$ B cells is not well defined, but it is believed to be the yolk sac, omentum, and fetal liver *(281)*.

HSCs, from which B cells arise, are present in the fetal liver, cord blood, and later in bone marrow. Apparently, the CD45$^+$ that express B-cell progenitors are retained in the fetal liver and bone marrow until differentiation into IgM$^+$/CD79 cells. Data showing that CD34$^+$ B-cell precursors are undetectable in cord blood support this concept *(282)*. However, another study that found B cells that express CD34 and CD10 or CD19 in the blood challenged this concept *(283)*. The differentiation of B cells from CD34$^+$ B-cell progenitors was studied in vivo in severe combined immunodeficiency (SCID) mice infused with human fetal cells and in vitro in stromal-dependent culture systems detailing development of HSC from cord blood or bone marrow.

In these systems, it was shown that in humans, similarly to mice, B-cell development is a genetically programmed stepwise process characterized by (a) the expression of regulatory genes; (b) occurrence and disappearance of certain membrane antigen; (c) somatic rearrangements of germline genes containing the information for the specificity of Ig receptor; and (d) signaling molecules associated with the BCR, such as Ig β-B29, Ig α-mb-1, and B-lymphoid tyrosine kinase (Blk). The prevailing concept of human B-cell differentiation consists of progressive changes to the genetic program during the differentiation of CD35$^+$ multipotent HSCs that represent the most primitive HSCs from which CD34$^+$, CD38$^+$ B-cell progenitors are derived *(284)*. From these progenitors arise pre-pro-B cells expressing CD10 and CD19. Pro-B cells express a surrogate light chain receptor encoded by two very homologous *V-pre-B* genes and the λ5 gene. Pro-B cells do not exhibit any rearrangement of V_H and V_L genes but have the enzymes that mediate the recombination of V-gene segments such as RAG1 and RAG2. Progression to the pre-B1 stage is associated first with the somatic rearrangement of D-J gene segments of the V heavy chain gene and with the expression of CD29 and mb-1 required for the transduction signals. In the next stage of the development, the large dividing pre-B1 cells bear an in-frame productive VDJ μ chain and maintain the expression of pseudo λ, CD10, and CD19. However, the pre-B1 cells downregulate the expression of CD34, RAG, and TdT enzymes *(284–286)*. In the pre-B2 small cells, the CD34 gene is completely silenced and the rearrangement of light chain genes is completed, allowing for the expression of IgM-CD79 complexes on the surface of immature B cells *(287)*.

As we have seen, in both lower and higher vertebrate species, B-cell development is a stepwise process composed of various stages, which are irreversible after the beginning of the differentiation process. This process is characterized by the activation of certain genes expressed in all the stages of maturation, the activation of new genes or silencing of other genes in certain stages, and the activation in early stages of enzymes that mediate the rearrangement of V genes and a large number of proteins composing pre-B- and B-cell receptors (IgL pre-B λ5, mb1, B29, Blk). All of these processes follow a genetic program controlled by some genes, which are specifically required for B-cell development, and by transcription factors involved in transcriptional control of the promoters of various genes expressed or silenced during B-cell development.

The expression of some genes such as *Ikaros*, and some transcription factors such as E47, E12, EBF, BSAP, PAX-5, and PU.1 are required for the survival of HSC-common lymphoid precursors and are critical for B-cell differentiation.

The critical role of *Ikaros* gene expression in early B-cell development in mice was demonstrated by two distinct Ikaros-targeted mutations. These mice lack not only B cells but also T cells, NKs, and dendritic cells *(288,289)*. The *Ikaros* gene encodes a zinc-finger transcription factor that acts as a master regulator of the development of the B lineage *(288)*. A mutation that deletes the N-terminal zinc-finger DNA-binding domain blocks B-cell development in early stages *(288)*. The Ikaros protein has two C-terminal zinc-finger domains that interact with four N-terminal zinc-finger domains. The homo- or heterodimerization of Ikaros proteins with DNA-binding activity requires the interaction of at least three zinc-finger domains *(290)*. A second strain of mice with Ikaros-targeted mutations was obtained by making different deletions of the C-terminal domain that prevent dimerization. These mice lack both fetal B1 and adult B2 cells. The differentiation of B cells in these mice is blocked at the level of fetal and postnatal HSCs *(289)*. A third strain was obtained via homologous recombination by introducing an in-frame β galactosidase sequence into exon 2 of the *Ikaros* gene. These mice lack B cells in the fetal liver and display a marked reduction of pre- and pro-B cells but also have B1 cells (B220$^+$, CD5$^+$ IgM$^+$, and Mac-1$^+$) in the peritoneal cavity *(291)*. B cells from these mice exhibit a defect in IL-7-dependent proliferation and the progression of IgM$^-$ to IgM$^+$ B cells. Taken together, the results strongly suggest that the *Ikaros* gene is required for optimum proliferation and differentiation of B cells.

High expression of *Ikaros* was observed in the pronephros and mesonephros of Atlantic cod and rainbow trout *(292)*. In these species, the kidney is the major source of B cells. The expression of Helios, another member of the Ikaros family, was detected during the neural stage in 15-d-old embryos of Mexican axolotl, and both Helios and Ikaros transcripts were detected in the ventral area containing HSCs at d 38. This observation indicates that during lymphoid development of Mexican axolotl, the expression of Helios precedes the expression of Ikaros *(293)*.

Ikaros genes exert a positive and negative regulatory effect on various genes expressed during multiple stages of the differentiation of B cells. Thus, it was shown that Ikaros binds to regulatory elements in the promoters of TdT and λ5. *Ikaros* also binds to the 5'-upstream regulatory region of the pre-*VB1* and pre-VB2 genes *(294)* and to the TATA-less promoter of B28 *(295)*.

This information strongly suggests that the Ikaros gene family plays a critical role in the development of lymphoid precursors and of pro- and pre-B cells in lower and higher vertebrate species.

Other transcription factors, including E2A and EBF, also play an important role in the early stages of B-cell development. The *E2A* gene encodes two factors, E12 and E47, which arise through alternative splicing. *E2A* belongs to the basic helix–loop–helix family of transcription factors, which is not B-cell specific *(296)*. However, E2A knockout mice exhibit a complete block at the pro-B-cell stage because of a lack of expression of RAG1 and RAG2 and the structural components of the pre-B receptor *(297)*. Binding sites for these factors were identified on the promoter of various genes—on the111bp promoter of the *RAG1* gene, which can bind to E47 and E12, and on the λ5 TATA-less promoter/enhancer, which may bind to E47 *(297)*.

Early differentiation B factor (EBF) is another transcription factor that exhibits a broad regulatory effect on the expression of various genes during B-cell development. Mice bearing EBF-targeted mutations exhibit a blockage at the pro-B-cell stage *(298)*. EBF is a B-cell restricted factor that binds as a homodimer via a large binding domain motif containing a zinc-coordination element *(299)*. EBF binding motifs were identified in the upstream segment of the λ5 promoter, 5'-upstream region of V-pre-B1 and V-pre-B2 promoters, and the promoter of B29 and mb1 *(300)*. Recently, the promoter of human V pre-B was cloned and sequenced. It shows 56% homology with its mouse counterpart and has three binding sites for EBF. The ectopic expression of the human V-pre-B promoter in HeLa cells induces the activity of a reporter gene under the control of V-pre-B promoter. This effect is enhanced by E47, suggesting a synergistic effect between EBF and E47 on V-pre-B-promoter activity *(300)*. In human B cells, E47 also controls the expression of the *mb-1* and *B29* genes that encode proteins required for the signaling pathways induced by BCE *(300)*.

B-cell-specific activator protein (BSAP) transcription factor plays a role in the regulation of antigen expressed on the membrane of B cells in various stages of differentiation. Thus, BSAP may be involved in the expression of CD19 because a promoter fragment of 280bp of *CD19* gene contains a binding site for BSPA and Ets *(301)*. Similarly, the promoter of the *CD72* gene contains a segment located between −162 to −196, which has putative BSPA and PU.1 binding sites *(302)*. In contrast, the expression of CD20, which is a pre-B-cell specific factor, may be regulated by PU.1 because the 280bp promoter of this gene contains binding sites for the PU.1 and Oct transcription factors *(303,304)*. Finally, the 5'-upstream region of the promoter of CD22 that is associated with the BCR contains binding sites for BSAP and NF-κB *(305)*.

PAX5 is another essential transcription factor for B-lineage commitment. The absence of PAX5 arrests B-cell development at the pre-B and immature B-cell stages *(306)*. In these mice, pro-B cells express CD43, c-Kit, HSA, and IL-7R but fail to express CD25 and BP-1 required for the expression of a surrogate pre-B receptor. In addition, they do not exhibit V (D) J rearrangements. Studies in PAX-5-deficient embryos showed that the fetal liver B-cell development is blocked at the pro-B-cell stage. It noteworthy that HSCs from PAX 5-deficient mice retained a broad lymphomyeloid differentiation capacity *(307,308)*. During the late phase of the maturation of B cells, PAX-5 is involved in the expression of CD19 and the switching of IgM-producing cells to IgE-producing cells. DNA-binding motifs for PAX-5 were identified in the promoter of CD19 *(308)* and the promoter of IgE *(309)*.

PAX-5 and EBF are expressed in prebursal committed B-cell progenitors prior to colonization of the embryonic bursa of Fabricius *(310)*. These observations demonstrate that PAX-5 and EBF play an important role in the differentiation process of the B-cell lineage in various vertebrate species.

Table 14 summarizes the effect of various transcription factors on genes during B-cell development.

B-cell development is a stepwise differentiation process in which some genes are activated whereas others are silenced in various stages. Both the activation and silencing of genes is genetically regulated by genes that encode transcription factors specific for B lineage and others that exhibit pleiomorphic effects. A certain degree of redundancy among the transcription factors exists because the DNA-binding motifs for a given transcription factor might be shared by various genes expressed at multiple stages of the differentiation of B cells. Table 14 illustrates the role of various transcription factors in the expression of various genes during B-cell development.

3.2. Thymus Organogenesis and Embryonic Development of α/β T Cells

In all vertebrate species, T cells arise from the common lymphoid progenitor (CLP), which can be located in different tissues in different species. The Ikaros gene family plays a crucial role in the differentiation of CLPs. This concept is supported by a seminal observation showing that Ikaros knockout mice lack T cells as well as other cells derived from CLPs such as B cells, NKs, and dendritic cells. The CLPs migrate to the thymus, where T lymphocytes mature and differentiate. The generation of T cells is under the strict control of nonlymphocytic thymic cells comprised mainly of epithelial and mesenchymal cells. The thymus gland is derived from endoderm and associated mesodermal tissue of the pharyngeal pouches and the ectoderm of the brancheal clefts. The ontogeny of the thymus gland is best studied in higher vertebrate species. Thymic organogenesis can be divided into five sequential stages: (a) formation of the thymic primordium; (b) colonization by CLPs, which migrate from various tissues in different species; (c) proliferation of thymocytes; (d) location of thymocytes in different zones of the thymus; and (e) apoptosis of thymocytes as the result of negative selection and migration of mature T cells to peripheral lymphoid organs.

Table 14
Transcription Factors Involved in the Development of B-Cell Lineage

A. Transcription factors required for transition in various stages of differentiation

Transition	Transcription factor
HSCs->common lymphoid precursor	Ikaros, PU.1, AML-1, NFkb-RelA, Myb, GATA-2, E2A SCl-Tal
Common lymphocyte progenitor-> pro-B	Ikaros, E2a,EBF
Pro-B-> pre-B	Ikaros, EBF
Pre-B-> immature B cells	BSAP, Sox-4

B. DNA binding motif for transcription factor identified on the promoter of various genes present in B cells in various stages of development

Promoter of gene	Transcription factors
IgH	Oct-2, OCA-B, NFIL-6
Igκ	EBF, OCA-B
λ5	Ikaros, BSAP, EBF, E47, PU.1, elf-1, ets-1
Vpre-B	Ikaros, E47, BSAP, EBF
mb1	PAX-5, EBF, BSAP, elf-1, ets-1
B29	Ikaros, EBF, Oct, elf-1, ets-1
RAG	Ikaros, PU.1, NF-Y/CBf, E47, E12, elf-
TdT	Ikaros, E47, E12, elf-1
BLK	BSAP, NFκB
CD19	PAX-4, BSAP, E47
CD20	PU.1, Oct
CD22	BSAP, NFkB
CD72	BSAP, PU.1

In mice, the epithelial cells in the thymus primordium are formed at d 10.5 of gestation from the pharyngeal endoderm of the third pharyngeal pouch and neural crest mesoderm *(311–313)*.

Early studies suggested that thymic epithelial cells of the cortex are derived from ectodermal stem cells, whereas those from the medulla are formed from the endoderm of third pharyngeal pouch *(313)*. Gill et al. provided direct evidence for thymic progenitor cells, giving rise to both medullary and cortical epithelial cells *(314)*. These authors generated the monoclonal antibody MTS24, which detects a mucin-like glycoprotein on the surface of epithelial cell progenitors. These cells are characterized by their capacity for self-renewal and differentiation potential into other lineages. The MTS24[+] cells from thymi of 15.5-d-old embryos coexpress cytokeratins-5 and -8, which are markers of adult cortical and medullary thymic epithelial cells. Ectopic grafts of purified

MTS24$^+$ epithelial cells can differentiate into cortical and medullary epithelial cells. The epithelial compartment in the thymus is unique, because it cannot be classified as stratified layers as can the skin. Based on the expression of keratin genes, a genetic marker of epithelial cell progenitors was divided into two subsets. The subset K8$^+$K18$^+$ K5$^-$ is located in the cortex; and the subset K5$^+$, K14$^+$ is restricted to the medulla *(315)*. The epithelial cell progenitors were competent and sufficient to support the development and maturation of T cells within the thymus.

In the thymus, the T cells exhibit a major expansion phase from days 11 to 15 of embryonic life. At this stage, the undifferentiated T cells (pro-T cells) localized in the cortex do not express CD3, CD4, or CD8 (triple-negative). Later, they express Pgp-1, Thy1, CD5, and CD25 (IL-2R). At d 13 of ontogeny, CD4$^-$CD8$^-$ cells (double-negative) begin to rearrange the genes that encode the TCR, a process preceded by the activation of *RAG* genes. In mouse thymocytes, T cell receptor *(TCR)* genes are in the germline configuration until d 14, when the first rearrangements of V γ and δ are detectable and the *CD3* gene is transcribed. The TCR heterodimer, which consists of V γ/δ and CD3, can be detected on the surface of cortical thymocytes at days 14–15. The Vβ and Vα gene transcripts are detectable at ds 16 and 17 *(316,317)* and of fetal life, respectively. TCR$^-$ or TCR$^-$ low double-negative thymocytes move from the cortex to the medulla at ds 17 and 18 and express both CD4 and CD8 (double-positive). Between d 18 and birth (d 21), they differentiate into two major mature subsets: TCR^{high} CD4$^+$ CD8$^-$ and TCR^{high} CD4$^-$ CD8$^+$ T cells, which emigrate from the thymus and colonize peripheral lymphoid organs.

In fish, the thymus is the first organ to become a lymphoid, followed by the kidney and the spleen. However, there are distinct organogenesis patterns of thymus development between marine and river fish species.

In trout embryo, a thymic primordium is evident between d 5 and 8 prehatching *(318,319)*. It appears as a thickened area of pharyngeal epithelial cells containing few T cells *(314)*. At hatching, the thymus consists of a few layers of epithelial cells, and at d 1 prehatching, the lymphocytes expressing Ikaros and RAG proteins become predominant *(320)*. Complete rearrangement of the *TCR-V2* gene and the presence of TdT are detected at d 15 postfertilization, a time that coincides with the occurrence of a thymic analog *(320)*. In trout embryos, the T cell is probably derived from the yolk sac and ventral aorta.

In zebrafish, a thymic primordium lacking lymphocytes and consisting of two layers of epithelial cells is observed as early as 60 h postfertilization. The first lymphoid cells in the thymic analog were observed at 65 h postfertilization, and at d 4 postfertilization, the number of lymphocytes increased considerably *(321)*. It noteworthy that in zebrafish the thymus becomes colonized with lymphocytes before the pronephros becomes a hematopoietic organ. It is likely that the T lymphocytes in zebrafish derived from HSCs located in the ICM and dorsal aorta *(320)* that express the *Ikaros* and *RAG* transcripts *(331)*.

In *Xenopus*, the thymus primordium is evident at d 3 postfertilization, and 1 d later, it is seeded with lymphoid cells. At this embryonic stage, the lymphocytes express RAG, and 1 d later, *TCR* genes are rearranged. Sometime during d 4–12 postfertilization, a second seeding takes place, which extends into the juvenile and adult periods *(322)*. The T-cell progenitors derive from fetal liver colonized by HSCs from VBI and DLP mesodermal tissues proper to embryo *(323)*. After the first wave of colonization of the thymus with lymphoid progenitors, 20% of thymocytes express XTLA-1 T-cell-specific antigen, and at 12 d postfertilization, 65% express CD8 and the vast majority expresses CD5 antigen *(324)*.

There is little information of thymus organogenesis in reptiles. El Deeb and Zada, using an anti-T-cell antibody, reported the presence of T cells in 40- to 41-d-old embryos *(258)*.

Similar to amphibians, the thymus primordium in birds is colonized by several waves during embryonic life. T cells derive from HSCs beginning on d 4 of embryogenesis in the para-aortic mesenchymal tissue *(325)*. The first and second waves of colonization of the thymus with HSCs occurs at d 6 and 7 of embryonic life, respectively *(326,327)*. In birds, the rearrangement of V genes that encode the TCR occurs exclusively in the thymus. Whereas *Vb1* gene rearrangements were observed at d 12 in thymocytes, the Vb2 rearrangements were observed at d 14 of embryonic life *(328)*.

In pigs, as in birds, the thymus primordium, which appears at the end of the first trimester of intrauterine life (d 38 of gestation), is sequentially colonized by T-cell progenitors that express CD45 antigen. The T-cell progenitors do not express CD3, CD4, or CD8 (triple-negative). The differentiation of thymocytes expressing the α/β TCR occurs progressively from $CD3^-$, $CD4^+$, $CD8^+$ during the first 10 d of embryonic life. At d 55 of embryonic life, the T cells are fully mature and express CD25 *(329)*.

In humans, the thymus develops from the third brachial pouch at about 6 wk of gestation *(330)*. The pathway of the differentiation T-cell progenitors in the human thymus was studied by various methods that consisted of phenotypic analysis of the expression of various membrane markers and transcription of genes that encoded the TCR in thymus samples harvested from fetuses, the infusion of fetal liver, thymus, cord blood cells in NOD-SCID mice, and the growth and differentiation of cells in fetal thymus organ culture on thymic stromal cells. The most primitive T-cell progenitor expresses high levels of CD34 and CD45RA and lacks expression of CD38, CD2, and CD5 *(331,332)*. Important phenotypic changes occurring during the early stages of $CD34^+$

CD38⁻ fetal liver cells in fetal organ cultures showed that they differentiate into two populations: CD4⁺ CD3⁻ CD7⁻ and CD4⁻ CD7⁻ CD3⁻. Although the CD4⁺ subset differentiates into dendritic cells, the other subset differentiates into CD4⁺ CD7⁺ CD3⁺ cells. After 11 d of culture, they are CD2⁺ and the expression of CD1a is upregulated. At this stage, the rearrangement of TCR genes is initiated *(332)*. In the thymus, CD34⁺ CD1a⁺ T cells become double positive, expressing CD4 followed by CD8α before the acquisition of CD8β. This double-positive subset is the subject of positive selection, and the cells that do not die express activation markers (CD69 followed by CD27) *(333)*. Productive rearrangements of the TCR *V*β gene were detected in CD34⁺ CD1a⁻ cells, whereas pre Tα and CD3 leading a functional TCR were present in double-positive T cells *(334–336)*. In vitro studies of the differentiation of CD34⁺ cells isolated from human and Rhesus monkey cord blood cultured on thymic stromal cells showed that the differentiation of HSCs into mature T cells recapitulates T-cell in vivo ontogeny *(337)*.

3.3. Fetal Development of δγ/δ T Cells

A minority of T cells in the lymphoid organs expresses an alternative TCR that is encoded by Vγ and Vδ genes. These T cells have been found in many species. The γ/δ T cells display various functions, such as cooperation with α/β T cells in the immediate hypersensitivity reaction, secretion of cytokines, Ig subclass switching, non-MHC-restricted cytotoxicity, and antimicrobial defense reactions. They accumulate at the site of infections by bacteria, viruses, and parasites and in granulomas *(338)*.

In birds, the γ/δ T cells are the first T cells generated in the thymus during ontogeny, and, in adult life, they represent about 50% of blood T lymphocytes *(339)*.

In mice, cells that express γ/δ TCR transcripts are detectable in the fetal thymus at d 14 of gestation *(340)*. The analysis of the expression of Vγ genes in the murine fetal thymus suggests the ordered and selective occurrence of distinct γ/δ T-cell subsets *(341)*. In mice, γ/δ T cells predominate in the skin, gut, lungs, and female reproductive organs.

A discrete subset expresses a TCR encoded by Vγ3 and Vδ4. In fetal life, mature Vγ3^high HSA^low T cells mature from immature thymic Vγ3^low HSA^high *(342)*. Interestingly, these cells, found in fetal thymus and in the skin of adult mice, express the Ly49E and CD94/NKG2 inhibitory receptors of NK cells *(344)*. The expression of NK inhibitory receptors correlates with the expression of CD44, 2B4, and IL-2R and the absence of CD25 *(343)*. This observation clearly shows that γ/δ T cells do not derive from a common precursor of T cells because no α/β T cells expressing inhibitory receptors of NK cells were identified in α/β T cells. Thus, the concept is strengthened by other observa-

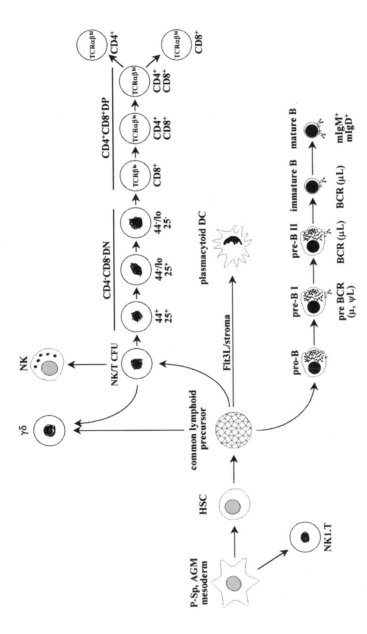

Fig. 27. Development of lymphoid lineage during ontogeny, leading to the generation of B and T cells and plasmatoid dendritic cells.

tions that demonstrate that γ/δ T cells develop normally in α/β TCR and β2-microglobulin knockout mice *(345)*. The γ/δ T cells might develop extrathymically because, in nude mice, they constitute the majority of gut intraepithelial lymphocytes *(346)*.

Human cells expressing γ/δ TCR and CD3 transcripts were identified in fetal liver at 6–8 wk of gestation, before the occurrence of the thymus primordium *(348)*. McVay et al. found transcripts of V genes in primitive gut between 6 and 9 wk of gestation, whereas they were detected in the fetal thymus at a later stage of gestation *(347)*. This raises the hypothesis of extrathymic origin of some TCR-γ/δ TCR T cells.

Taken together, these studies provide evidence that in various vertebrate species, different fetal tissues support the development of γ/δ T cells.

3.4. Ontogenetic Development of NK T Cells

In mice, a discrete subset of T cells called NK1 T cells express α/β TCR and the NK1.1 antigen characteristic for NK cells. The TCR of NK T cells is encoded by an invariant $V\alpha$ gene, resulting from the recombination of $V\alpha14$ and $J\alpha28$ segments. The invariant $V\alpha$ gene can pair with $V\beta8$, $V\beta7$, or $V\beta2$ genes. These cells recognize peptide in association with CD1 molecules *(110)*. Whereas the vast majority of T cells expressing α/β TCR develop around day 15 of gestation in the thymus, NK T cells preferentially develop extrathymically. Makino et al. have found transcripts of invariant $V\alpha14$ in embryos at d 9.5 of gestation and in the yolk sac and fetal liver at d 11.5–13.5 of gestation, respectively *(349)*. Fluorescent phenotypic analysis of these cells showed that they express a TCR composed of $V\alpha14$ and $V\beta8$ chains and CD3. It is believed that NK T cells are derived from the AGM at d 8.5–9 of embryogenesis and migrate later to fetal liver and then to thymus around day 15 of gestation.

Figure 27 illustrates the differentiation of B, T, and plasmacytoid dendritic cells from common lymphoid progenitor.

3

Phenotypic Characteristics of Neonatal B Cells

1. INTRODUCTION

Macromolecules associated with the membrane of B cells mediate three major functions of B cells. The first function is recognition of antigen, leading to the activation and proliferation of resting B cells as well as the differentiation of plasma and memory cells. The second function is binding and internalization of antigen, followed by its processing for presentation of peptides to T cells in association with MHC molecules. The third function consists of delivering signal via cytokines and costimultory molecules.

Repetitive epitopes comprise T-independent antigen, which are recognized by the B-cell receptor (BCR), resulting in crosslinking of the BCR and subsequent activation and differentiation of B cells. Stimulation of B cells by T-dependent antigen requires not only the binding of antigen to BCRs but also the interaction of costimulatory molecules with their counterparts on T cells.

Polyclonal activators (B-cell mitogens) can induce the activation and differentiation of resting B cells by circumventing the binding of antigen to BCRs, subsequent to activator binding to mitogen or Tol receptors.

2. MOLECULES ASSOCIATED WITH B-CELL MEMBRANE

2.1. Structure and Function of the BCR

The BCR is composed of a macromolecular complex with surface Ig (sIg) that is able to bind the antigen and macromolecules involved in signal transduction, which leads to the activation or repression of B-cell genes. CD79a and CD79b, which are encoded by *mb-1* and *B29* genes, respectively, are directly associated with sIg, whereas other molecules such as CD19, CD21, CD22, and CD81 are associated with the sIg/CD79 BCR complex.

CD79 is a disulfide-bonded heterodimer, composed of CD79a (Igα) and CD79b (Igβ), which mediates signal transduction via the pre-BCR during the development of B cells and via the BCR in immature and mature B cells. Both molecules are type I transmembrane proteins belonging to the Ig superfamily *(350)*.

From: *Contemporary Immunology: Neonatal Immunity*
By: Constantin Bona © Humana Press Inc., Totowa, NJ

In the BCR, one sIg is always paired with one CD79a and one CD79b molecule at a stoichiometry of 1:2. The ITAM motifs found in the intracellular domain of CD79a and CD79b are critical for the transduction signals. The first step in BCR signal transduction is the activation of protein tyrosine kinase (PTK) family members phosphorelays, which phosphorylate CD79. At least four PTKs act as BCR phosphorelays: Src9 Lyn, Fyn, Syk p85, and Btk. Btk is critical at the pre-B-cell stage in humans but not in mice. In humans, null mutations in Btk cause X-linked agammaglobulinemia. SLP-65 has been identified as the immediate downstream substrate of Syk and contains an SH2 domain *(351)*. SLP-65 belongs to a family of adaptor proteins including Grb2, Vav, Nck *(351,352)*, and CrkL *(353)*. Fully activated CD79 is required for the coordinate synthesis of second messengers (PI3 and PIP3), which are generated by enzymatic activation of phospholipase C and PI3K. P13K is required for the production of PIP3 and the recruitment of Btk on the membrane via the PH domain. Btk also contributes to PKCβ activation The Bkt-PKCβ pathway is a significant survival factor for B cells subsequent to ligation of the BCR by increasing the production of growth factors such as c-rel and Bcl-X$_L$. Bkt is also required for the activation of PLCγ on BCR crosslinking and mediates the production of diacylglycerol (DAG) and IP3.

These second messengers (P13, PIP3, and DAG) trigger the downstream activation of mitogen-acivated protein (MAP) kinases *(354,355)* and nuclear translocation of transcription factors such NF-κB and NF-AT. SLP-65 and BLNK adaptor proteins regulate this process and appear to be master elements in the signals transduced subsequent to the binding of antigen to the BCR *(356)*.

BCR signaling in mature B cells induces translocation of the BCR into cholesterol and sphingolipid membrane microdomains (rafts) that harbor the Src family kinase Lyn, which becomes phosphorylated upon BCR crosslinking *(357)*. Multiple coreceptor molecules are associated with the BCR and are expressed throughout B-cell differentiation and maturation; these factors typically upregulate the threshold of BCR signaling.

2.1.1. CD45

CD45 is a transmembrane protein tyrosine phosphatase that deactivates the Src family of kinases. CD45 is required for normal B-cell development and antigen stimulation by maintaining Src kinases in a partially activated state. This concept is well-supported by studies with two strains of CD45 knockout mice; one strain possesses a targeted mutation in exon 6 and the other in exon 9. B cells of these mice display phenotypic alterations characterized by a decreased number of IgD^{high}, IgM^{low}, CD23, and class II molecules *(358,359)*. B cells from the CD45 mutant mice cannot proliferate subsequent to crosslinking of the BCR with anti-IgM or anti-IgD antibodies, whereas they respond normally to lipopolysaccharide (LPS), IL-4, and anti-CD40 antibody *(359,360)*.

Loss of CD45 results in hyperphosphorylation of Src kinase and a concomitant decrease in its function. Hyperphosphorylation of Lyn prevents binding to the CD79a cytoplasmic domain. Therefore, CD45 is required to maintain Lyn and other Src kinase family members in a partially phosphorylated state, enabling the BCR to respond optimally to antigen stimulation. Finally, CD45 is required for the activation of ERK-MAP kinase pathway *(358)*.

2.1.2. CD19

CD19 also is associated with the B-cell membrane and contains nine highly conserved tyrosine residues in its cytoplasmic domain. CD19 is phosphorylated at low levels in basal state and forms a complex with Lyn and Vav *(361)*. The antigen ligation of BCRs leads to increased Lyn phosphorylation and thereby to activation of CD19 and CD79. Phosphorylated CD19 enhances the activity of other members of the Src kinase family, such as PCLγ2, which is downstream of Syk and PI3K *(362–365)*. CD19 also appears to be a phosphorelay to Grb2, Sos, C-Abl, and PTK *(366–368)*. Thus, CD19 is central to regulation of intrinsic and BCR-induced Src family PTK activity *(362)*.

2.1.3. CD22

CD22 is a transmembrane glycoprotein restricted to the B cell but present in the cytoplasm of pro-B , pre-B, and IgD⁺ B cells. CD22 controls signal transduction thresholds initiated upon antigen binding to the BCR. CD22 is associated with the BCR *(369)* and its natural ligand, which is a sialic protein. The cytoplasmic domain of CD22 contains six tyrosine residues, which are rapidly phosphorylated following ligand binding to the BCR. Phosphorylated CD22 physically interacts with positive regulatory molecules such as Syk, PI3K, PCLγ2, Grb2, and Sos *(370–372)*. Lajaunias et al. *(373)* showed that the expression of CD22 in conventional B2 cells is downregulated after crosslinking of the BCR with anti-IgM antibodies but is upregulated after stimulation with LPS, interleukin (IL)-4, or anti-CD40 antibody. By contrast, CD22 expression is barely altered in B1 cells after incubation with anti-IgM antibodies. These observations suggest that CD22 is differentially regulated subsequent to activation of B1 and B2 subsets of B cells.

In summary, current evidence demonstrates that the ligation of the BCR induces several specific phosphorelays, leading to activation of coreceptors and various transcription factors that activate B-cell-specific genes. Mutations affecting components of BCR signaling (e.g., CD79a, SLP-65, BTK, PKTβ p85, PI3 kinase, Vav, CD45, and CD19) have been reported to affect development of the B1 subset *(374–376)*.

2.1.4. LCK

LCK is another enzyme involved in BCR signaling. It is expressed only in B1 cells *(377)*. In LCK knockout mice, impaired phosphorylation and activation of the MAP kinase ERK was observed during BCR crosslinking in B1 cells, whereas no differences were observed in the frequency of CD5⁺ IgM⁺ B1 cells *(377)*. The impairment in BCR signaling in B1 cells of LCK knockout mice suggests that LCK is required for BCR mediated signaling in this B-cell subset.

2.2. Costimulatory Molecules Associated With the B-Cell Membrane

Binding of antigen to the BCR activates signaling cascades that induce transcription of genes for B-cell activation and differentiation. However, except for ligands that crosslink the BCR (such as anti-IgM antibodies and T-independent antigen) the engagement of BCRs by T-dependent antigen or hapten-carrier complexes alone is not sufficient to activate B cells. Full activation requires the interaction of T cells with costimulatory molecules (e.g., *CD80, CD86*, and CD40) associated with the B-cell membrane. *CD80* and *CD86* bind *CD28* and CTLA-4, which are associated with the membrane of T cells, respectively, and the CD40 with CD40L (CD154).

2.2.1. CD80 and CD86

Both *CD80* and *CD86* belong to the Ig gene superfamily and are composed of an extracellular domain of 220 amino acids, a hydrophobic transmembrane domain of 23 amino acids, and a tail of 60 amino acids. Both are expressed on the surface of B cells as well as other antigen-presenting cells, such as dendridic cells or macrophages.

CD80 and *CD86* genes display only 26% structural homology *(378)*, which may explain their differential binding to CD28 and CTLA-4. For example, *CD80* displays 20 times higher binding affinity to CTLA-4 as it does to CD28. A large body of information is related to the activation/inhibition and signaling pathways in T cells subsequent to binding of *CD80* and *CD86* to *CD28* and CTLA-4 coreceptors, but few data concern the molecular alterations in B cells. Utilization of monoclonal antibodies specific for *CD80* and *CD86* recently permitted revealing experiments. Crosslinking of *CD86* enhances the proliferation of B cells and promotes the synthesis of IgG2a and IgG2b. The crosslinking of CD80 blocked the proliferation of B cells. Thus, whereas *CD80* provides a negative signal for the proliferation of B cells, *CD86* stimulates the activity of B cells *(379)*.

CD80 and *CD86* possess markedly different cytoplasmic domains. The cytoplasmic domain of CD80 has a short tail that lacks tyrosine residues, whereas CD86 contains three tyrosine residues as potential protein kinase C phosphorylation sites *(381)*. The cytoplasmic tail of *CD80* contains a tetrapeptide motif called RRNE at position 275–278 and a highly conserved serine at position 284 that can be phosphorylated. *CD80* from cells stimulated with ionomycin coprecipitates with a 39 kDa phosphoprotein that can contribute to the phosphorylation of *CD80 (382)*. Thus, *CD80* and *CD86* can mediate differential signal transduction and regulate the function of B cells differently *(379)*.

The negative signal transduction induced by ligation of *CD80* inhibits B-cell proliferation by upregulating proapoptotic genes such as *caspase-3*, *caspase-8*, *Fas*, *Fas ligand*, *Bax*, and *Bac*. In contrast, the signal delivered via *CD86* enhances B-cell proliferation and activates antiapoptotic genes such as *Bcl-x(L)* *(379)*.

2.2.2. CD40

CD40 is a member of the nerve growth factor family and is expressed on B cells and dendritic cells. The binding of CD40 to the CD40 ligand expressed on T cells (called CD154) exerts various effects, including increased interaction between adhesion molecules LFA1/ICAM-1, proliferation of B cells, enhanced expression of costimulatory molecules CD80 and CD86 *(382–385)*, and class switching to IgE and IgG1 *(386)*. Optimal activation of B cells requires a synergistic effect between the activation of BCRs and CD40. CD40 does not possess intrinsic kinase activity, probably because of absence of conserved tyrosine residues in its cytoplasmic tail. However, CD40 does possess several residues potentially available for serine and threonine phosphorylation, allowing for interaction with tumor necrosis factor (TNF)-receptor-associated factor (TRAF), which serves as an adaptor protein in the CD40 signaling pathway *(386)*.

In B lymphocytes, cooperation of multiple signaling pathways initiated by the binding of CD40 to CD154 leads to the activation of transcription factors and subsequently to gene expression.

Both BCR and CD40 signaling stimulate MAP kinase modules, leading to the activation of transcription factors such as c-Jun NF-κB, NFAT, and AP-1 *(387,388)*. Among three MAP kinase modules studied by Dadgastor et al. *(389)*, it appears that the ERK-MAP kinase pathway has a minor role in CD40-mediated gene expression. The role of the p38 MAP kinase pathway appears to be small and almost entirely cooperative with other pathways. The p38 pathway may contribute to the downregulated expression of *Ndr1*, *Rb2*, and *SPA-1* genes, which inhibit cell growth. By contrast, the PI3K pathway contributes significantly to the gene induction of CD40 via downregulation of *Rb1* and *BTG-2* genes with antiproliferative properties.

CD40 plays an important role in the expression of CD80 and CD86 costimulatory molecules. Two functional domains in CD40, threonines at position 227 and 234, regulate induction of CD80 expression *(390)*. The phosphorylation of threonine in the PXQXT motifs of TNFR-2 is necessary for the synergy between BCRs and CD40 *(391)*. TRAF molecules associated with CD40 are required for class switching because they induce *IgG1* and *IgE* promoter transcription activity. This concept is supported by experiments demonstrating that mutation of TRAF-binding motifs within the CD40 cytoplasmic tail lead to significant decreases of promoter activity within *IgG1* and *IgE* constant region genes *(392)*.

Taken together, these data demonstrate that the binding of specific ligands to costimulatory molecules *CD80, CD86,* and CD40 triggers the activation of B-cell growth, cell interaction, Ig synthesis, and class switching, which augments the binding affinity of antibodies.

2.3. Fc and Complement Receptors Associated With the B-Cell Membrane

The receptors that mediate antigen internalization are the FcγR (CD16, CD32, CD64), FcεR (CD23), and complement (CD21 and CD35) receptors. Among the receptors expressed on various cells, CD32, CD23, and CD21 are expressed on B cells.

2.3.1. CD32

FcγIIRB is an inhibitory, single-chain, low-affinity receptor with an extracellular and a cytoplasmic domain containing a tyrosine inhibitory motif (ITIM) *(393)*. CD23 is encoded by a single gene, but alternative splicing of pro-messenger RNA (mRNA) generates two isoforms: FcγRIIb1 and FcγRIIb2 *(394)*. FcγRIIb1 is preferentially expressed on B cells and is involved in the negative regulation of antibody response, BCR-generated calcium mobilization, and cell proliferation. The inhibitory activity is related to an inhibitory sequence of 13 amino acids (AENTITYSLLKHP) embedded in the cytoplasmic domain *(395)*. Co-ligation of BCRs and CD23 leads to tyrosine phosphorylation but also rapid abrogation of ITAM activation signaling by hydrolyzing membrane inositol phosphate PIP3, a product of CD23 activation. In the absence of PIP3, the protein bound to the PH domain is released, leading to a blockage of calcium signaling and to arrest of B-cell proliferation triggered by the BCR *(394)*.

2.3.2. CD21 and CD35

These receptors for complement bind to C3b, C3d, or C3g. They are expressed on B cells and follicular dendritic cells. CD21 contains an extracellular domain of 15–16 repetitive units called SCR, a transmembrane domain, and a 34-amino acid cytoplasmic domain. The cytoplasmic domain is devoid of signaling motifs, but it is required for the internalization of polymerized C3b and C3g *(365)*. CD35 serves as cofactor for the hydrolysis of C3b-antigen complexes, allowing the binding of C3b to CD21. CD21, the receptor for C3d fragment of complement, is associated with CD19 and CD81 (TAPA-1), forming a signaling complex that can activate BCR signaling. The role of CD21 and CD53 in B-cell development is supported by data indicating a 40% reduction of peritoneal B1 cells, a 30–60% reduction of serum levels of IgG, and a reduction of germinal center formation in CD21/CD35 knockout mice (reviewed in ref. *362*).

3. EXPRESSION OF THE BCR AND OTHER MEMBRANE-ASSOCIATED RECEPTORS IN NEONATAL B LYMPHOCYTES

Classically, newborns were considered deficient in mounting a humoral immune response as a result of immaturity in their B cells. The immaturity of neonatal B cells implies difficulties in the induction of B-cell differentiation as a result of genetic and phenotypic differences between neonatal and adult B lymphocytes. More recently, a thorough analysis of the BCR and the phenotype of neonatal B cells did not reveal important differences, indicating that the poor responses of neonatal B cells to T-dependent antigen might be related to the immaturity of T cells and antigen-presenting cells in neonates.

3.1. Expression of the BCR Complex on Neonatal B Cells

As described earlier, the BCR exists as a protein complex on the B-cell surface. This complex is composed of surface Ig associated with CD79a and CD79b. Surface Ig differs from secreted Ig, because surface Ig contains two additional segments: a transmembrane domain and a cytoplasmic region. The Ig receptor and secreted Ig are encoded by V_H and V_L ($V\kappa$ or $V\lambda$) genes. Several exons comprise these genes: V_H (D) J_H (V_L, J_L), and constant region (Cκ or Cλ). The surface Ig component of the BCR contains a transmembrane domain and a cytoplasmic region encoded by two additional exons: M1 and M2. CD79a is encoded by the *mb-1* gene, and CD79b is encoded by the *B29* gene.

In the common lymphocyte progenitor from which B-cell progenitors derive, the exons encoding surface Ig are in germline configuration. During B-cell development, the exons encoding Ig are assembled by a process of somatic recombination *(396)*, leading to a complete surface IgM molecule expressed on immature B cells, which are predominant in the neonatal immune system. After birth, the immature B cells mature and express both surface IgM and IgD. With subsequent antigen stimulation, the V_H genes can recombine with other constant region exons, leading to the surface expression of IgG, IgA, or IgE. The somatic recombination is mediated by RAG enzymes, which are activated during various stages of B-cell development.

The VDJ recombination process is of fundamental importance to the generation of antibody diversity because of multiple possible combinations of joining events and also because of allelic exclusion, because the VDJ of a single chromosome can be productively rearranged.

VDJ recombination is a site-specific recombination process that occurs only between exons flanked by conserved recombination signal sequences (RS), each of which is composed of a conserved palindromic heptamer and an AT-rich nonamer separated by a 12- or 23-bp spacer. These two sequence blocks comprise the recognition sites for the joining of the D segment to J_H, the V_H to DJ, and the V_L to J_L exons *(397–399)*. Joining results either from inversion or deletion of intervening sequences, depending on the relative orientation of the recombining exons *(396)*. The recombination process is initiated and mediated by RAG enzymes, which bind to RS. The recombination process is initiated via double-strand DNA breaks between Ig exons and RS. Then, RS ends are joined, and TdT can modify the coding ends by addition or deletion of nucleotides, which contributes to the diversity of BCRs (reviewed in ref. *400*). In addition to RAG enzymes, other proteins participate in the repair of RAG-initiated double-strand breaks. Three proteins are subunits of DNA-dependent protein kinase consisting of the Ku70 and Ku80 subunits and a catalytic subunit related to PI3 kinase *(401)*.

The recombination process during development of the B-cell lineage begins in pro-B cells expressing V-pre-BCR and then continues with the rearrangement of D and J exons of heavy chain in pre-B1 cells, which exhibit the phenotype $B200^+$ $CD45^+$ $CD25^-$ c-kit^+ *(402,403)*. The joining of V_H exon to rearranged DJ segment and to μ-constant region exons occurs in pre-B-II large cells. The pre-B cells have cytoplasmic IgM heavy chain and express B220, CD43, CD25 c-Kit markers, and TdT. In the pre-B-II small lymphocytes, the rearrangement of exons encoding the light chain occurs. These cells express sIgM but cease to express CD45, CD25, c-kit, and TdT. From pre-B-II small cells arise the immature lymphocytes ($B220^+$ $sIgM^+$), which are predominant during the first weeks after birth. The *RAG* genes are first expressed in the pro-B cell ($CD220^+$ $CD43^+$ HSA^- $CD4^-$) and increase as B cells mature and the VDJ recombination process occurs. Their expression decreases in pre-B-II large cells and reoccurs in pre-B-II small cells during recombination of V_L and J_L exons but ceases in immature B cells *(404,405)*. CD79a and CD79b comprise an integral component of BCRs that is required for both surface expression and signaling. In particular, they play a role in the transition of immature IgM^{high} IgD^{low} B cells to mature B cells. Mice expressing the IgM/CD79b transgenic receptor exhibit normal maturation. However, mice harboring a truncation of the CD79d intracellular domain exhibit impaired B lymphopoiesis, in particular during the transition phase of $B200^+$ c-kit^+ to $B220^+$ $CD25^+$ pre-B cells, with a three- to sixfold reduction of IgM^+ immature B cells. In these mice, the immature B cells exhibit a reduced migration efficiency, resulting in an over 100-fold reduction of mature B cells in peripheral organs *(406)*.

A major characteristic of the neonatal immune system consists of induction of an immune response to a restricted range of antigen, producing largely IgM antibodies. In humans, neonatal B cells differ from adult B cells by a series of phenotypic features. Phenotypic analysis of cord blood B cells showed a predominance of CD5$^+$ B cells and more consistent expression of high levels of IgM than adult cells. Whereas the adult B cells expressed 12,000 to 48,000 IgM molecules per cell, the cord blood B cells express 63,000 to 240,000 IgM molecules per cell. No quantitative differences were observed in the sIgM density between cord blood B1 and B2 cells. In contrast to adult B cells-in which the majority of IgM is located within cytoplasm-most of the IgM for cord blood cells is located on the membrane *(407)*. The high density of IgM BCRs in neonatal B cells may increase the sensitivity of the response to polymeric antigen, causing the crosslinking of BCRs. This concept is supported by observations that neonatal B cells can make antibodies subsequent to stimulation with trinitrophenyl (TNP)-*Brucella abortus*, a TI-1 independent antigen *(408)*.

CD22 is a molecule associated with BCRs and is known to be a negative regulator of BCR signaling. Comparison of the expression of CD22 on cord blood and adult peripheral lymphocytes showed a significantly lower percentage of CD22$^+$CD5$^-$ B cells in the neonatal lymphocyte population. The stimulation of neonatal lymphocytes with anti-IgM antibodies (which crosslink the BCR) resulted in a dramatically reduced number of both CD22$^+$ CD5$^+$ and CD22$^+$ CD5$^-$ B cells. Meanwhile, the T-cell-dependent stimulation with anti-CD40 monoclonal antibody and IL-4 resulted in a dramatically increased number of CD22$^+$ neonatal B cells *(409)*. These data suggest that whereas polyclonal stimulation of neonatal B cells lowers the threshold of BCR signaling after crosslinking, the T-cell-dependent stimulation might increase the inhibiting effect of CD22 on BCR signaling of neonatal B cells.

The binding of antigen to BCR induces a rapid translocation into cholesterol and the sphingomyelin-rich microdomains, called lipid rafts. Lipid rafts provide the platforms for BCR signaling and the phosphorylation of Src kinase family members such as Lyn. These events lead to the internalization of BCR in mature B cells *(357)*. Comparison of BCR crosslinking by anti-IgM antibody on two B-cell lines (WEHI-231, an immature B-cell line, and CH27, a mature phenotype) revealed strikingly different responses to BCR crosslinking. After crosslinking, the cell lysates (obtained by incubation with Triton X-100 detergent) were subjected to density gradient centrifugation. In the case of CH27, about 40% of the BCR was present within lipid raft, whereas in the case of WEHI-231 only 3% of BCR was present. This result clearly showed that in the case of immature B cells, the BCR and CD79a did not translocate significantly in the lipid rafts subsequent to the crosslinking with anti-IgM antibodies. Both BCRs and CD79a were detected in the soluble fraction. In contrast to CH27 cells, which exhibited a significant internalization of BCRs on crosslinking (25% by 40 min), in the case of WEHI-213 cells, the constitutive internalization was not affected by crosslinking *(410)*. These elegant experiments provided evidence that the lipid raft in immature B cells may be different compared to mature B cells in either ability to translocate BCRs or to stabilize BCR localization in lipid rafts.

The transition from immature to mature B cells is associated with a series of signaling processes through BCRs. The signaling via IgH is necessary for allelic exclusion and differentiation of pro-B cells in pre-B cells. This concept is supported by data originating from transgenic mice harboring an IgM-bearing mutation in the transmembrane domain. These mice cannot express sIgM and lack pre-B cells and allelic exclusion *(411)*. The same effect was observed in mice expressing an IgM heavy chain and also with mutation in transmembrane domain that prevented the association of BCRs with CD79 *(412)*. Crosslinking of BCRs triggers sequential activation of at least three phosphorelays required for the generation of second message.

Study of syk phosphorylation and Src-related kinases (Lyn, Fyn, fgr, Blk, and LCK) did not show differences between adult and neonatal lymphocytes isolated from 2- to 3-d-old mice. By contrast, purified neonatal B cells, consisting of more than 90% IgM$^+$ cells, expressed low levels of p59 Fyn and p55 fgr. These two elements attain the levels found in adult B cells by 2–4 wk after birth *(413)*. The reduced expression of Fyn and fgr in neonatal B cells might account for the differences in IgM signaling noted in immature B cells. Neonatal B cells are deficient in the expression of p56, which is another BCR-associated protein *(414)*.

Another difference between neonatal and adult B cells is their ability to hydrolyze phospholipids in response to crosslinking of BCRs.

Hashimoto et al. *(415)*, using a gene-targeted approach, generated phospholipase C-γ2-deficient mice with an interferon (IFN)-induced Cre recombinase transgene. The inactivation of *PLC-γ2* gene in these mice 2 d after birth resulted in a two- to threefold reduction of B220$^+$IgM$^+$ cells in all peripheral organs as well as defects in B-cell development at the pre-B-cell stage. Taken together, these results demonstrated that there are subtle differences in the BCR signaling pathways between neonatal and adult B cells, which may also explain the meager neonatal response to immunization.

3.2. Costimulatory Molecules Expressed on Neonatal B Cells

The BCR and the majority of antigen associated with the membrane of immature and mature B cells are not expressed on hematopoietic stem cells (HSCs) or B-cell progenitors. However, CD80 and CD86 are expressed on CD45$^+$ and embryoid bodies by d 12 of gestation. HSCs were stained with antibodies specific for CD80 and CD86, and stain data were confirmed by reverse transcriptase polymerase chain reaction (RT-PCR) and Northern blotting. These experiments showed the presence of corresponding transcripts of both genes. CD80 and CD86 are expressed on 10–20% and 30–50% of CD45$^+$

HSCs, respectively. In addition, it was shown that CTLA-4-Ig, but not CD28-Ig fusion protein, binds to CD80 *(416)*. The binding of CTLA-4 to *CD80* indicates that the CD80 molecule is functional on HSCs. Presently, there is no information regarding the function of CD80 and CD86 molecules during the embryonic development.

Comparing expression of CD80 and CD86 on lymphocytes from cord blood, young children (2–20 mo), and adults showed no detectable CD80 expression on resting B cells. By contrast, CD86 was expressed at the same level of density on neonatal and adult B lymphocytes. Stimulation of neonatal B cells with PMA and ionomycin induced CD80 expression. No significant differences were observed in the fluorescence intensity of the expression of CD80 and CD86 on stimulated neonatal and adult B cells *(417)*.

The limited ability of neonatal B cells to respond to T-dependent antigen and to generate memory cells can be related to the defective expression of CD40 or other costimulatory molecules. CD40 expression is equivalent between neonatal and adult B cells *(418)*. Elliot et al. *(419)* studied the expression of CD40 in peripheral blood lymphocytes (PBLs) from cord blood, young children (2–12 mo), and adults. They reported that in some healthy neonates, the expression of CD40 was higher than in adults. However, the fluorescence intensity after stimulation with PMA and ionomycin was identical on cord blood and adult lymphocytes. Therefore, reduced synthesis subsequent to binding of CD40L by neonatal B cells cannot be related to the expression of CD40 but rather to differences in CD40 signaling pathways in neonatal B cells.

These observations taken together show that limited response of neonatal B cells is not related to lack or poor expression of costimulatory molecules but possibly relates to immature signal transduction.

3.3. Expression of Fc Receptors on Neonatal B Cells

Binding of immune complexes to B cells (by co-engaging the BCR and FcγRII-CD32) induces inhibitory pathways that may lead to apoptosis *(420,421)*. This action may be beneficial for neonatal B cells, because the maternal antibodies (IgG) can form immune complexes with environmental antigen after birth. Jessup et al. *(422)* compared the expression of two CD32 isoforms (FcγRIIa and FcγRIIb) in neonatal and adult B lymphocytes. Most cord blood and adult B lymphocytes expressed both isoforms, yet cord blood lymphocytes expressed lower levels of CD32. The reduced expression of CD32 on neonatal B cells may make them more resistant to the Fc-mediated inhibition seen in adult B cells.

The production of IgE is very low in neonates, although VDJCε transcripts can be detected in fetal liver by 20 wk of gestation *(423)*. However, the increased concentration of IgE specific for allergens or parasites *(424,425)* indicates that neonatal lymphocytes are able to synthesize IgE. It has been shown that CD23 and CD21 have an important role in IgE production *(426)*. CD23 is a low-affinity receptor for IgE that is constitutively expressed on B cells. CD21 expressed on B cells and follicular dendritic cells is a high-affinity receptor for CD23. CD23 downregulates IgE production *(427)*, which may partially explain the poor synthesis of IgE in neonates. Studies of the expression of CD21 and CD23 on cord blood and adult B lymphocytes demonstrated that the percentage of CD23$^+$ and CD21$^+$ B cells was comparable in neonatal and adult B cells *(428)*. Therefore, equivalent expression of CD23 and CD21 on neonatal and adult B cells cannot explain the poor IgE synthesis subsequent to downregulation by CD23.

3.4. Expression of CD72 and CD38 in Neonatal B Cells

CD72 is a C-type lectin receptor that binds CD5, a ligand expressed on all T cells as well as the B1 cell subset. CD72 ligation plays an important role in the induction of primary response by naïve B cells and increases the sensitivity to IL-10 stimulation (implicated in class switching and apparently defective in newborn B cells). Strong support for these conclusions came from observations that combined stimulation with anti-CD72 and IL-10 increased the synthesis of Ig by neonatal but not adult B cells *(429)*.

CD38 is an ectoenzyme marker expressed on the surface of B cells. Its extracellular domain mediates the conversion of nicotinamide adenine dinucleotide (NAD) to cyclic- adenonine dinucleo-phosphate (ADP)-ribose, producing nicotin acid dinucleotide and nicotinic acid. Both products are powerful calcium messengers in various cells *(430,431)*. Anti-CD38 induces the proliferation of B cells *(432)*. Immature B lymphocytes from young (1-wk-old) mice that express significant levels of CD38 still fail to proliferate with anti-CD38 plus anti-IgM antibodies. Proliferation was observed only in older mice (2 wk old) and reached adult levels by age 4 wk *(433)*. The role of CD38 in the development of B cells is not known, but possibly, CD38 delivers signals that are integrated in transduction pathways initiated by the ligation of BCRs.

The data illustrated in Table 15 summarizes the major phenotypic differences between neonatal and adult B cells.

Analysis of phenotype of neonatal and adult B cells shows some important differences that may explain why neonates produce mainly IgM antibodies, which display low affinity for antigen, multispecificity, and high connectivity. The major B-cell species in neonates is the B1 cell, whereas in adults, the B2 subset constitutes the majority. The B2 subset is able to synthesize high-affinity antibodies and exhibits class switching and somatic mutations. Lack of anti-

Table 15
Phenotypic Characteristics of Neonatal and Adult B Cells

Trait	Neonatal	Adult
Predominance of B-cell subset		
	B1	B2
Surface Ig	IgM	IgM IgD
Ig synthesis	Mmainly IgM	All subclasses
CD80	Not expressed	Not expressed
CD86	Comparable	
CD32	Expressed	Lower expressed
CD40	Expressed	Higher expressed
CD21	Comparable	
CD22	High CD22+ CD5⁻	Low CD22⁺ CD5⁻
CD72	Normal ligation	Defective ligation
p50 ^{fyn}, p55^{frg}	Normal	Low level

body diversity may be related to low expression of TdT, which is responsible for the increase of diversity resulting from N-addition process, low expression of molecules associated with BCRs, and activation of BCR signal transduction.

Apparently, the inability of neonatal B2 cells to mount a vigorous response to T-cell-dependent antigen is not related to low expression of costimulatory molecules but rather to immaturity of T cells. Neonatal B cells do produce antibodies after stimulation with polyclonal activators such as Epstein–Barr virus, pockweed mitogen, *Nocardia opaca* mitogen, protein A, and LPC in murine B cells. Neonatal B cells do not exhibit class switching, a defect related perhaps to defective expression of activation-induced cytidine deaminase, an RNA-editing enzyme involved in the process of class switching and somatic mutation *(434)*. Finally, subtle differences in Src-tyrosine kinases noted in neonatal B cells, as compared to adult B cells, may explain differences in signaling pathway resulting from BCR occupancy.

Investigations of the development of the B1 subset, carried out in transgenic mice, suggest that specific transcription factors and enzymes are critical for the neonatal development of this B-cell subset. B1 cells were not detected in mice bearing null mutations of CD45, CD19, Btk, PKCβ, or the p85a subunit of PI3K (reviewed in ref. *374*). A decreased number of B1 cells were observed in CD21/CD35 or CD81/TAPA-1 knockout mice. However, an increased number of B1 cells was observed in moth-eaten mice, which lack functional SHP-1 *(435)* or CD22 *(436)*, the recruiter of SHP-1 to the BCR that leads to enhanced proliferation of B1 cells.

4. POSITIVE AND NEGATIVE SELECTION OF B CELLS DURING DEVELOPMENT

After birth, the bone marrow generates approx 100 million B cells daily, *(437)* and about 5×10^7 exhibit the phenotype of immature B cells *(438)*. The majority of neonatal immature B cells display a short half-life between 2 and 4 d, and approx $2–3 \times 10^6$ are found in the peripheral lymphoid organs, where they mature into antigen-responsive B cells. These B cells have a longer half-life *(439)*.

These quantitative differences suggest that only a small fraction of B cells produced in the bone marrow survive to colonize peripheral lymphoid organs after birth. B cells arising from the differentiation of B-cell progenitors display BCRs that can recognize the entire antigen dictionary (about 1 billion epitopes) of foreign and and slef-antigen.

Ehrlich *(43)*, a classic immunologist, proposed that the immune system must avoid the response to self-antigen, a concept he termed as *horor autotoxicus*. This concept implies that the immune system possesses the intrinsic ability to distinguish self from nonself. Ehrlich's concept implies that during the development of immune system, the B cells are censored. Those bearing a BCR specific for foreign antigen are positively selected, but those bearing a BCR specific for self-antigen are negatively selected.

During B-cell development, the first positive selection takes place in the bone marrow at the level of pre-B cells. Only pre-B cells displaying in-frame rearrangements of the V_H gene survive and eventually differentiate into immature B cells. Thus, the BCR expressed on the pre-B and immature B cells, which predominate after birth, is involved in the positive selection. The concept of positive selection is supported by two groups of findings. First, the repertoire of neonatal peripheral B cells is more limited vs adults *(440)*. Second, only a small proportion of B cells produced in the bone marrow emigrate and colonize the peripheral lymphoid organs *(439)*. This suggests that the immature B cells, which leave the bone marrow after birth and later during adult life, were properly and positively selected and received adequate signals that permitted their survival.

Two factors influence positive selection of B cells during primary development. One factor is the level of expression of BCRs at the B-cell surface. This was elegantly demonstrated by a study of the expression of BCRs in IgHμδ transgenic mice containing various numbers of copies of transgene *(441)*. The mice having 1–15 copies of transgene exhibited an increased number of a subset of B2 cells in marginal zone of the germinal center. This B2 subset, called MZ/T2, exhibits the following phenotype: sIgD^{high}, sIgM^{high}, CD21/CD35^{high}, CD23^{low} CD1d$^+$ CD24$^+$. By contrast, mice containing 20–30 copies of transgene have a reduced number of cells in bone marrow and spleen and essentially no B cells in the lymph nodes.

The form and localization of antigen also play an important role in the process of positive selection of B2 cells. This was shown in double transgenic mice containing VH-VL transgenes specific for hen egg lysozyme (HEL) plus lysozyme gene encoding for soluble or cell-bound HEL. In these mice, the B cells bind to HEL with affinities ranging from 10^{-5} to 10^{-9}. When HEL was expressed at concentration of 1 nM in soluble form in blood, the B cells with HEL low-binding affinity were positively selected, whereas those with high-binding affinity were deleted. Both B cells with low- or high-binding affinity were deleted in mice expressing the cell-bound form of HEL *(442)*.

Apparently, the mechanisms of positive selection of B1 subset are different. This subset expresses BCR specific for multivalent self-antigen such as immunoglobulins, erythrocytes, thymocytes, cytoplasmic antigen, DNA (reviewed in ref. *271*), and phosphatidyl choline *(443)*, or environmental antigen such as phosphoryl choline *(444)*. Binding specificity of antibodies produced by hybridomas expressing CD5 transcript *(445)* (obtained from moth-eaten mice, a strain in which more than 90% of cells are CD5$^+$) *(446,447)* were compared to other strains prone to autoimmune diseases *(445)* or B-cell lymphoma *(448)*. This study confirmed the differences in positive selection of the B1 subset across antigen/antibodies.

The idea of positive selection of B1 cells is based on the observation that the majority of murine antibromelin-treated red blood cell (RBC) autoantibodies produced by B1 cells are encoded by the restricted set of V_H and V_L genes (V_H11–V_k 9, V_{H12}–V_{k4}) *(449)*. Human cold agglutinin produced mainly by CD5$^+$ B cells are encoded by a single gene member of the V_{H4} family (data reviewed in ref. *109*). B1 cell precursors probably are positively selected by the self-antigen mentioned earlier, which induce the expression of CD5. The ligation of CD5 to CD75, as well as low-affinity binding of B1 BCRs to multimeric antigen, downregulates the BCR signaling and allows the survival of B1 cells. It is noteworthy that in B1 cells, the STAT3 is constitutively phosphorylated *(450)*. The autophosphorylation of STAT3 by unknown environmental stimuli may contribute to positive selection, because it was shown that targeted mutation of STAT 3 results in embryonic death.

The concept of negative selection has its roots in Burnet's clonal theory, which proposed that self-reactive B cells are deleted during B-cell development, leading to central tolerance. Central tolerance occurs during lymphocyte ontogeny as a result of negative selection in bone morrow. The concept of negative selection of B cells is well-supported by studies carried out in transgenic mice. In mice expressing V_H and V_L genes encoding antibodies specific for allogeneic MHC class I molecules *(46)*, HEL *(47)*, or an allelic form of the CD8 self-antigen *(451)*, B cells specific for these antigen are deleted. Deletion occurs in the bone marrow during the differentiation of pre-B (sIg⁻) to immature (sIgM⁺) B-cell stages *(451)*. Deletion of self-reactive clones may also occur in peripheral lymphoid organs, particularly in immature HSA⁺ B cells exported from bone marrow to enter into the marginal zone of the white pulp of spleen *(452)*. Negative selection operates at the cellular level through alteration of signaling pathways or by apoptosis initiated by the interaction of high-affinity BCRs with antigen *(453)*.

Current evidence supports several conclusions about positive and negative selection of B cells during development.

First, positive selection of B2 cells occurs in the bone marrow at pre-B and immature B cells, which express BCRs with low affinity for unknown antigen. In contrast, the B1 subset is selected by virtue of their BCRs to interact with multivalent microenvironmental or self-antigen. The positive selection may be associated with downregulation of signaling pathways initiated by the binding of ligands to BCRs and associated molecules.

Second, central clonal deletion occurs in bone morrow during the transition from pre-B to immature B cells as a result of exposure to self-antigen. Central clonal deletion can also occur in the peripheral lymphoid organs and, in particular, within the marginal zone of white pulp. Negative selection depends on the threshold of BCR occupancy, either because of an increased density of membrane-associated BCRs or because of exposure with membrane-bound antigen.

Thus, the neonatal B cells found in peripheral lymphoid organs arise from both positive and negative selection.

4

Molecular Characteristics of the Neonatal B-Cell Repertoire

1. INTRODUCTION

Development of the neonatal repertoire occurs through a process in which antigen-specific B-cell clones are generated and maintained during adult life or are eliminated early after birth.

Based on the possible random combinations of germ line gene segments (V[D]J and VL-JL) and the random pairing of heavy and light chains that take place in pre-B cells, the potential neonatal B-cell repertoire is greater than 100 million distinct B-cell receptor (BCR) specificities. During the early antigen-independent phase, the repertoire is largely synchronous. However, after birth it quickly achieves an asynchronous pattern because clonal specificity in the neonatal repertoire emerges in a nonrandom fashion. This is based on multiple rearrangements of gene segments encoding the BCR, which will exhibit different specificities.

In addition to genetic elements encoding the BCR, the neonatal repertoire results from the interaction of many other genetic elements, including some that are linked to an Ig allotype and others that are not. This conclusion arises from a study carried out in inbred murine strains *(454–457)*. Studies in F1 mice analyzed antigen-specific clones that induce a polyclonal response and showed that they are codominantly expressed *(454–456)*. Other studies analyzed the oligoclonal responses for certain epitopes and showed that the expression of clonotype is controlled by allotype or other genes. Thus, analysis of influenza hemagglutinin (HA)-clonotype showed that the neonatal repertoire of F1 mice differed from both parents because many parental clonotypes were absent, and novel clonotypes not expressed in the parents had emerged *(457)*. In Balb/c mice, spectrotype analysis of anti-β2-1 fructosan antibodies showed five bands, three of which were predominant. By isoelectrofocusing (IEF) gel analysis, these bands focused in the pH 6.3–6.8 range. In Balb/Cx C57Bl/6 F1 mice and B.C8 mice, the spectrotypes were more heterogeneous than that of either parent, indicating that the expression of *VH* genes encoding β2-1 fructosan-spe-

From: *Contemporary Immunology: Neonatal Immunity*
By: Constantin Bona © Humana Press Inc., Totowa, NJ

cific clonotypes is under the influence of genes encoding allotype-, major histocompatibility (MHC)-, sex-, or color. The gene controlling the diversity of the anti-β2-1 fructosan response was designated *Sr1*. It maps to chromosome 14 in mice *(458)*.

There is some degree of stability and plasticity in the neonatal B-cell repertoire. The stability of the neonatal repertoire can be related to maternal antibodies that clear the antigen to which the newborn is exposed or to intrinsic properties of some neonatal clones to proliferate during postnatal life. This concept is supported by idiotype analysis of B cells producing anti-hen egg lyzozyme (HEL) antibodies after immunization with an lipopolysaccharide (LPS)-HEL conjugate. This experiment showed that the idiotypes of antibodies were similar in newborn mice and adult mice *(459)*, indicating that the development of some neonatal clones is fixed throughout life. In contrast, the analysis of HA-specific clonotypes present after birth showed a lesser degree of diversity at 6 d of age compared to 12–14 d of age. Several clonotypes found in 6-d-old mice were absent in 13-d-old mice, and others were found at high frequency in 13-d-old mice that were not detected in 6-d-old mice *(460)*. These findings could be explained by suppression of some clonotypes soon after birth by maternal antibodies, whereas the occurrence of new clonotypes may be to the result of antigen-dependent expansion of B cells emerging from the bone marrow. Alternatively, the stability or rapid change in the neonatal repertoire may result from genetic programs favoring the extinction or expansion of certain clonotypes during neonatal life.

Antigen exposure of the newborn may result in further development of the neonatal repertoire, leading to diversification of neonatal B cells by other somatic mechanisms such as somatic hypermutation, gene conversion, *N*-region nucleotide deletion, or addition mediated by TdT and receptor editing. The ligand-driven events may have a net effect of preserving and fixing some clones expanded by antigen exposure.

These observations indicate that the neonatal B-cell repertoire should exhibit different molecular characteristics compared to the adult B-cell repertoire. Such differences may consist of alternative utilization of V_H and V_L gene families, biased pairing of V_H and V_L genes, frequency of *N*-addition and/or somatic mutation, and class switching and temporal expression of some *V* genes after birth.

It is noteworthy that these molecular characteristics may be species-specific and may take place in different lymphoid organs in various species. Species-specific differences were identified in comparative immunology studies.

2. DIVERSIFICATION OF THE NEONATAL REPERTOIRE IN THE ANURANS

The anurans and mammals diverged at the end of the Devonian period (370 million yr ago). Thus, the study of the diversification of the neonatal repertoire may shed light on what is essential for the immune system of vertebrates in general and what is specific for mammals. For instance, differences in antigen exposure of mammalian embryos, which develop in an antigen-free environment in the uterus, compared to larvae soon after hatching and the transition at the metamorphosis stage when the larval immune system becomes immunocompetent provide precious information for understanding the neonatal B-cell repertoire.

In Xenopus, there are about 100 V_H genes. In larvae, the V_H genes, based on structural homology, were classified into 11 families. The V_H genes recombine with more than 19 D_H and 9 J_H genes. In early stages, the $V[D]J$ genes recombine with the $C\mu$ *constant* gene but later can switch to IgY, a homolog of mammalian IgG, and IgX, preferentially produced in the gut. Three genes encode the constant light chain: π, σ, and λ (data reviewed in ref. *254*).

The development of larval B cells is divided into two phases: one starts at d 4 when the V_H genes are rearranged and the first RAG transcripts can be detected. The second phase starts at d 12 and extends to the end of metamorphosis. During this period, the V_L genes are rearranged and the B-cell repertoire begins to diversify. The diversification of the larval B-cell repertoire probably contributes to the ability of the larval immune system to produce antibodies against various antigen. From the time that the spleen becomes visible (d 12), the majority of B cells express sIgM *(461)* and differ from adult B cells in re-expression of the BCR after capping *(462)*.

The diversity of the larval B-cell repertoire through metamorphosis results from recombination of germ line exons encoding the *V* genes rather than via antigen selection. Very few DJ recombinations are abortively rearranged in larvae *(463)*. The diversity of the repertoire results from the utilization of all V_H gene families with the exception of V_H11, which is rarely used in adult pre-B cells. A biased rearrangement of D_H12 and D_H16 with J_H6 was observed in pre-B cells, but sequence analysis of the V_H genes of the tadpole at d 30–35 showed that all the rearrangements were different *(464)*. Although no *N*-diversity was observed in the larval repertoire *(464)*, the CDR3 of the developing Xenopus were quite diverse. Most larval and neonatal V_H genes sequenced contain CDR3s encoded by 3–10 codons *(465)*, which is much shorter than in mammals, suggesting that the shorter length may explain the more limited diversity of the neonatal B-cell repertoire. No receptor editing leading to a second rearrangement of V_L genes has been reported in Xenopus *(466)*.

This information strongly suggests that the diversification of larval and neonatal repertoires in amphibians results mainly from somatic recombination of germ line sequences with little additional somatic diversification by *N*-nucleotide addition or receptor editing.

3. DEVELOPMENT OF THE AVIAN B-CELL REPERTOIRE

In birds, repertoire diversification is generated by recombination of a single copy of the V_H ($V_H 1$) gene with a D segment that exists as a multigene cluster *(467)*. The V_H gene pairs with a single copy of the V_L ($V\lambda 1$) gene. The V_L exhibits rapid diversification by a gene conversion process using a group of pseudogenes as a donor. The first rearrangement occurs during embryogenesis in the pre-B cell. During prebursal rearrangement of D→J and V→DJ, no *N* additions were observed *(467)*. Whereas in mammals there are genetically programmed sequential rearrangements of gene segments (D-J, V-DJ, and V_L-J_L), in birds the rearrangement of *V* genes is stochastic rather than sequential. Among 100 clones analyzed, several had V_H-V_L rearrangements, others only V_H, and 5 clones only V_L genes. In these cells, the V_H genes were in the germ line configuration *(468)*. Diversification occurs in the bursal stage after birth, and only the rearranged V genes undergo gene conversion *(469)*. Therefore, although *V[D]J* and $V_L J_L$ recombination and sIg expression are bursa-independent events, the bursa is required for the diversification of the B-cell repertoire after birth, and at hatching, 90 to 95% of bursal B cells express a BCR. During the bursal stage, after birth, and later in adult life, both V_H and V_L genes undergo gene conversion by transfer of a block of information from pseudo-V genes *(470)*. The frequency of successful gene conversion occurs every 10–15 cell cycles.

A single *V* gene can undergo 4–10 conversion events in the bursa before the B cells emigrate to peripheral lymphoid organs *(471)*. Recently, it was shown that the activation-induced cytosine deaminase enzyme is required for the gene conversion process *(472)*.

It is not clear how the B-cell repertoire is positively selected in the bursa posthatching. The bursa is a gut-associated lymphoid tissue (GALT) and a site of antigen trapping. Thus, exogenous and gut-derived antigen can be actively transported across the bursa epithelium into bursal lymphoid follicles *(473)*. Arakawa et al. studied the percentage of productive V-J joints in posthatch bursa from normal chickens and from chickens injected into the bursa lumen with an NP-BSA conjugate *(474)*. They found a significant increase in productive V-J joints in the V_L gene after injection of antigen. These results strongly suggest that after hatching, the diversification of the B-cell repertoire in bursa can be shaped after exposure of B cells to environmental antigen.

The process of B-cell repertoire diversification in birds shows that the basic genetic mechanisms have been conserved during the evolution of vertebrates but that the avian evolved different mechanisms governing B-cell repertoire diversification after birth.

4. DIVERSIFICATION OF THE MURINE NEONATAL REPERTOIRE

As in all mammalian species, the murine neonatal repertoire results from the random combinatorial association of gene segments ($V[D]J$, $V_L J_L$) encoding the specificity of the BCR.

The functional V_H gene results from the recombination of 100–500 V_H, 12 D, and 4 functional J segments located upstream of *constant region* genes. V_H genes located on chromosome 12 tend to cluster and map contiguously to one another with some interspersions, particularly for those located closest to the D_H cluster *(475)*. Based on nucleotide sequence homology and chromosome position, the V_H genes were classified into 12 V_H gene families *(476)*. The number of V_H genes composing each family varies considerably from one *($V_H X24$)* to several hundred *($V_H J558$)* related members.

V_K genes located on chromosome 6 result from the combinatorial association of 300 V_K and 4 functional J_K gene segments. Like the V_H genes, based on nucleotide sequence homology, the V_K genes were classified into 20 V_K families; each family contains from 1 to 25 related members *(475,477,478)*. In mice, 95% of immunoglobulins express the κ light chain.

The Vλ locus is the smallest. It is located on chromosome 16 and is composed of four units: Vλ2-Jλ2, VλX-Jλ2, Vλ1-Jλ3, and Vλ1-Jλ1). The Vλ genes encode 5% of murine immunoglobulins.

Table 16 illustrates the position of V_H, V_K, and Vλ families on mouse chromosomes 12, 6, and 16, respectively.

Three major methods were used to study the expression of V gene families in fetal, neonatal, and adult B cells. These consisted of Northern blot assay using RNA extracted from cells or hybridomas, single cell *in situ* hybridization, and complementary DNA (cDNA) library analysis.

Study of the utilization of V_H and V_K gene families might shed light on the mechanisms that play a critical role in the generation of the antibody repertoire. In principle, the antibody repertoire is optimized for efficient protection and defense of the host against microbes, whereas the host is protected from danger by elimination of B cells that produce pathogenic autoantibodies.

In adult mice, the V_H gene family usage is random and correlates to the complexity and the size of a given family *(479–481)*. For example, whereas the $V_H J558$ family, which contains more than 50 members, is expressed in 40–50% of B cells, the $V_H X24$ gene family, which contains 1 member, is expressed

Table 16
Position of *VH* and *VK* Gene Families on Heavy and k-Light Chain Loci

V_H locus

5'-J558-3606-V_H10 J606-V_H12-3609N-VGAM-3660-S107-VGAM-V_H11-X24-SM7-S107-Q52-7193-3'

V_K locus

5' (VK11-VK24-VK9-VK26)-(Vk1-VK9)-(VK4-VK8-VK10-VK12-VK13-VK19)-(VK28-RN7S)-VK23-VK21 JK 3'

in 1–2% of B cells *(482)*. It is noteworthy that there are strain variations in the utilization of V_H gene families. For instance, up to a threefold difference has been observed in the case of V_HJ558 gene family (most distal) usage vs V_H7183 family (most proximal to the D_H gene cluster) usage *(483)*. In sharp contrast, a biased usage of V_H gene families was observed in the early phases of embryonic development, specifically in pre-B cells. Analysis of V_H gene family expression in Abelson murine leukemia virus (MuLV)-transformed pre-B-cell lines *(484)* or fetal liver pre-B-cell hybridomas *(485)* obtained from Balb/c mice showed that the V_H7283 gene family and in particular one of its members, V_H81X (located closest to the D locus), was preferentially rearranged. In Abelson MuLV-transformed pre-B-cell lines obtained from the NIH/Swiss outbred strain of mice, the V_HQ52 locus, also located proximally to the D_H locus, was highly utilized *(486)*. These data showed that there is a position-dependent expression of V_H gene families biased toward the utilization of proximal V_H gene families during the development of B cells. It is interesting to note that, whereas in pre-B cells the frequency of V_H81X gene rearrangements are functional (>80%), in the adult they are virtually nonfunctional, and this gene is rarely expressed in B cells producing antibodies *(487,488)*.

The expression of the rearranged V_H81X gene as a transgene blocks B-cell development at the CD43$^+$ pre-B-cell stage *(489)*. This can be related either to inhibition of both productive and nonproductive rearrangements of endogenous V[D]J genes or to an inability to associate with the Vλ5 surrogate light chain.

In CD43$^+$ pro-B cells, the surrogate λ5 is necessary for the assembly of an Ig-like μ/λ5 transmembrane complex that is necessary for activation of signaling transduction pathways leading to differentiation and proliferation of pro-B and pre-B cells. Studies carried out on transformed pre-B-cell lines showed that two $V_H81X/μ$ chains, exhibiting different V_H-D-J_H joining sequences, do not assemble covalently with a λ5 light chain *(490)*. Therefore, the blockage of B-cell development observed in V_H81X transgenic mice can be related to formation of a V_H $\mu/\lambda5$ complex required for triggering proliferation and/or differentiation at key checkpoints during the development of B cells. The high utilization of the V_H7183 family observed before the expression of the BCR during the earliest stages of the development of B cells that express a surrogate $\mu/\lambda5$ receptor indicate that this phenomenon does not result from antigen selection but is a consequence of programmed rearrangement.

A decline of V_HX81 utilization was observed in fetal liver B cells at days 16 and 18 of gestation *(491)*. It is interesting to note that targeted mutation of the V_H81X gene does not alter the development of the B-cell repertoire in spite of the fact that expression of the V_H7183 gene is affected. This may result from a compensatory effect by utilization of other members of the V_H7183 family, which is composed of 12 different but highly homologous gene segments *(492)*. Alternatively, it may be because of the presence of the neo^r gene used for disruption of the V_H81X gene. Such a disruption can affect other members of the V_H7183 family located in proximity to V_H81X or can prevent V_H gene replacement of V_H7183 genes that preferentially use V_H81X joints *(492)*.

The simplest interpretation of position-dependent biased usage of proximal V_H gene families is V_H gene accessibility to rearrangement. The recombinational machinery works via a one-dimensional "tracking" mechanism that scans upstream from the DJ_H complex for V_H segments located at the 3'end *(493)*.

The neonatal repertoire is not different from the fetal liver repertoire and is characterized by high utilization of the V_H7183 and V_HQ52 gene families *(491,494–496)*. However, Malynn et al. have found high levels of transcripts of the V_H3660 gene family in livers of 1-d-old and in the spleen of 3- and 7-d-old Balb/c and C57BL/6 mice *(495)*. The V_H3660 family is located more distally to the D_H locus between the $VGAM$ and V_HS107 families in the center of the murine V_H locus. This suggests that the expression of the V_H gene family in the neonatal repertoire is not strictly position-dependent.

The V_H7183 gene family is composed of 14 different germ line genes *(496)*. Apparently, biased usage among the members of the V_H7183 family exists in neonatal B cells. Thus, the 7183.2 and 7183.6 genes were expressed solely in neonates, whereas the 7183.9 and 7183.11 genes were preferentially expressed in B cells from adult mice *(496)*. This observation suggests that the utilization of different members of the V_H7183 gene family in the neonatal repertoire also is developmentally programmed. This explanation will be strengthened when the position of various members of the V_H7183 gene family are mapped, because it is known that various members of the V_H7183 family are interspersed.

It is probable that neonatal B cells that use V_H7183 produce antibodies that exhibit low-affinity and multispecific binding activity, because it is well known that such antibodies predominate in the neonatal repertoire *(497)*. Indeed, analysis of the binding specificity of monoclonal antibodies produced by hybridomas obtained by fusion of LPS-stimulated cells from Balb/c, New Zealand (NZB), and MRL mice and selected for the expression of V_H7183 genes showed that they exhibited multispecific activity. Such antibodies bound to various self-antigen such as myelin basic protein, thyroglobulin, cardiolipin, Sm, mitochondria smooth muscle, and nuclear and glomerular basement membrane antigen *(498)*. However, it should be noted that biased expression of the V_H7183 family was observed not only in neonatal B cells producing multispecific antibodies but also in neonatal B cells producing influenza virus HA-specific antibodies *(499)*.

Targeted recombination may play an important role in biased expression of proximally (V_H7183, V_HQ52) vs distally located (V_HJ558) family members. The opportunity for targeted recombination in most D-J combinations is owing to the fact that all the D_H genes have AC nucleotides at the 3'-end, and J_Hs have a TAC near the 5'-end. Targeted recombination using AC overlap will result in a D-J combination that is in-frame *(500)*. Analysis of the 3'-end of the nucleotide sequence of V_H7183 and V_HQ52 genes showed a sequence that overlaps with the 5'-end of D_H segments. This implies that all rearrangements will be productive and that the final V[D]J rearrangements will be in-frame *(484,501)*. Because most neonatal D-J rearrangements have the D region in reading frame 1 *(502)*, this should allow preferential expression of V_H7183 vs V_HJ558 genes in neonatal B cells. This concept is supported by the results obtained in competitive recombination substrate assays demonstrating that the recombinant signal sequence (RSS) for V_H81X is preferred over the consensus for the V_HJ558 RSS. These findings suggest that RSS differences may play an important role in biased expression of proximal V_H gene families in neonatal B cells *(503)*.

Study of the structure of D and J_H segments expressed in neonatal B cells showed additional differences compared to adult B cells.

In contrast to fetal B cells, in which a relative increase in the utilization of $DQ52$ (the most 3' J_H proximal D segment) was noted, in neonatal B cells two different observations were made. In one reported experiment, the preferential utilization of *Dfl16.1*, 5', and *Q52*, the most J_H-proximal segments, were highly expressed in immature B cells *(504)*. In 1-d-old mice, a high usage of *Sp2* and *Q52* D segments was observed *(505)*. These differences may be because of RSS of various D segments preferentially targeted recombination of certain D segments.

In contrast to fetal B cells in which a distinct preference for J_H4 and a relative increase in J_H1 usage was observed *(505)*, in 1-d-old mice decreased usage of J_H4 and almost identical usage of J_H1, J_H2, and J_H3 were noted *(502)*.

The most striking difference between neonatal and adult B cells consists of the length and extent of diversity of the *CDR3*, which can explain why the neonatal repertoire is more restricted compared to the adult repertoire.

Shorter CDR3 segments characterizing neonatal V_H genes can be related to a lack or paucity of addition of P and N nucleotides. The N-region addition is a template-independent process that is mediated by TdT *(506)*, whereas P nucleotide addition is template dependent *(507)*. The role of TdT in template-independent N-region diversity was clearly demonstrated by comparing the sequences of $V[D]J$ junctions in TdT knockout and TdT+/- mice. In contrast to TdT+/- lymphocytes, the sequences of $V_H S107$ and $V_H 81X$ $D_H J_H$ junctions in lymphocytes from TdT–/– mice did not contain N regions *(508)*.

Sequence analysis of $V[D]J$ rearrangements showed that the N-region in neonatal B cells are almost totally lacking *(494,500,509,510)*. Therefore, lack of N region may explain the reduced diversity of the neonatal B-cell repertoire.

A shift in biased usage of $V_H 7183$ and $V_H Q52$ gene families leading to normalization of adult-like usage was observed between one to two weeks after birth *(494,495)*.

The mechanisms of normalization are not well understood. Normalization can be the result of changes in genetically programmed recombinational or intercellular constraints affecting the repertoire *(493)*. Alternatively, they can result from cellular selection *(511)*. Among various factors, one may consider negative selection of B cells in the periphery because $V_H 81X$ is very rarely used in antibodies or by endogenous or foreign antigen to which young animals are exposed. The role of foreign antigen exposure should be taken into consideration in light of the results of V_H gene usage in adult axenic mice. In these mice, less frequent usage of the $V_H J558$ family and increased usage of $V_H 7183$ were observed at a frequency expected from random usage *(512)*.

However, it can not be excluded that V_H gene replacement also may play a role in normalization of the V_H repertoire, because V_H replacement events involving $V_H 7183/V_H Q52$ genes were observed *(513)*.

In adult mice, B1 cells are localized mainly in the peritoneal and pleural cavities, and very few (1–2%) are found in spleen. B1 cells display a very restricted repertoire for some autoantigen and a few microenvironmental antigen because of highly biased expression of V gene families. For example, antibodies specific for phosphatidyl choline (PtC), which is a major component of cell membranes, are encoded by $V_H 11$-$V_K 9$ or $V_H 12$-$V_K 4$ *(448,449)*. The more accepted view is that B1 cells arise from distinct progenitors that are committed to generate B1 cells but not B2 cells *(271)*. The generation of the B1 neonatal repertoire was studied in transgenic mice expressing $V_H 12$ and $V_K 4$ transgenes. The development of B1 cells that express the transgenes that encode antibodies specific for PtC was studied in newborn livers and spleens in two transgenic lines bearing a low- or high-copy number of transgenes. In the first 120 h of postnatal life, the number of PtC-specific B cells was increased 20-fold compared to nontransgenic mice, doubling about every 24–30 h and becoming predominant at 6 d after birth. These mice do not have PtC-binding B2 cells in spite of the fact that 30% of total B cells are CD5[-], namely, B2 cells *(514)*. This observation suggests that V_H12 and V_K4 can rearrange only in B1 cells, or if this rearrangement also occurs in B2 cells, the B2 cells cannot express a BCR encoded by two V genes. This is in agreement with other observations suggesting that B1 and B2 cells use different V_H genes *(506)*. Antigen-driven selection mechanisms may be responsible for restricted usage of V gene families in neonatal B1 cells because selection proceeds rapidly after birth. Lack of B cells expressing the transgenes in adult bone marrow indicates that the selection occurs in the periphery and is initiated after Ig gene rearrangement and the expression of the BCR. It is noteworthy that the majority of B cells expressing V_H12 are excluded from the peripheral repertoire in adults, with the exception of cells expressing a CDR3 composed of 10 amino acids including a glycine in position 4 (designated as 10/G4). Thus, in contrast to the neonatal repertoire, the adult V_H12 is restricted by clonal expansion of a minute subset that has a particular CDR3 and binds PtC.

Taken together, these findings show that there are important differences between the usage of V_H genes in neonatal B1 and B2 cells and between neonatal and adult B2 cells.

In mice, the V_K light-chain genes contribute significantly to antibody diversity because 95% of murine Ig molecules bear a κ chain. In adult mice, all V_K gene families are expressed without evident biased usage of a given family. Study of V_K gene family expression in neonatal B cells showed, similarly to adult mice, that all families are expressed *(515,516)*. It is particularly important to note that usage of the V_K21 family, which is located the most proximal to J_K, is not increased in the fetal *(515)* and neonatal *(516)* repertoires. This finding demonstrates that V_K gene expression does not follow the V_H paradigm, which consists of the skewed V_H gene family expression in the neonatal repertoire.

Thus, if a position-related process is involved in the expression of V_H gene families in pre-B- and neonatal-cell repertoire until 7 to 14 d after birth, then a similar mechanism is not operating at the V_K locus.

Table 17 shows the complexity and the expression of the V_K family in newborn and adult LPS-stimulated B cells. An important factor in the generation of antibody diversity consists of the pairing of V_H with V_L genes. For example, the random association of 10^4 V_H and V_K would give 10^8 different antigen-binding sites. The analysis of the pairing of V_H with V_K genes in polyclonally activated B cells shows that the pairing is stochastic, with a few exceptions: V_K1 and V_K8 with V_HQ52, $S107$, and $X24$ in adult mice and V_K1 with V_HQ52 in neonatal B cells *(517)*.

Table 17
Expression of V_K Gene Families Among LPS-Stimulated Splenocyte Colonies From Neonatal and Adult C57BL/6 Mice

Gene family	VK2	VK22	VK24	VK1	VK9	VK4	VK9	VK10	VK19	VK21
Gene complexity	5	7	2	3	11	8	12	5	10	10
V_K expression in										
Neonatal	4.7[a]	0.2	0	40.1	23	5.4	13.8	0.3	1.2	0
Adult	1.7	4.3	0.3	25.8	5.1	3.3	9.0	1.4	6.1	2.6

[a]Percentage of total C_K^+ colonies.
Neonatal mice were 4 to 6 d old and adult mice were 14 to 24 wk old.

Besides somatic recombination and pairing of various *V* gene segments and *N*-addition, two other processes, somatic hypermutation and receptor editing, play an important role in diversification of the repertoire.

In *V* genes, somatic hypermutation generates mutations at a rate six orders of magnitude higher than the rate of spontaneous mutations in other mammalian structural genes *(518)*. One of most interesting aspects of the process of somatic mutation in *Ig* genes is its targeting to rearranged heavy- and light-chain *V* genes, whereas the genes encoding the constant region of heavy and light chains are stable.

The majority of somatic mutations in *V* genes are base pair mutations resulting in replacement or silent mutations *(518)*. Small insertions or deletions were observed only rarely *(519)*. Point mutations begin to appear near the *V* gene at a frequency of 10^{-2} mutations/bp/cell generation *(520)*, and then in *V* genes at a frequency of 10^{-3} to 10^{-4} mutations/bp/cell generation *(521,522)*. Somatic mutations are antigen-dependent events that arise during the immune responses against T-cell-dependent antigen that occur in germinal centers (GCs). Somatic mutations in Ig genes contribute to the increased affinity of antibodies and to better and more efficient defense reactions.

Antibody responses against T-cell-dependent antigen can be induced in neonatal life. Structural analysis of *V* genes expressed in antibodies specific for (T,G)A-L polymer and NP-CGG conjugate showed that somatic mutation, memory generation, and repertoire shift occurred subsequent to priming of neonates with these antigen *(523)*. Primary antibody responses to synthetic polymers are restricted to side chain T and G and, in A/J mice, are dominated by B cells expressing the V_H, *H10* gene, which is from the small $V_H SM7$ family, and the $V_K 1$ light chain. Like adults, neonates immunized with (T,G)A-L make a primary response to side-chain amino acids and to the A-L epitope only when immunized with synthetic polymer coupled to methylated BSA in Freund's complete adjuvant (FCA) at age 5 to 7 d *(523)*. Sequence analysis of 48 neonatally rearranged $V_H H10$ genes showed that 34% of $V_H H10$ gene had 1, 17% had 2, 10% had 3, and 2% had 6 bp nucleotide changes. A closed rate of mutation was observed in the V_H genes from mice immunized with NP-CGG conjugate at d 1 to 2 after birth and analyzed 14 to 28 d after priming *(523)*.

These elegant studies demonstrated that in neonatal mouse B cells, the DNA replicative machinery, a prerequisite for the induction of somatic mutations, is active within 1 d of birth.

BCR engagement may lead either to elimination of autoreactive cells during B-cell development or to increased diversity in peripheral B cells by a receptor editing process. The process leading to elimination of autoreactive cells takes place in pre-B cells and is called "receptor editing." In peripheral B cells, the process contributing to increased diversity of the repertoire is called "receptor revision" to distinguish it from receptor editing leading to tolerance.

Both processes consist of the capacity of V_L or V_H to undergo successive rearrangements. The receptor editing process was explored in several strains of transgenic or knockin mice. The first detailed demonstration of V_L chain editing was provided by a study of anti-DNA heavy-chain transgenic mice in which it was shown that a receptor editing of the double-stranded DNA (dsDNA)-specific BCR. This resulted from the secondary rearrangements of V_K-J_K *(524)* that reduced the diversity of the observed V_K repertoire in the periphery and biased usage of J_K5 segment *(525)*. Studies of four separate *Ig* knockin mouse strains showed that about 25% of light chains expressed in the BCR of developing B cells in vivo were produced by receptor editing *(526)*. Magari et al., using a knockin mouse strain expressing a rearranged *V[D]J* gene, showed that light-chain rearrangement in peripheral B cells contributed to the generation of high-affinity antibodies *(527)*. This finding strongly suggested that in addition to the somatic hypermutation process, the receptor revision process can contribute to the diversification of the repertoire. For receptor editing or receptor revision processes to operate, a signaling of the BCR expressed in pro-B and pre-B cells is required to retain active recombination machinery, namely RAG enzymes. The fact that *RAG* genes are expressed in pro-B and pre-BII cells explains the high frequency of receptor editing in these cells *(526)*. The re-expression of *RAG* genes is required in neonatal or adult B cells for a secondary rearrangement to occur. The possibility of the re-expression of *RAG* genes in mouse peripheral B cells was demonstrated in activated mature GC B cells *(528)* occurring after antigen stimulation *(529–531)*. To investigate possible receptor revision in newborn mice, we studied expression of the *RAG2* gene in 7-d-old mice immunized with an empty plasmid as control (pC) or with a plasmid containing the *HA* gene of the WSN strain of the influenza virus (pHA). Figure 28 shows the occurrence of GCs 7 d after immunization, which disappeared by 28 d as assessed by staining of spleen sections with anti-PNA antibodies. Centrocytes were detected in GCs 7 to 28 d after immunization with monoclonal anti-GL7 antibody, and their presence paralleled the detection of *RAG1* activity in GCs as assessed by staining with anti-*RAG1* monoclonal antibody. The absence of GL7$^+$ and *RAG1*$^+$ cells in the spleen of a mouse immunized with empty plasmid indicated that the induction of *RAG1* activity did not result from CpG motifs in empty plasmid but from the viral peptide encoded by the gene expressed in pHA plasmid. The data presented in Table 18 show a significant increase of B200$^+$ GL7$^+$ cells in the spleen of mice 7–21 d after immunization with pHA but not in mice immunized with control plasmid. Figure 29 demonstrates that the expression of *RAG1* was limited to sorted B220$^+$

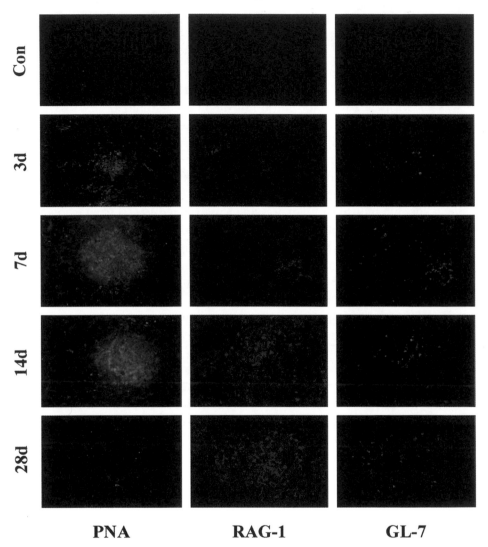

PNA   **RAG-1**   **GL-7**

Fig. 28. Expression of RAG-1 protein in splenic germinal centers of 7-d-old Balb immunized with a empty plasmid (pC) and a plasmid-counting influenza virus hemagglutinin gene (pHA). Spleen specimens from 1-d-old mice immunized with empty plasmid or with pHA were harvested 3, 7, 14, and 28 d after immunization. The spleens were embedded in 10 × 10 mm cryomolds (Fisher Scientific, Springfield, NJ) using Histp Prep. Serial 7 μm sections were fixed for 10 m at –20 C in acetone, methanol (1:1) and stained with 10 μg/mL FITC-anti-PNA (left panel), R-PE anti-RAG-1 (center panel), or FITC anti-GL-7 monoclonal antibodies. After extensive washings with 1% BSA in PBS, the sections were coverslipped with Vechtashield and examined in a Zeiss Axinphot microscope (×100).

Table 18
Percentage of B220+, GL7+, B220+GL7+ Cells in Spleen After Injection with Empty Plasmid (pC) or a Plasmid Containing Hemagglutinin of WSN Infuenza Virus Strain pHA

Day after injection	pC			pHA		
	B220+	GL7+	B220+GL7+	B220+	GL7+	B220+GL7+
3	53.3[a]	0.2	0.9	61.2	0.2	0.9
7	47.8	0.6	1.4	53.3	7.1	6.4
14	44.5	1.5	1.7	47.5	9.5	16.5
21	41.6	1.5	1.3	48.1	2.8	5.2

[a] Percentage of B220+, GL7+, B220+GL7+ cells was analyzed in lymphocyte population gate.

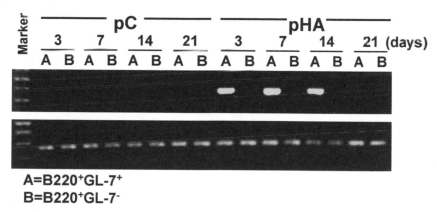

A=B220⁺GL-7⁺
B=B220⁺GL-7⁻

Fig. 29. Detection of RAG-2 transcripts in spleens of 7-d-old Balb/c mice immunized with pC and pHA plasmids. Single cell suspension of B200+GL-7+ and B220+ GL-7- cells sorted from spleens of animals harvested d 3, 7, 14, and 21 after immunization were used to extract cellular RNA. 8 µl of total RNA obtained from 5×10^6 sorted cells was treated with DNaseI and was reverse transcribed with primers specific for RAG-2 and β-actin. PCR products were separated onto 1% agarose gel and visualized with ethidium bromide. pC or pHA stand for RNA extracted from spleens of 7-d-old Balb/c mice immunized i.m. with 100 µg of pC or pHA. 3, 7, 14, and 21 stand for days of harvesting the spleen after injection of plasmids. A, RNA extracted from BB220+GL-7+ sorted cells; B, RNA extracted from B220+GL-7- sorted cells.

GL7⁺ B cells in spleens harvested 3,7, and 14 d after immunization with pHA plasmid but not in B200⁺ GL7⁻ B cells. (Data not published.)

Taken together, these results demonstrated that GCs are induced by the immunization of 7-d-old mice with a plasmid containing a viral gene. The occurrence of a GC is associated with an increased number of B cells expressing the GL7 marker. The RAG1 transcript was detected in B200⁺ GL7⁺ before the occurrence of organized GCs and lasted for 14 d, whereas the RAG1 protein was detected 7 d after immunization and lasted until d 28. These findings strongly suggest that the immunization of neonates with naked DNA induced the expression of RAG1, which, via secondary rearrangements, can contribute to the diversification of the neonatal repertoire.

5. DIVERSIFICATION OF THE B-CELL REPERTOIRE IN RABBITS

In rabbits, the IgH locus, as in other mammalian species, consists of multiple V_H, D, and J_H segments. It contains a minimum of 100 V_H genes separated from each other by 5 kb. Among approx 100 V_H genes, 50% are functional. Because they exhibit high nucleotide homology, they are considered members of the same V_H gene family. The V_H1 gene is the most proximally located. It appears that, among a large variety of V_H genes, only four are used in $V[D]J$ rearrangements, and V_H1 is used in about 80% of functional rearrangements.

The D gene locus contains 11 segments spanning over 20 kb of DNA, and there are 5 functional J_H segments *(532)*. The constant heavy-chain locus contains 16 C_H genes: $C\mu$, $C\gamma$, $C\varepsilon$, and 13 $C\alpha$ genes. Like mice, in rabbits, 80–90% of *Ig* express the κ light chain. The κ locus in rabbits is more complex than in mice because it contains two distinct $C\kappa$ genes: $C\kappa1$ and $C\kappa2$. Each $C\kappa$ gene is associated with one cluster of $J\kappa$ and two clusters of $V\kappa$ genes. The rabbit λ locus also is more complex than in mice and more closely resembles the human λ locus, containing four $V\lambda$ genes and as many as eight $C\lambda$ genes (reviewed in ref. *272*).

B lymphopoiesis in rabbits begins at days 17–19 of gestation, when pre-B cells can be detected in fetal liver. B-cell lymphopoiesis late in fetal life and at the first day after birth switches from the liver to bone marrow. Most B cells that develop early in ontogeny migrate soon after birth to the GALT system, which in rabbits is composed of appendix, *sacculus rotundus*, and Peyer's patches. After birth, in rabbits, few B cells develop because they exhibit a long half-life. Somatic diversification of the B-cell repertoire occurs in the GALT system. Exposure of B cells from the GALT system to bacteria may play a role in the diversification of the repertoire because the GALT system in germ-free rabbits is poorly developed, and these rabbits are highly immunocompromised *(533)*.

There are some similarities and differences between the molecular pattern of development of murine and rabbit fetal and neonatal repertoires.

First, $V[D]J$ rearrangements were detected in 14-d-old fetuses, and V_H1 (the most proximal V_H gene) was found preferentially rearranged in 14-to 28-d-old fetuses *(534)*. In newborn and 1-wk-old rabbits, V_H1 was found in 80% of $V[D]J$ rearrangements *(535)*. This indicated that, similarly to mice, there are position-dependent rearrangements of V_H genes. High usage of V_H1 in the neonates may explain the restricted rabbit neonatal repertoire and minimal antibody response to various antigen, even in 2- to 3-wk-old rabbits *(536,537)*.

In contrast to mice, in which the D-J segments are first rearranged in pro-B cells, in rabbits, the V_H-D_H rearrangement is a more frequent initial rearrangement among V_H gene segments *(538)*. Also, whereas in mice DQ52 (the 5'-most D_H gene) is preferentially expressed in the neonatal B-cell repertoire, the rabbit *DQ52* gene was not used in *V[D]J* rearrangements in 19- to 28-d-old fetuses or in the bone marrow from a 28-d-old fetus. This may result from the fact that, in rabbits, the 3'-RSS of *DQ52* shows an atypical nonamer. The *Df* gene located in the center of the D_H locus was preferentially used in *V[D]J* rearrangements from 15- to 28-d-old fetuses *(539)*.

In rabbits, the *V[D]J* genes do not diversify until after birth. Actually, Short et al. found that in 3 wk-old rabbits, the majority of *V[D]J* genes were not diversified, whereas at 9 wk of age they were highly diversified *(540)*. This diversification resulted from *N*-addition and to a high frequency of gene conversion in V_H genes. Gene conversion was observed in both the CDR and the framework segments *(532)*. Although the *N*-addition was observed starting at d 14 of gestation *(272)*, the diversification by gene conversion occurs later during the first few weeks of life mainly in the GALT system, namely, in the appendix of 6-wk-old rabbits *(541)*.

In summary, these findings show that there are some particular molecular features that contribute to the establishment of the B-cell repertoire in rabbits. First, neonatal B cells that developed during ontogeny have a long half-life, and very few B cells develop in adults. Second, the restricted neonatal repertoire is related to biased usage of the V_H1 and *Df* segments localized to the center of the D_H locus. Third, diversification of the repertoire resulting from *N*-nucleotide addition occurs in embryonic life, whereas the diversity resulting from gene conversion occurs later in postnatal life, mainly in the GALT system.

6. DEVELOPMENT OF THE B-CELL REPERTOIRE IN SHEEP AND CATTLE

In sheep, the majority of immunoglobulins bear the λ light chain. The sheep *Ig* variable repertoire consists of nine different V_H genes, six of which are functional. Based on the high sequence homology of functional V_H genes (>80), it was considered that all six V_H genes belong to a single V_H gene family. The V_H segments combine with a large set of very heterogeneous *D* segments and with a small number of J_H segments *(542)*. In sharp contrast, the λ locus is composed of greater than 100 germ line genes that recombine with only two Jλ segments, Jλ1 and Jλ2, among which Jλ1 is more frequently used than Jλ2 *(543)*. Among numerous V_L genes, only a few (20–30) were used and found to be rearranged.

Six different V_K genes were identified that, based on sequence homology, were classified into four V_K families. V_K3 and V_K4 families each contain a single member. The V_K genes recombine with two J_K segments.

The most fascinating aspect of the development of the sheep B-cell repertoire consists of two distinct features. First, the establishment of the repertoire in fetal lambs is completely independent of antigen exposure because ovine placenta is impermeable to macromolecules. Second, mature IgM$^+$ B cells appear early in ontogeny, around d 45 of gestation. They migrate and colonize the spleen at d 40 of gestation and then the ileal Peyer's patches, where the B-cell repertoire is rapidly expanded at 70–100 d of gestation. Third, the B-cell compartment matures during fetal development, as demonstrated by the ability of fetal lambs to produce antibodies after immunization with various antigen. Fourth, structural analysis of sheep V genes demonstrated that no new rearrangements occur after the initial colonization of the ileal Peyer's patches during the second half of fetal life *(545)*. Although there are no data on the structure of V_H genes expressed in fetal lambs, analysis of a genomic DNA library from an adult sheep showed that rearranged *V[D]J* exhibits large nucleotide variation in *CDR1* and 2, extensive *N*-nucleotide addition, and D segments of various lengths and sequences *(542)*. Thus, the V_H diversity results from somatic mutation rather than combinatorial mechanisms. In addition, no indication of gene conversion was noted. In early stages of embryonic life (61- to 90-d-old fetuses), all V_K family members were more or less equally represented. Meanwhile, in older fetuses, a biased usage was observed because nearly all V_K-J_K rearranged genes exclusively used V_K3, V_K4, and J_K2. Sequences of V_K3 and V_K4 showed little variation in either CDRs or framework segments *(546)*.

Diversification of the Vλ repertoire results from combinatorial rearrangements of multiple functional Vλ genes with a marked absence of *P*- or *N*-nucleotide addition *(547)*, as well as from antigen-independent hypermutation processes *(548)*. Comparison of the sequences originating from fetal or 1-d-old lambs to those of adult animals indicates little diversification in young lambs. The striking nucleotide differences between the neonatal and adult Vλ repertoires strongly suggest that they result from accumulation of mutations with age *(547)*. Taken together, these findings show that the diversity in the fetal and neonatal repertoires is the result of limited V_H and V_K usage to few mutations and to the absence of *P*- and *N*-nucleotide addition in V_L genes. The diversification process takes place mainly in ileal Peyer's patches that may represent the equivalent of the Bursa of Fabricius in avians.

In cattle, the primary source of B-cell progenitors is the fetal liver and spleen. No B cells were found in the bone marrow in the third trimester of gestation or in 2- or 12-d-old calves *(549)*. After birth, the spleen is likely to be the organ of gene rearrangement because *RAG1* gene expression was found in the spleen of 14-d-old calves and disappeared in 32-wk-old cattle *(550)*. Similarly to sheep, in cattle, the B cells might migrate to ileal Peyer's patches where they undergo proliferation and the diversification of *Ig* genes.

Restriction fragment length polymorphism (RFLP) analysis of bovine genomic DNA indicated the V_H locus contains many V_H genes. However, comparison of germ line gene sequences with the V_H sequences from adult splenic cDNA indicated that the B-cell repertoire is dominated by a single V_H family comprised of as few as 15 members and closely related to the human V_H2 or murine *Q52* V_H families. The *D* segments are of greater length, and at least two J_H segments are used *(551,552)*.

The majority of bovine Ig bears a λ light chain. The λ locus contains 20 *V*λ germ line genes. Among them are 14 pseudogenes that exhibit various structural defects, including a lack of RSS at the 3'-end, stop codons, truncations, insertions, or deletions resulting in the loss of reading frames. Two *J*λ segments were identified in genomic DNA, but all the expressed *V*λ genes examined contained a single *J*λ segment. The *V*λ-*J*λ can associate with four different *C*λ genes *(553)*. Apparently, in cattle, the V_K locus is complex but not well studied.

In fetal livers, only the transcripts of the bovine V_H1 family were detected *(551)*. The diversity of the V_H probably lies in the length of *CDR3*, which ranges from 13 to 28 codons. The putative *D* genes are read in one reading frame. One J_H segment seems to be used throughout life, because it was found in cDNA sequences of V_H genes from both fetal and adult cattle. The diversification of the *V*λ repertoire was studied by comparing the complete *V*λ cDNA sequences obtained from ileal Peyer's patches from 11-d-old and 32-wk-old calves. This analysis demonstrated that diversification had occurred by 11 d after birth, when the majority of rearranged *V*λ genes used the *V*λ B4 gene family. This gene usage was found in the majority of cDNA sequences of older animals, indicating that *V*λ genes expressed in the neonatal repertoire are maintained in adult life. Structural differences were clustered in CDR segments with a few scattered changes in framework regions. The same V-J junction was observed in all clones analyzed, indicating that rearranged *V*λ gene segments recombined by a single predominant rearrangement *(553)*. These observations suggest that combinatorial mechanisms are unlikely to be significant in the generation of antibody diversity in calves. In contrast, there are several findings strongly suggesting that gene conversion soon after birth is the major mechanism leading to antibody diversity. The major argument is that the variation observed in rearranged *V* genes compared to germ line genes showed that there are clusters of nucleotide changes and that they can originate from the *V*λ pseudogenes, which function as sequence donors.

In ileal Peyer's patches, the fact that the $V\lambda$ genes already exhibit sequence variation suggests that significant diversification of the repertoire occurs in fetal spleen and within a few days after birth in the GALT system.

7. DEVELOPMENT OF THE HUMAN NEONATAL REPERTOIRE

In humans, 60% of immunoglobulins bear a κ light chain, and 40% bear a λ light chain.

The V_H locus located on chromosome 14 represents a region of 957 kb of DNA containing 123 V_H genes, among which 39 are functional, 29 are pseudogenes, and others have non-rearranged open reading frames *(554)*. Based on >80% DNA homology, the V_H genes are grouped into seven families. The D_H locus consists of 9.5-kb tandem repeat units that contain 29 germ line genes; of these 25 are functional and are classified into 6 D_H families. There are nine J_H segments, of which six are functional.

The V_K locus located on chromosome 2 contains 76 germ line genes; of these, 32 are functional. They are organized into two cassettes: the first, composed of 40 genes, is located in the J_K proximal region; the second, composed of 36 genes, is located in the distal inverted region. The V_K genes were classified into seven families or subgroups. All five J_K segments are functional *(555,556)*. V_H and V_K genes may be found at other chromosomal locations where they are not expressed. The loci containing these nonexpressed genes are called orphons. It is believed that orphons arise by inversions and conversions that have been maintained during evolution. A V_H orphon was identified on chromosome 16, and a V_K orphon was found located close to the centromere on chromosome 2.

The $V\lambda$ locus located on chromosome 22 is composed of 70 $V\lambda$ genes, of which 30 are functional, and 7 $J\lambda$ segments, of which 4 are functional *(557,558)*.

Generation of the neonatal repertoire results from random combinatorial events of the segments encoding V_H, V_K, and $V\lambda$ genes.

The rearrangements of *V* genes in humans during embryonic life begin at 7–8 wk of gestation in the fetal liver when the first wave of pre-B cells is detected. The pre-B cells are characterized by the presence of cytoplasmic *IgM* and a $V\lambda$-like chain and lack of surface *IgM*. The pseudo-light-chain cluster contains three genes *(14.1, Fl1,* and *16.1)* located on chromosome 22 close to the $V\lambda$ locus. Structural analysis of the pseudo-λ genes shows similar organization and high nucleotide homology, suggesting that the two systems,(λ and λ-like, diverged after duplication of a common ancestor *(559)*. In fetal livers (8 wk of gestation), only transcripts of the *16.1* λ-like gene were detected in the large cDNA library analyzed *(559)*.

Immature B cells (sIgM$^+$), followed by mature B lymphocytes (sIgM$^+$, sIgD$^+$), were detected at 7–8 and 12 wk of gestation, respectively. During intrauterine development, Ig class switching occurs only in a few B cells, indicating that this process is independent of antigen exposure because the intrauterine environment is sterile.

Analysis of the expression of sIg and CD5 showed that 88% of neonatal CD19+ B cells express sIgD, and about 80% expressed both IgD and IgM. Only a few (<10%) are IgM+IgD−. About 50% express CD5 and sIgD and may be considered B1 cells.

Like mice, the rearrangement of V gene segments follows a similar genetic program of rearrangements:

$$D_H \rightarrow J_H, \ V_H \rightarrow DJ_H \ C\mu \ \text{and} \ V_L\text{-}J_L$$

A study of V[D]J rearrangements in human fetal liver at 7, 13, and 18 wk of gestation showed a preferential usage of the *VH3, DQ52*, and *Dxp* gene families from 30 estimated D segments and J_H3 and J_H4. The diversity of CDR3 in fetal liver B cells is limited by the absence of *P* junctions and fewer *N* additions in D-J junctions. Meanwhile, the D_H reading frame appears to be randomly used. The rearrangements of D elements occur by inversion and D-D fusion that could result from unequal crossing over *(560)*. In contrast, other investigators have found preferential expression of V_H5 and V_H6 in 7-wk-old fetal livers, suggesting a position-biased usage because the V_H6 gene is the most J_H proximally located *(561)*. A biased usage of V_H6 also was found in fetal livers from 16- to 24-d-old fetuses *(562)*. Sequence analysis of heavy-chain transcripts obtained from fetal livers at 104 and 130 d of gestation identified by hybridization with a $C\mu$ probe showed the same pattern of usage of V_H gene segments, because three highly conserved V_H3, DQ52, and J_H3 and J_H4 genes were highly expressed, whereas transcripts from V_H1, V_H2, V_H4, V_H5, and V_H6 genes were expressed at a low frequency *(563)*. The preferential use of D_HQ52 in sterile and mature V[D]J transcripts indicates that nonrandom usage of some gene segments in fetal B cells reflects a genetic regulatory program intrinsic to B cells in this stage of development and that the V_H3 genes play an important biological role *(564)*.

Study of the expression of V_H genes in the neonatal repertoire, particularly in cord blood lymphocytes, showed that all V_H, D_H families and J_H segments are expressed, with a higher frequency of utilization of the V_H3 and V_H1; D_H2, D_H3, and D_H6 families; and J_H6, J_H4, and J_H5. A shift in the utilization of J_H segments is evident, because in fetal livers, J_H3 was frequently used. Another study reported the frequent use of the V_H7 gene family in cord blood B cells *(565)*.

It is known that B1 CD5+ cells predominate in cord blood. Analysis of V_H gene family expression in cord blood-derived Epstein–Barr virus (EBV)-transformed B-cell lines showed frequent usage (30%) of the V_H4 gene family. It was shown that the V_H4 gene family encodes for self-reactive and multispecific antibodies *(566)*.

One may ask whether the shift in use of V_H gene segments during transition from the fetal to neonatal repertoire is because of exposure to antigen after birth. This question was addressed by studying the expression of V_H genes in preterm neonates (gestational age: 25–29 wk) vs full-term neonates. This study showed that the exposure of preterm neonates to antigen resulted in a higher frequency of class switching to IgG and a higher number of somatic mutations within 2 wk of postnatal life. In contrast, premature exposure to extrauterine environmental antigen did not alter the pattern of V_H expression and did not lead to a switch to an adult-like repertoire. In addition, the length of CDR3 was not increased by N-nucleotide addition. This observation clearly indicates that V_H region diversity is mainly developmentally regulated and that the repertoire restrictions persist in spite of premature exposure to antigen *(567)*.

Sequence analysis of the V_H6 gene from cord blood B cells showed no mutations; however, almost all sequences from 10-d-old newborns with acute infections had mutations *(568)*. The V_H6 gene of 2- and 10-mo-old healthy children exhibited mutations, and the frequency of mutation increased with age *(569)*. Comparison of the V_H6 gene sequence expressed in newborns and young children with the V_H4 germ line gene showed a mutation frequency of 4.3% with a range from 1 to 24 mutations in the 241-bp gene segment analyzed. The mutation frequency was higher in the CDR (1.6%) compared to the framework region (0.9%) with a replacement:silent ratio of 4 for CDR and 2.9 for framework segments. Comparison of CDR3 length in different infant age groups did not show a significant difference *(569)*. These results show that mutation in the V_H6 gene is a rare event in newborns and children younger than age 6 mo and that the frequency of mutation increased after age 6 mo, indicating an antigen-driven process. This explanation is supported by the paralleled increased of the frequency of mutations and the replacement:silent mutation ratios.

Study of the neonatal κ repertoire was carried out using cDNA obtained by unbiased polymerase chain reaction (PCR) amplification of nonproductive and productive rearrangement of V_K genes. Initial studies suggested that the V_K gene family is nonstochastically used, because genes belonging to the V_K1 and V_K3 families located in the distal half of the locus were predominantly expressed *(570,571)*. A finer analysis was carried out using a single-cell PCR technique, purified sIgD$^+$ CD5$^-$, and CD5$^+$ sIgD$^+$ B cells purified from cord blood *(572)*.

In this study, the expression of V_K families was analyzed in productive and nonproductive rearrangements, which affords the opportunity to understand the molecular mechanisms before the repertoire is shaped by positive and negative selection. This study demonstrated that six out of seven V_K families were rearranged in the neonatal repertoire. In the nonproductive repertoire, the members of V_K1, V_K3, and V_K6 occurred as frequently as expected from genome complexity, whereas the occurrence of V_K2 was less frequent than expected. V_K4

and V_K5 were more frequently used than expected from random use in the productive repertoire. A member of the V_K3 family gene, A27, was overrepresented.

Roughly the same pattern of V_K gene family expression was observed in the productive repertoire: V_K1 and V_K5 were expressed significantly more often in neonatal than adult repertoires. V_K3, V_K4, V_K6, and V_K7 gene expression did not differ between the neonatal and adult repertoires, and V_K2 was less frequently expressed. Thus, V_K genes from both the proximal and distal cassettes were found in the neonatal repertoire, but those from the distal cassette were found less frequently. With respect to individual V_K genes, genes *B2, L9,* and *O12/O2* were expressed more significantly, accounting for 79% of productive rearrangements in the neonatal repertoire.

Compared to the adult repertoire, the junctional diversity was less marked (28% neonatal vs 57% adult productive rearrangements contained *N*-nucleotide), whereas CDR3 length was comparable (average: 27 nucleotides). In neonatal B cells, J_K2 was predominantly used, J_K5 was used at the expected frequency, J_K1 was used less, and J_K3 and J_K4 were significantly less used than expected. Seventeen mutations were found in all neonatal V_K rearrangements, indicating an overall mutational frequency rate of 3.27×10^4 per base pair.

In contrast to CD5$^-$IgD$^+$ B cells, CD5$^+$ B1 cells showed some important differences. Only productive rearrangement of V_K genes from the distal cassette was found. Meanwhile, no differences in J_K usage and *N*-nucleotide insertions were observed in CD5$^+$ B1 cells compared to neonatal IgD$^+$CD5$^-$ B2 cells.

These results demonstrated that there is a molecular preference, based on chromosomal position, in the selection of V_K gene families and J_K segments in the neonatal repertoire, leading to a more restricted and uniform repertoire in neonates compared to adults. Limited variability in the generation of V_K-J_K joints, less receptor editing, and the shorter length of CDR3 also are important factors that contribute to a more restricted V_K repertoire in neonates. Higher expression of some individual members of the proximal V_K gene families suggests positive selection by exposure to self-antigen rather than to foreign antigen because the intrauterine environment is sterile. High usage of the distal cassette in neonatal B1 cells suggests positive selection by self-antigen, which explains why these cells produce multispecific and self-reactive autoantibodies.

There are no extensive studies of the $V\lambda$ neonatal repertoire, which in humans represents 40% of immunoglobulins.

A study of $V\lambda J\lambda$ rearrangements in IgM$^+$ B cells from fetal spleens at 18 wk of gestation showed an overrepresentation of the distal $J\lambda$ cluster recombining with the $J\lambda7$ segment. $V\lambda$ genes paired stochastically with V_H genes in fetal spleen IgM$^+$ B cells *(573)*.

In conclusion, the major molecular characteristic of the human neonatal repertoire consists of preferential usage of V_H and V_K families located in the proximity of the J clusters. The restricted and more uniform repertoire is related to less frequent P and N addition and shorter CDR3 length. The frequency of mutation is considerably lower than in adults because B cells are not exposed to antigen during gestation.

5

Genetically Programmed Temporal Ordered Activation of Neonatal B-Cell Clones

1. INTRODUCTION

Several molecular factors contribute to the restricted neonatal repertoire. Among them, the most important are position-dependent usage of a few V gene families, shorter length of CDR3, lack of region diversity, and low frequency of somatic mutation. The ordered emergence of B-cell clones after birth is an additional, important factor. This may be because of the fact that some B-cell clones appear or mature at different rates rather than they do in concert. Studies using inbred animal strains demonstrated that the temporal pattern of B-cell clone emergence is similar in all individuals, indicating that a heritable genetic program determines the development of clones producing antibodies with various antigen specificities.

Two approaches were used to study sequential activation of B-cell clones after birth: (a) the study of the antibody response after immunization of the fetus at various periods of gestation or of the newborn at various intervals after birth, and (b) the study of the antibody response in lethally irradiated adult mice reconstituted with syngeneic fetal or neonatal cells and immunized with foreign antigens at various intervals after reconstitution.

Hierarchical B-cell activation during fetal life and after birth was initially characterized in lambs. This study was facilitated by three factors: (a) early B-cell maturation during fetal life (mature B cells are detected at d 40 of the 150-d gestation period), (b) lack of maternal antibody influence because the placenta of a pregnant sheep does not allow IgG transfer from mother to fetus, and (c) the relative ease of surgical procedures for intrafetal immunization.

Fetal lambs immunized by d 60 with ϕX phage or at 65–70 or 80–101 d of gestation with ovalbumin and ferritin produced specific antibodies detected 6–52 d after immunization. The majority of antiphage antibodies produced by the fetus were IgM. In sharp contrast, immunization with BCE failed to induce antibody production. Antibody responses against these three antigens were observed only after immunization of 40-d-old lambs.

From: *Contemporary Immunology: Neonatal Immunity*
By: Constantin Bona © Humana Press Inc., Totowa, NJ

The sequential activation of B-cell clones also was described in the opossum. At birth, the opossum enters the maternal pouch, newborns can be immunized directly, and antibody responses can be studied at various intervals after immunization. Antibodies to the following antigens appeared in a temporal order: bovine serum albumin-dinitrophenol (BSA-DNP) or hemocyanin-DNP conjugates in embryos age 8 to 19 d; bacteriophage F2 in embryos age 15 d: ϕX-174 and T4 phage in embryos age 29 d: RNAase in embryos age 40 to 49 d; and lysozyme in embryos age 50 d. It is interesting to note that the response to ϕX-174 bacteriophage was first seen at day 15 when the thymus had defined cortical and medullary zones, whereas the response to T2 was found in 20-d-old embryos immunized when the spleen had begun to acquire perivascular lymphoid elements.

Although a distinct hierarchy of responsiveness against various antigens was clearly demonstrated in these pioneering studies in the lamb and opossum, an analysis of antigen specificity of clones was not possible because these animal models lack adequate methodology to study responses at the clonal level.

2. SEQUENTIAL ACTIVATION OF B-CELL CLONES IN LETHALLY IRRADIATED MICE RECONSTITUTED WITH FETAL LIVER CELLS

The study of B-cell ontogeny in mice was precluded by the difficulty of immunizing the early fetus   as was done in fetal lambs. This difficulty was overcome by grafting fetal liver cells into syngeneic lethally irradiated adult mice. Grafted cells proliferate in the irradiated host and give rise to distinct spleen colonies. Subsequent transfer of a spleen colony into lethally irradiated mice is capable of repopulating lymphatic tissue with cells derived from a single progenitor cell. These mice were immunized at various times after reconstitution with various antigens, and antibody responses were measured at various intervals after antigen injection. This experimental model allowed for the determination of the time course of occurrence of B-cell clones that produce antibodies specific for various antigens.

Such a model was used to establish the onset of immunocompetence against and sheep red blood cells in 12-d-old fetal cells.This study showed that the ability to recognize foreign antigens was established between 19 and 20 d, reaching the level of adults by 25–32 d of development. In contrast, recognition of the erythrocyte antigen became significant over a period of 26 to 33 d, corresponding to 7 to 14 d after birth. The results of this experiment were the first to indicate sequential acquisition of immune reactivity during B-cell development in fetal liver precursors.

In another set of experiments, the hierarchy of antigen responsiveness was determined in lethally irradiated mice reconstituted with cells obtained from the livers of 18- to 19-d-old fetal or newborn mice. After reconstitution, the recipient mice were immunized at various times. In this experiment, the response against F2 and ϕX-174 phages occurred between 3 and 7 d after reconstitution. Meanwhile, the T4 phage-specific response occurred after 14 d, anti-DNP and antilysozyme responses occurred after 21 d, antifluorescein and anti-RNase responses were detected after 28 d, and antibodies specific for myoglobin occurred 6 wk after reconstitution. The ordered maturation of these responses was independent of major histocompatibility complex (MHC) and allotype because a similar pattern was observed in C3H/HeJ, AKR, and Balb/c mice. The sequential acquisition of responses against these antigens cannot be explained by the immunogenicity of the antigens because different patterns were observed for different haptens coupled to the same carrier, such as DNP-BSA and FTC-BSA. The response pattern also cannot be explained by the lack of T-cell maturation because the responses induced by phages, lysozyme, RNase, and myoglobin are all T-cell-dependent responses. The most likely explanation of these results is that there is a genetically programmed maturation of B-cell clones derived from fetal or neonatal liver precursors. This is in spite of the fact that environmental factors may affect the circulation and migration of fetal cells in irradiated hosts.

The absence of environmental influences and the genetic control of sequential acquisition of fetal cell responsiveness were demonstrated in another experiment. Fetal tissues from 14- to 19-d-old embryos were cultured in vitro for 4–5 d and then injected into KLH-primed irradiated recipients. The recipients were scarified 14–16 d later, and the frequency of hapten-reactive B cells was determined by splenic focus assays after stimulation of cultures with KLH-hapten conjugates at a concentration of 10^{-6} of hapten. In this experiment, it was shown that DNP-specific B cells were found in the fetal liver at d 16 of gestation, whereas fluorescein-specific B cells were found at 16–18 d of gestation. NP or phosphoryl choline-reactive B cells were detected in the fetal liver at any age. This experiment demonstrated that the maturation of B-cell precursors from fetal livers followed a genetically controlled temporal order.

3. FREQUENCY OF HAPTEN-SPECIFIC B CELLS IN NEONATAL MICE DETERMINED BY SPLENIC FOCUS ASSAY

The frequency of hapten-specific B cells can be enumerated accurately by combining adoptive transfer of a limited number of cells in carrier-primed irradiated mice with in vitro culture of spleen fragments with antigen or hapten-carrier protein conjugates. This technique, called the splenic focus assay, permits assessment of the reactivity pattern of monoclonal antibodies determined by isoelectric spectrum or idiotype expression as markers of V region genes encoding antibody specificity.

This method was used to determine the frequency of neonatal clonotypes for several haptens such as DNP 2,4,6-trinitrophenol (TNP), fluorescein, p-azophenylarsonate dimethylaminoapthalene-sulfonyl (Dansyl), and PR8 influenza virus.

The frequency of DNP clonotypes from 1-d-old mice ranged from 1 to 2 foci/10^6 spleen cells. The number was somewhat higher from 3- to 5-d-old donors ($2.3/10^6$), indicating that in the neonatal spleen the frequency of B cells producing anti-DNP antibodies remained constant during the first week after birth. The same frequency was observed for B cells producing anti-TNP antibodies, whereas the frequency of fluorescein-specific B cells was five- to six-fold lower. Whereas the frequency of DNP- and TNP-specific precursors at birth is almost identical to the frequency in adults, the analysis of reactivity patterns of DNP and TNP antibodies by isoelectric focusing showed that during the first 4 d of neonatal life, three clonotypes were dominant with three distinct pH isoforms (pIs) (5.05, 5.25, and 5.55 for DNP-specific antibodies and 5.00, 5.15, and 5.40 for TNP-specific antibodies). The frequency of these clonotypes decreased by half by d 6 and represented a small minority by d 9, having been replaced with new clonotypes. Dansyl-specific precursors were found at a high frequency at birth, reaching the level of adults during the first week of life, whereas the frequency of p-azophenylarsonate-specific prescursors appeared to decrease during the first week of life.

In adult mice, the frequency of influenza virus hemagglutinin (HA)-reactive B cells was substantially lower than the frequency of hapten-specific B cells. Analysis of the reactivity pattern of clonotypes in adult mice showed that it contains a minimum 100–200 unique specificities. Analysis of the HA-specific B-cell repertoire of 12- to 14-d-old mice showed that the clonotype reactivity pattern was considerably less diverse and that some neonatal clonotypes were rapidly replaced by others during postnatal life. These results argue again for a temporally ordered diversification during postnatal life. From these observations, several conclusions can be drawn:

a. The precursors for hapten-specific B cells are present soon after birth in peripheral lymphoid organs.
b. The clonotype pattern constantly and rapidly changes during postnatal life.
c. A genetic mechanism may account for early expression of some clonotypes and late expression of others.
d. The scoring of hapten-specific precursor frequency can be determined more accurately in focus spleen assay, which maximizes T-cell help even in the absence of fully mature antigen-presenting and T helper cells.

4. TEMPORALLY ORDERED ACTIVATION OF B-CELL CLONES AFTER IMMUNIZATION OF NEWBORN MICE WITH VARIOUS ANTIGENS

The T-cell dependence of the immune responses elicited by polysaccharide antigens represent the best model to investigate sequential activation of B-cell clones for several reasons. First, the majority of polysaccharide antigens are T-cell independent and, therefore, B cells expressing a BCR specific for these antigens are stimulated after interaction with the BCR. Second, in contrast to responses induced by T-cell-dependent antigens (hapten-protein conjugates or proteins) the responses elicited by polysaccharides are generally oligo- or pauciclonal. Third, as illustrated in Table 19, antipolysaccharide antibodies are encoded by a limited number of V genes and may exhibit a particular $V_{H^-}V_L$ gene pairing. Fourth, V genes that encode antipolysaccharide antibodies expressed cross-reactive idiotypes (IdX) that are phenotypic markers of V germ line genes.

4.1. Antibody Responses Induced in 1-d-Old Mice

One-day-old Balb/c mice immunized with gum ghatti, grass or bacterial levan, or lipopolysaccharide (LPS) can develop antibodies specific for β2-6-D-galactan, β 2-6 fructosan, and α methyl-D-galactoside, respectively. Antigalactan antibodies produced by Balb/c mice in response to immunization with gum ghatti share the X24 IdX with the XRPC24 galactan-binding myeloma protein. The immunization of 1-, 7-, 14-, or 21-d-old mice showed development of a significant immune response as assessed by scoring the number of plaque-forming cells (PFCs). PFCs are reduced by approx 30% on addition of rabbit anti-X24 IdX antibodies to the assay. The magnitude of PFC response did not vary substantially in 1- to 21-d-old mice.

The antilevan antibody response is induced after immunization with polyfructosans such as grass and bacterial levan. Grass levan consists of a linear backbone of β 2-6 fructosan, whereas bacterial levan consists of a backbone of β 2-6 fructosan with β 2-1 branch points. The immune response against β 2-6 fructosan is T-independent, because it can be induced in nude mice. Anti-β 2-6 fructosan antibodies do not share IdX of ABPC48 and UPC10 myeloma proteins that bind to levan. This indicates that the B cells able to produce anti-β 2-6 fructosan antibodies bearing ABPC48 or UPC10 IdX are silent in Balb/c mice. Anti-β 2-6 fructosan antibodies can be elicited following immunization of 1-d-old Balb/c mice with bacterial levan, as assessed by both plaque-form-

Table 20
Anti-Polysaacharide Responses Elicited by the Immunization
of 1-d-Old mice

Anti-galactan response

Age of mice	anti-galactan PFC/10^6	% expressing X24IdX
1 d-old	130+/–24	44
7 d-old	150+/–12	42
14 d-old	148+/–12	31
21 d-old	115+/–42	51

PFC response was measured 5 d after the immunization with 50 μg gum ghatti

Anti-α-methyl-D-galactoside response

Age of mice	immunization with	HA titer* of anti LPS Ab	HI titer:* of 348Id
1-d-old	saline	1.2+/–0.3	0
1-d-old	10 μg S.tranaroa LPS	4.1+/–1.8	2.0+/–0
32-d-old	saline	2.8+/–0.5	1.2+/–0.3
32-d-old	10 μg S.tranaroa LPS	8.7+/–1.2	4.4+/–0.3

*expressed as $\log_2$ units
Antibody response was tested 5 d after immunization.

Anti-β 2-6 fructoasan antibody response

Age of mice	immunization with	HA titer*	PFC/10^6
1-d-old	saline	0.3+/–0.3	5+/–2
1-d-old	10 μg levan	1.8+/–0.4	46+/–7
9-d-old	saline	2.0+/–0.3	14+/–7
9-d-old	10 μg levan	5.1+/–0.8	89+/–13
56-d-old	saline	3.8+/–0.4	21+/–5
56-d-old	10 μg levan	9.5+/–0.9	156+/–25

Adapted from ref. *596*.

ing cell (PFC) and hemmaglutination assays. The magnitude of the response gradually increases during postnatal life reaching the adult level by 8 weeks.

LPS from Salmonella tranaroa, Salmonella tel-aviv and Proteus mirabilis has D-methyl D-galactoside as the immunodominant sugar. The myeloma protein MOPC384 binds to this dominant sugar, providing a tool to investigate the expression of its idiotype (i.e., 384 IdX) on the response induced by LPS. We showed that the immunization of 1-d-old Balb/c mice induced an anti-methyl-galactoside response expressing 348 IdX. The magnitude of the response induced in 1-d-old mice was about half of that observed in 8-wk-old mice.

The experimental results illustrating the observations described earlier are depicted in Table 20. These results clearly demonstrate that the precursors of

B-cell clones that produce antibodies specific for some polysaccharides are present early after birth.

4.2. Antibody Responses Induced During the First Week After Birth

The sequential activation of neonatal B cells implies that antibody responses specific for other antigens may be induced by the immunization of young mice rather than that of newborns.

Several reports showed that the B cells stimulated by phosphoryl choline (PC), phenyl arsonate, and DNP or TNP conjugates can be induced only in 1-wk-old mice.

Balb/c mice immunized with microbes containing PC in their cell wall, such as Streptococcus pneumonia or Proteus morganii, develop T-independent anti-PC responses, whereas those immunized with PC that is conjugated with carrier proteins develop T-dependent responses. In both cases, the majority of anti-PC antibodies express a germ line gene-encoded idioype called T15, which is shared with PC-binding myeloma proteins such as TEPC15 or S107.

Using splenic focus assay, analysis of the frequency of T15 IdX-dominant PC-specific precursors showed that they appear quite late in neonatal development. Although no PC-specific foci were detected in the spleens of 1- to 5-d-old mice, a significant number were detected in 6- to 7-d-old mice. Sixty-six percent of monoclonal antibodies produced by PC-specific foci expressed T15 IdX, and the percentage of B cells producing T15 IdX^+ antibodies increased further by d 9 after birth. Whereas the T15 IdX-dominant precursors occur late after birth, an anti-PC antibody response lacking T15 IdX can be elicited in 1-d-old mice immunized with PC-LPS conjugate. These results showed that during the first week of postnatal life, the mice acquire a sequential responsiveness to different PC antigens. Only TI1 antigens such as PC-LPS induced the earliest response. This response consists of the activation of B cells producing T15 IdX^- anti-PC antibodies, whereas the dominant T15 IdX^+-producing B cells are activated later, by the end of first week after birth. It is noteworthy that the *xid* gene plays an important role in the activation of B cells that produce anti-PC antibodies. For instance, CBA/N females exhibiting a defect in B-lymphocyte maturation are unable to respond to PC that is conjugated with various carriers.

The immunization of mice with phenyl arsonate conjugate induces antiphenyl arsonate antibodies of which 30–50% expressed an IdX. The expression of IdX is allotype linked. Transfer experiments to study the neonatal development of B cells that produce antiphenyl arsonate antibodies showed that B cells that produce dominant IdX antiphenyl arsonate antibodies are present by d 9 after birth.

Table 21
Ontogeny of Anti-TNP Antibody Response and the Expression of 460Id

Age of mice	Immunization	PFC/10^6	% of 460 Id
1-d-old	Saline	2±2	0
1-d-old	TNP-LPS	112±21	0
1-d-old	TNP- Ficoll	7±4	0
3-d-old	Saline	4±3	0
3-d-old	TNP-LPS	179±11	0
3-d-old	TNP-Ficoll	16±7	0
7-d old	Saline	24±6	0
7-d-old	TNP-LPS	211±44	16±3
7-d-old	TNP-Ficoll	18±5	0
14-d-old	Saline	26±9	0
14-d-old	TNP-LPS	280±31	20±7
14-d-old	TNP-Ficoll	345±26	8±2
28-d-old	Saline	82±34	0
28-d-old	TNP-LPS	506±124	35±6
28-d-old	TNP-Ficoll	613±16	6±2

Adapted from ref. *601*.
Abbreviations: TNP, trinitrophenyl; LPS, lipopolysaccharide, PFC, plague-forming cells.

In contrast to the responses elicited by PC, which are pauciclonal, the responses induced by DNP and TNP conjugates are polyclonal and are encoded by V genes belonging to various V_H and V_L gene families. Precursors of B cells producing anti-DNP or anti-TNP antibodies were identified in fetal and neonatal livers in adoptive transfer experiments in irradiated mice or by spleen focus assay. The results of these experiments suggested that newborn mice must be able to mount a response against TNP or DNP haptens. A fraction of anti-TNP antibody-producing cells share 460IdX expressed on MOPC460 and MOPC315 DNP and TNP-binding myeloma proteins. Whereas Ig molecules expressing 460IdX are not detected in naïve mice, anti-TNP antibodies bearing 460IdX were noted in mice immunized with T-dependent or -independent antigens. Based on this information, we have studied the anti-TNP response and the expression of 460IdX in mice immunized with TI1 (TNP-LPS and TNP-B.abortus conjugates) and TI2 (e.g., TNP-Ficoll) antigen. Immunization of 1-d-old mice with TNP-LPS or TNP-B.abortus conjugates elicited a substantial anti-TNP response, but B cells producing 460IdX$^+$ anti-TNP antibodies were detected only in 7-d-old Balb/c mice. These results clearly demonstrate the sequential activation of B-cell clones producing anti-TNP antibodies, because the clones producing antibodies and expressing 460IdX occurred 1 wk after the clones producing anti-TNP antibodies lacking 460IdX. The experimental results supporting this conclusion are presented in Table 21.

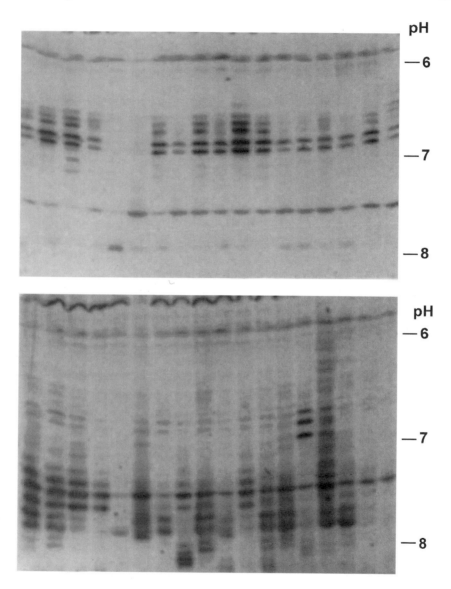

Fig. 30. Isoelectrofocusing (IEF) pattern of Balb/c antibacterial levan antibodies. Sera obtained from 18 individual Balb/c mice 10 d after immunization with bacterial levan. The upper panel shows anti-β2, 1)-fructosan antibodies reactive with ^{125}I-inulin-BSA and the lower panel shows anti-β (2,6)-antibodies reactive with ^{125}I-bacterial levan. (From Stein K, et al. J Exp Med 1980;151:1088–1102.)

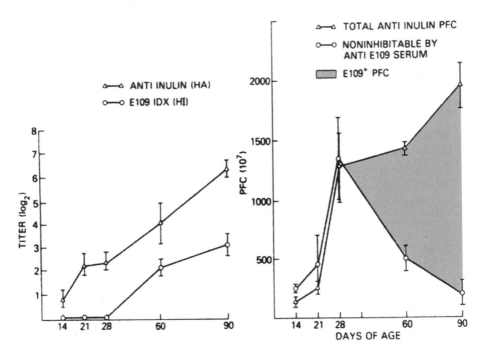

Fig. 31. Age dependence of anti-inulin response in Balb/c mice. Left panel, serum antibody response 5 d after immunization of BALB/c mice of various ages with bacterial levan. Right panel, anti-inulin PFC response and expression of E109 IdX 5 d after immunization of Balb/c of various ages with bacterial levan. (From Bona C, et al. J Immunol 1979;123:1484–1490.)

4.3. Antibody Responses Induced Late in Postnatal Life

Study of the ontogenic development of anti-β 2-1 fructosan and anti-α 1-6 dextran antibody responses showed that they could be induced late in postnatal life.The β 2-1-linked fructose linear polymer is found in inulin, but β 2-1 fructosan also represents the branch points of the β 2-6 fructosan backbone of bacterial levans. Although levans can induce a T-independent antibody response, inulin by itself is not immunogenic without being coupled with a protein carrier.

The anti-β 2-1 fructosan antibody response induced by inulin-BSA conjugate is very restricted compared to that induced by bacterial levan. This was demonstrated by analysis of the isoelectrofocusing (IEF) pattern. In Balb/c mice, anti-inulin antibodies display a characteristic IEF pattern that is essentially identical in all individuals, consisting of a single spectrotype comprised of five bands, of which three predominate and focus in the pH 6.3 to 6.8 range. Figure 30 illustrates the IEF pattern of anti-inulin and antibacterial levan antibodies in adult Balb/c mice. Anti-inulin antibodies share three distinct IdXs (IdX G, IdX A, and

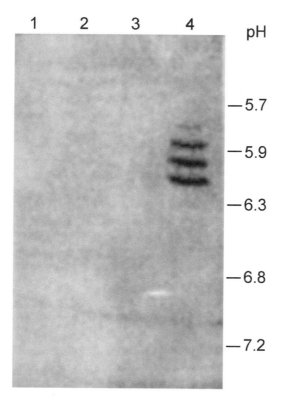

Fig. 32. IEF pattern of anti-inulin antibodies of various ages. Serum from Balb/c mice of various ages was electrophoresed and the blots were incubated with ^{125}I-inulin-BSA. Lane 1 serum from mice immunized at 7-d of age; lane 2 serum from mice immunized at 14 d of age; lane 3 serum from animals immunized at 21 of age; lane 4 serum from mice immunized at 12 wk of age. (From Bona C et al. J Immunol 1979;123:1484–1490.)

IdX B) with 11 β 2-1 fructosan-binding myeloma proteins. Study of the ontogeny of anti-β 2-1 fructosan antibodies by hemagglutination, PFC, and IEF assays indicated that they occur long after birth. A weak PFC response was first observed in 21-d-old mice, followed by a substantial increase at 28 d (Figs. 31 and 32). As can be seen in Fig. 31, the dominant anti-inulin clones expressing IdX D-E109 were detected only in mice older than 4 wk. Several experimental findings support the concept that the late occurrence of anti-β 2-1 fructosan is related to a genuine ontogenic delay. First, it was found that polyclonal activation by a B-cell mitogen, NWSM, which is known to induce the proliferation of B cells in their early stages, induced an increased in 3H-thymidine incorporation in spleen cells of 1-wk-old Balb/c mice. The cells producing anti-β 2-1 fructosan antibodies stimulated by NWSM were not detected until the donors were age 4

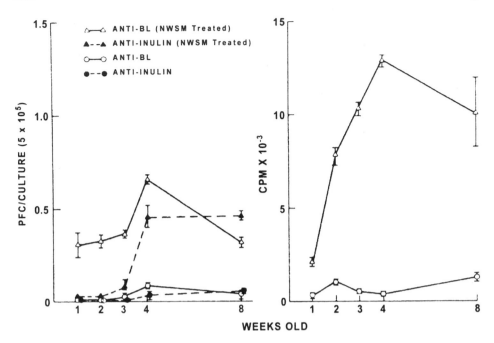

Fig. 33. Age dependence of PFC response and proliferation induced by NWSM. Left panel, anti-inulin and antilevan PFC response after 3 d of stimulation of splenic cells from Balb/c mice of various ages. Right panel, 3H-thymidine incorporation of spleen cells from Balb/c mice stimulated for 3 d with NWSM. (From Bona C, et al. J Immunol 1979;123:1484–1490.)

wk (Fig. 33). Second, we have shown that the ontogenic delay was not caused by the absence of environmental antigens because bacterial levan is produced by various bacterial species present in normal flora. In adoptive transfer experiments, it was shown that the infusion of B cells from 1-wk-old Balb/c mice into irradiated CAL.20 adult mice developed a response 7–14 d after the transfer, thereby corresponding to the time required for the maturation of the response in Balb/c mice (600). Third, the ontogenic delay of the antibody response correlates with a very low frequency ($1–2/10^6$ B cells) in the spleens of 3-wk-old mice. Taken together, these observations clearly demonstrated a significant ontogenic delay of the anti-inulin antibody response.

A longer delay was observed in the case of the anti-α-(1,6)-dextran antibody response. In Balb/c mice, the response induced by B512 dextran is characterized by a predominant idiotype-QUPC52. Howard and Hale reported that α-(1,6)-dextran-specific antibodies were observed particularly late. For example, at age 55 d, they represented only 10% of the amount of antibodies produced by 3-mo-old mice. This observation is supported by other observations in which the response for α-(1,6)-dextran was studied following immunization with B512 dextran and a six-sugar hapten, isomaltohexose, in which structure is homologous with the antigenic determinant of α-(1,6)-dextran. Immunization of mice at various ages from 1 d to 12 wk after birth showed that antidextran antibodies after immunization with B512 dextran or isomamaltohexose-KLH conjugate were not detected until the mice were 12 wk old.

The data reviewed in this chapter clearly demonstrate that there is a temporally ordered and sequential activation of the antigen-specific B-cell precursors during fetal development and postnatal life that appears to be antigen-independent. Several explanations can be put forth to support this concept.

First, the position-dependent rearrangement of the most proximal V_H and $V\lambda$ gene families during B-cell development restricts the fetal and neonatal repertoire. Although this possibility should be considered for lack of antibody responses during the first week after birth, it cannot explain entirely the late responses because the preferential expression of proximal V_H gene families after birth switch and normalize by d 7–14. In addition, this cannot explain the usage of V_K families, which does not follow the paradigm of position-dependent expression of V_H families, because in newborn mice the V_K families located in the center of the V_K locus are highly expressed.

Second, the delayed ontogenic response can not be the result of induction of tolerance because the precursors of B cells activated late after birth were detected in fetal livers and in neonatal spleens by very sensitive methods such as splenic focus assay. In addition, adoptive transfer experiments of cells from newborns into irradiated adult mice showed, in the case of inulin-specific B cells, that they can respond to antigen stimulus only several weeks after transfer, a time corresponding to natural maturation in normal mice.

Third, the long ontogenic delay may be related to tolerization of immature B cells by environmental antigens. This explanation is not likely, because polysaccharide antigens that were present early in life did not induce tolerance except when they were administered in very high doses. Furthermore, this cannot explain the delayed response to haptens or to inulin, which are not naturally present in environment.

Fourth, the delayed response cannot be related to maternal antibodies, because the vast majority of antibodies specific for polysaccharides are IgM, which does not cross the placenta.

Finally, the most plausible explanation is that an "internal clock" genetically programs the sequential acquisition of the neonatal repertoire by mechanisms that are not yet understood.

It is of importance that these mechanisms be elucidated in the future, because it would help to produce better vaccines for newborns and young children.

6
Antibody Responses in Fetuses and Newborns

1. INTRODUCTION

The paradigm of neonatal unresponsiveness resulting from the immaturity of the neonatal immune system and the high susceptibility to tolerance of newborn lymphocytes was derived from an experiment carried out in mice. This experiment showed that newborn mice injected with high numbers of allogeneic hematopoietic cells failed to reject the allograft (607).

This paradigm was challenged by findings generated from comparative immunology studies demonstrating substantial differences among mammalian species regarding the maturation of the immune system during fetal and postnatal life.

In the case of the antibody response, mature B cells were identified in the fetal liver during the last trimester of gestation and in the spleen and cord blood after birth in some mammalian species such as rabbits, lambs, swine, cattle, monkeys, and humans.

Accurate experimental and/or clinical studies demonstrated that in these species, both fetuses and neonates were able to mount responses induced by foreign antigens.

2. THE FETAL ANTIBODY RESPONSE IN MAMMALIAN SPECIES

The demonstration of induction of an antibody response after fetal immunization was determined in species in which the transfer of maternal antigens is impeded by placental structure. Simple surgical procedures permitted direct immunization of the fetus or injection of antigens into the amniotic fluid.

Because these maneuvers are not feasible or ethically acceptable in humans, the measurement of IgM and IgE antibodies, which do not cross the placenta, is used to ascertain the fetal origin of antibodies in newborns from infected mothers.

2.1. Antibody Responses in Fetal Lambs

The fetal lamb frequently has been used as a model to study early development of the immune response because the immune system reaches immuno-

From: *Contemporary Immunology: Neonatal Immunity*
By: Constantin Bona © Humana Press Inc., Totowa, NJ

competence in the last trimester of gestation. The immune responses induced in fetal lambs after *in utero* immunization can be considered authentic primary immune responses because of the syndesmochondrial placentation structure that prevents transplacental transfer of immunoglobulins from ewe to lamb. In fetal lambs, immunization can be carried out either by direct injection of antigen into fetal muscle *(574,608)* or following administration of antigen into the amniotic fluid. It was shown that the latter route of immunization was particularly efficient for genetic immunization and the induction of mucosal immunity *(609)*

In utero immunization of fetal lambs by intramuscular injection as early as 66–70 d into the 150-d of gestation period showed that the fetus is able to synthesize large amounts of antibodies. The highest titers of antibodies were obtained following immunization with bacteriophages, and slightly weaker responses were observed after immunization with ferritin and ovalbumin. The magnitude of the antibody response was not significantly different in fetuses injected between d 70 and 120 of gestation. It is noteworthy that in this study no antibody response was elicited after *in utero* immunization of fetuses with *diphtheria toxoid, Salmonella thyphosa,* or Bacillus Calmette-Guèrin (BCG) *(574)*. In another study, Fahey and Morris showed that the antibody response against various T-cell-dependent and -independent antigens could be induced at various stages of gestation *(608)*. Thus, antibodies specific for ferritin were detected at d 64; against chicken red blood cells, polymerized flagellin, and ovalbumin at d 72–76; against monomeric flagellin and dinitrophenyl (DNP)-conjugate at d 78; and against chicken γ-globulin at d 82 of gestation. After 90 d of gestation, animals responded to all antigens tested, with the exception of the somatic antigen of *S. thyphosa*. Interestingly, the lack of antibody response induced by fetal immunization with the somatic antigen of *S. thyphosa* was observed in experiments carried out independently by two groups of investigators *(574,608)*.

Fetal immunization by oral genetic immunization of fetal lambs was studied using two model systems: (a) plasmids containing genes encoding hepatitis B surface antigen (HBsAg), or (b) a truncated form of glycoprotein D of bovine herpes virus-1 (BHV-1)—(gP) *(608,609)*.

Oral immunization using DNA that encodes the BHV-1 gP protein injected once into the amniotic fluid induced detectable amounts of gP-specific antibodies in 80% of newborn lambs. It is important to note that this type of immunization induced not only systemic immunity but also mucosal immunity as assessed by viral shedding in newborn lambs challenged with BHV-l. More importantly, this immunization method induced memory B cells, because a strong anamnestic response was evident in 3-mo-old lambs challenged with BHV-1 *(610)*. Similar results were obtained with HBsAg. In this model, the efficacy of intra-amniotic immunization with a plasmid encoding HBsAg was compared to immunization with a recombinant purified HB surface protein.

Whereas all lambs immunized at d 123 of gestation with plasmid demonstrated protective antibodies, by comparison, 55-d-old lambs immunized with recombinant protein exhibited only a low titer of specific antibody *(610)*.

A possible explanation for the efficient induction of mucosal immunity by oral vaccination with naked DNA might be related to reduced turnover of intestinal epithelial cells during gestation, which could allow for longer persistence of the plasmid. The induction of mucosal immunity by fetal or oral administration is an important observation relevant to vaccination against enterotropic viruses or viruses causing infection of the respiratory tract.

2.2. Antibody Responses in Bovine Fetuses Infected With Leptospira

The ability of bovine fetuses to produce antibody was studied by injection of an attenuated *Leptospira* strain into the placentome (composed of maternal caruncle and fetal cotyledon) of 8- to 9-mo-pregnant cows (gestation period: 280 d). In this experiment, dams inoculated at 110 or 134 d of pregnancy aborted their fetuses. However, fetuses of dams inoculated between d 134 and 168 of pregnancy survived. Fetuses, which survived the acute phase of infection, displayed agglutinating antibodies against *Leptospira saxkoebing*. In addition, plasma cells were found in fetuses examined 41 d after infection *(611)*. Because in the bovine, antibodies are not transmitted from mother to fetus, this observation suggests that infection of the fetus in the late stage of gestation may elicit a humoral antibody response.

2.3. In Utero Naked DNA Gene Transfer in Fetal Piglets Induces Protective Immune Responses at Birth

B-cell lymphopoiesis during fetal development of piglets occurs in the bone marrow at d 45 of gestation when in-frame V[D]J rearrangements reach 70% *(612)*. Similar to ovines and bovines, maternal immunoglobulins are not transferred to the fetus via the placenta. Fazio et al. recently showed that a single intramuscular injection of a plasmid encoding HBsAg led to the production of protective antibodies in 50% of 1-wk-old newborns and in 90% of 21-d-old piglets *(613)*. This result suggests that naked DNA can be transferred from mother to fetus and is capable of stimulating B cells to produce antibodies in the last trimester of pregnancy.

2.4. Antibody Responses Induced by Fetal Immunization of Baboons

Baboons exhibit close similarity to humans with respect to maternal–fetal interactions and, like humans, only IgG antibodies are transferred via the placenta. Watts et al. have shown that intramuscular injection of fetuses at d 90, 120, and 150 of gestation with Recombivax HBsAg induced the production of protective antibodies in the fetuses but not in the pregnant mother *(614)*. The antibody response was maintained after birth up to age 40 mo. This response was significantly increased after virus challenge during neonatal life. This observation clearly demonstrated that fetal immunization primed B cells that were considerably expanded by neonatal challenge.

Experiments on fetal immunization with antigens or naked DNA in some mammalian species, including nonhuman primates, demonstrate three major findings. First, there are considerable differences among mammalian species regarding the maturation of B cells during gestation. In species that exhibit early maturation of the B-cell lineage, a fetal antibody response can be easily induced by injection of the antigen into the fetus or by oral immunization. Second, the early exposure to antigen during fetal life does not induce tolerance in the species mentioned above. Finally, these data may open new avenues for the improvement of vaccination in the case of vertically transmitted infectious diseases.

2.5. Antibody Responses in Human Fetuses Following Vertical Transmission of Infectious Agents

Vertically transmitted pathogens such as HIV, herpes virus, hepatitis B virus, *Treponema pallidum*, *Hemophilus sp. Chlamydia*, *plasmodium*, and *toxoplasma* are major causes of neonatal morbidity and mortality. However, the immune response in human fetuses after parenteral intrafetal immunization or infections with bacteria or viruses can not be studied because of ethical constraints. Currently, the presence of IgM or IgE antibodies in cord blood or serum is used to assess fetal immune responses in humans. In humans, neither IgM nor IgE cross the placenta.

The initial study suggesting a fetal immune response in humans was derived from the cytological analysis of spleens from fetuses with congenital syphilis or toxoplasmosis. The results of this study suggested that human fetuses are immunologically competent, showing precocious development of lymphoid organs and massive plasmocytosis *(615)*. The plasma cell represents the terminal differentiation endpoint of antigen-stimulated B cells. It should be mentioned that production of antibodies also was demonstrated in experimental models of congenital syphilis in rabbits and guinea pigs. In these experiments, it was shown that asymptomatic congenitally infected guinea pigs display, at the first day after birth, high levels of antitreponemal IgM *(616)*. Similarly, a humoral response was noted in congenital syphilis in rabbits infected with the Nicholas strain of *T. pallidum (617,618)*. Anti-rubella, *toxoplasma*, and cytomegalovirus (CMV)-specific IgM were found in babies born to mothers infected with these infectious agents.

Mumps virus infection of pregnant women may induce virus-specific antibodies and memory cells in the fetuses. This initially was shown in a study of 12 Eskimo children exposed to mumps virus during gestation. Exposure of the fetus to mumps virus evoked an immune response that persisted into childhood, as assessed by induction of an anamnestic response *(619)*. This study is relevant because infection with mumps virus in the Eskimos population is very rare.

Acquired immune responses to the *Plasmodium falciparum* merozoite surface protein-1 (MSP-1) antigen were described in infants born in an area of stable malaria transmission in Kenya *(620)*. The sensitization of fetuses results from the accumulation of infected red blood cells at the interface between maternal and fetal circulation, resulting in the adherence and sequestration of infected red blood cells in the placenta *(621)*. The induction of a fetal immune response in congenital malaria may result either from the subsequent exposure of the fetus to the malaria parasite or to soluble malaria antigens.

IgM specific for the MSP-1-derived peptide MSP$^{11-19}$, a vaccine candidate, was detected in the cord blood of 5.8% of newborns with congenital malaria. In addition, anti-MSP-1 IgM and IgG were identified in the culture medium of cord blood lymphocytes from 78% of newborns incubated with MSP-1-derived peptide. It is noteworthy that no antibodies specific for liver surface antigen LSA-1, an antigen expressed on the pre-erythrocyte hepatic form of malaria, were detected in these children. The results clearly show that some infants born in an area of coastal Kenya where malaria transmission is stable were primed to MSP-1 *in utero*.

In utero sensitization of fetuses also was described in infants born to pregnant women with helmintic infections such as Schistosomiasis and filariasis *(622)*. The priming of fetuses with antigens derived from these parasites was demonstrated by the presence of IgE antibodies specific for Schistosome and filarial antigens in the sera of newborns, as well as in the culture supernatant from cord blood lymphocytes stimulated with pokeweed mitogen, which is a T-dependent polyclonal B-cell mitogen.

Transplacental immunization of fetuses also was described in the case of pregnant women immunized with tetanus toxoid *(623)* and meningococcal serotype A and C vaccines *(624)*.

The capacity of the human fetus to produce antibody also was nicely illustrated in a rare case of *in utero* development of autoantibodies. This is the case of a few clinical observations of severe jaundice in newborns in which, during embryonic life, autoantibodies developed causing the hemolysis of red blood cells (RBCs) that was manifested by increased serum levels of bilirubin and reticulocytes, even without evidence of hemolysis *(625)*.

These results taken together strongly suggest that human fetuses, during the last trimester of gestation, have mature B cells that are capable of producing antibodies against antigens borne by infectious agents or that are transplacentally transmitted from mother to fetus. These findings may have practical implications leading to new ways of vaccination during pregnancy.

3. HUMORAL RESPONSES INDUCED IN NEWBORNS

The high degree of susceptibility to infection in newborns and protection against pathogens result from the presence of maternal antibodies. However, in addition to a protective effect, maternal antibodies may hamper responses early in ontogeny.

Previously, it was considered that the active immunization of newborns is affected by the immaturity of lymphocytes and, in the case of B cells, by defective or incomplete signaling following ligation of the BCR.

More recent data showed that newborn infants and animals are able to produce IgM and, in certain cases, IgG and IgA upon antigen exposure. Thus, the view of low competence or immune incompetence of newborns has gradually changed, in spite of the fact that the antibody response may be low. Antibody responses can be induced in neonates in certain conditions where there are notable differences among mammalian species with respect to maturity of the immune system during ontogeny.

3.1. Antibody Responses Induced in Newborn Mice

The ability of newborn mice to mount an antibody response depends on the type of antigen used. The response to T-dependent antigens requires the presentation of peptides derived from the processing of antigens by antigen-presenting cells (APCs), cognitive recognition of the major histocompatibility complex (MHC)-peptide complex by T cells, recognition of the antigen by B cells, and collaboration between T and B cells. The antibody response induced by T-independent antigens TI-1 and TI-2 does not require MHC-class-restricted presentation of antigen to T cells. However, the cytokines produced by T cells or APCs may influence the magnitude of the antibody response in neonates.

The antibody responses of newborn mice are genetically programmed with the sequential activation of clones specific for various antigens seen during postnatal life.

Howard and Hale were among the first to show that, in certain conditions, adult mice injected with small amounts of bacterial polysaccharides as newborns can mount an antibody response to that antigen *(604)*.

Antibody responses against some T-independent antigens such as galactan, levan, and lipopolysaccharide (LPS) can be induced after immunization of 1-d-old mice. However, the magnitude of neonatal antibody responses elicited by these antigens is 30–50% lower than the responses induced in adult mice *(586)* *(see* Table 22). Antibody responses specific for phosphoryl choline and T-dependent antigens such as phenyl arsenate and DNP and TNP conjugates, can be induced only in 5- to 9-d-old mice *(580–582,595)*. The unresponsiveness of neonates to TI-2 antigens can be restored by exogenous cytokine administration. Thus, Snapper et al. showed that highly purified neonatal B

Table 22
Effect of the Parenteral Administration of Anti-Idiotype Antibodies in 1-d-old Newborn Balb/c Mice

Amount of antibody given (μg)	Levan-specific PFC/spleen	%A48Id$^+$ PFC
Saline	3600±0.125 (3977)^a	6±3
0.01	3508± 0.123 (3218)	46±14
0.1	2855±0.218 (717)	65±17
1	2960± 0.127 (913)	73±20
10	2999±0.183 (997)	73±19

^{a}Mean ± SEM for $\log_{10}$ plaque-forming cell (PFC)/spleen, the geometric mean is in parentheses.
Five mice were studied for each group. Mice were immunized with bacterial levan at age 5 wk of age and the PFC response was measured 5 d after immunization.
Adapted from ref. *634*.

cells that are defective for IgM secretion, in response to stimulation by anti-Ig dextran conjugates, can synthesize IgM upon in vitro addition of CD40 ligand or polyclonal activators such as a recombinant protein-Osp or *E. coli* LPS *(626)*. Neonatal B cells, compared to adult B cells, show a relative enhancement in IgE and IgA synthesis. These results suggest that neonatal B cells are competent to synthesize Ig in response to TI-2 antigens if adequate stimuli are provided. Another report demonstrated that neonatal B cells are able to mount an adult-like antibody response to TNP-Ficoll, a TI-2 antigen, after the addition of interleukin (IL)-1 and/or IL-6. Anti-TNP antibodies that are secreted by neonatal B cells stimulated with TNP-Ficoll, IL-1, and IL-6 exhibit an avidity similar to antibodies produced by adult B cells *(627)*.

In vivo antibody responses specific for TNP-Ficoll *(590)* or type II pneumococcus *(628)* can be elicited only in 2- to 3-wk-old mice. However, the immunization of 1-d-old mice with these antigens must somehow prime the neonatal B cells, because stimulation with LPS or monophosphoryl Lipid A can overcome neonatal unresponsiveness and induce the differentiation of neonatal B cells into antibody-secreting cells *(629,630)*.

The antibody responses induced by the vast majority of proteins, with the exception of flagellin, are T-dependent and cannot be induced in newborns. However, immunization of animals with some proteins in the first weeks of postnatal life can elicit an antibody response. An antibody response against hen egg lysozyme (HEL) was elicited by the immunization of 7-d-old mice with HEL in FCA. These mice displayed 1013±303 HEL-specific PFC compared to 4717±2936 plaque-forming cells (PFCs) in adults. The expression of idiotypes of HEL antibodies (IdXE), which is characteristic of the adult response, also was present as early as age 10 d *(459)*. Protective antibody responses against influenza virus type A also were induced by immunization with purified hemagglutinin (HA) and neuraminidase (NA) coinjected with IL-12 on the first day after birth. The mice immunized simultaneously with soluble HA, NA, and IL-12 exhibited 100% survival after lethal challenge with infectious influenza virus compared to those immunized with the antigens alone. These mice produced higher levels of IgG1 and IgG2a antibodies. The higher protection observed in mice immunized with soluble antigens and IL-12 at birth was antibody-mediated, as demonstrated by the lack of a protective response in mice with B-cell deficiency resulting from a disrupted IgM gene *(631)*. In contrast, newborn mice immunized with the WSN strain of influenza virus exhibited a long-lasting unresponsiveness manifested by a very low concentration of anti-HA antibodies at 30 and 90 d before and after challenge with the virus *(632)*. These observations suggest that cytokines such as IL-12 exhibit an adjuvant effect on the response of neonates against influenza viral antigens.

The BCRs of neonatal B cells express idiotypes, which are the phenotypic markers of V genes that encoding the antigen specificity of the BCR as well as that of secreted antibodies.

Neonatal treatment with high amounts of anti-idiotypic antibodies induces the suppression of clones bearing corresponding idiotypes (reviewed in ref. *49*). However, neonatal treatment with minute amounts of idiotypic or anti-idiotypic antibodies can select and expand silent clones, which are not expressed during the immune response of adult mice.

Exposure of newborn mice to antibodies specific for Schisostoma soluble egg antigen (SEA) led to expression of IdX at age 9 wk. These mice produced significant SEA-specific IgG antibodies and showed prolonged survival after infection with *Schisostoma mansoni*. In the serum of mice injected with IdX anti-SEA antibodies as newborns, both idiotypes and anti-idiotypes were detected *(633)*. High levels of protective IdX antibody were explained by the induction of anti-idiotype antibodies bearing an internal image of the antigen, which led to expansion of the clones that shared similar idiotypes early in the neonatal life. This explanation is strongly supported by demonstration of the expansion of a silent clone following treatment with low doses of anti-idiotypic antibodies. In these experiments, 1-d-old mice were injected with various amounts of anti-A48 IdX antibodies. The A48 idiotype is expressed on the ABPC48 levan-binding myeloma protein but is not expressed on the antilevan antibody produced by adult mice. The data presented in Table 22 show that injection with 0.01–10 µg anti-A48IdX antibody after birth induced a strong antilevan PFC response and that 46–73% of B cells that produce antilevan antibodies displayed A48IdX. This response was levan-specific because the injection of 1-d-old mice with anti-M384 IdX antibodies that recognized an idiotype expressed on an LPS-binding myeloma protein did not induce an

Table 23
**Concentration of Anti-HA Antibodies Produced by Mice
Immunizedas Adult or Newborn With a Plasmid Containing WSN
Influenza Virus Hemagglutinin**

		Anti-HA antibodies	
Age of mice	Immunization	Before boost	7 d after boost
Newborn			
	Saline	<0.1[a] (30 d)	42±10
	WSN virus	0.1±0.1 (30 d)	2.2±0.3
	pC[b]	<0.1 (30 d)	48±12
	pHA[c]	0.5±0.18 (30 d)	55±17.5
	WSN virus	0.2±0.05 (90 d)	3.3±0.06
	pHA	2.0±1.2 (90 d)	30±27
Adult			
	Saline	<0.1	35.6±11.4
	WSN virus	33.6±11.4 (30 d)	273±21.6
	pC	0.2±0.3 (30 d)	51±28
	pHA	9.8±3.9 (30d)	118±58
	pHA	0.28±03 (90 d)	266±28.8

[a](μg anti-HA antibodies/mL; in parentheses the day of bleeding after completion of the immunization.
[b]Empty plasmid (control).
[c]Plasmid expressing WSN influenza virus hemagglutinin under the control of SV40 promoter.
Immunization was carried out as follows: i.p with 10 μg purified WSN virus; i.m. with 100 μg/mouse pC or pHA three times on d 1, 3, and 6 after births in the case of newborn mice and on d 0, 21, and 42 in the case of adult mice.
Adapted from ref. *632*.

A48IdX+ antilevan antibody response *(634)*. Similarly, injection of neonates with a monoclonal anti-idiotypic antibody specific for the idiotype of a myeloma protein induced protection against myeloma cell growth that lasted until adulthood *(635)*.

These observations indicate that anti-idiotypic antibodies can function as surrogate antigens and can stimulate the expansion and expression of clones bearing a BCR that expresses the corresponding idiotypes. Long-lasting responses into adulthood suggest the induction of memory cells.

3.2. Antibody Responses in Newborn Rabbits

In rabbits, immune competence develops gradually over the first weeks of postnatal life. However, splenic B cells from 1-d-old mice are strongly stimulated by antiallotype antibodies and are able to produce immunoglobulins upon in vitro stimulation with NWSM, a polyclonal B-cell mitogen *(273)*. The level of NWSM-induced synthesis of immunoglobulin by 1-d-old splenic B cells is 25% of that produced by 12-mo-old animals *(274)*. This result is in agreement with other observations that show anti-DNP IgG production within 12 h of birth. Isoelectric focusing analysis of anti-DNP antibodies obtained 8 d after immunization of neonatal rabbits with DNP-bovine gamma globulin (BGG) conjugates in saline, Freund's incomplete adjuvant (FIA), or FCA showed unique monoclonal or pauciclonal pattern differences in individual rabbits. This pattern was maintained for several weeks until a boost with antigen was performed that caused a more heterogeneous response *(636)*. These data indicate that newborn rabbits possess a large set of *V* genes that encode DNP-specific antibodies but that neonates differ from adults in their capacity to express a complete genetic repertoire for antibody diversity.

3.3. Antibody Response Development in Newborn Piglets

The immune responses of newborn piglets differ from other species, because piglets receive no maternal antibodies, and, therefore, at birth they are free from maternal protective factors. Butler et al. carried out interesting studies aimed at testing whether precosial newborn piglets can respond to a T-dependent (TD) antigen, such as FL-KLH, or a TI-2 antigen, such as TNP-Ficoll *(637)*. The results of this study suggest that bacterial colonization of the gastrointestinal tract results in a substantial increase of follicles in Peyer's patches and is associated with an increase of antibodies specific for the two antigens studied. The amount of antibodies generated depended on the nature of the colonizing bacteria.

Colonized piglets immunized at d 3 with FL-KLH exhibited a modest primary response by d 10, which was considerably increased 1 wk after challenge. No increase in anti-TNP antibodies was noted after booster immunization with TNP-Ficoll at age 4 wk *(637)*. The antibody response observed only after bacterial colonization of piglets is probably because of production of costimulatory molecules by macrophages and dendritic cells; by ligation of Toll-like receptors such as TollR2 and TollR4 by LPS, lipoprotein, and peptidoglycan; or by ligation of TollR9 by bacterial DNA that is rich in CpG motifs.

3.4. Infant B-Cell Responses

At birth, human newborns have a full repertoire of antigen-specific B cells in the bone marrow. However, the maturation of B-cell responses occurs gradually during the first years of life. The human newborn is able to produce IgM and even IgG and IgA at low concentrations. In vitro polyclonal activation of neonatal B cells with *Staphylococcus aureus* Cowan I or Epstein–Barr virus induces the synthesis of small amounts of IgM. Stimulation with pokeweed mitrogen (PKM) induces the production of IgM but not IgG, in spite of the fact that PKM is a T-dependent polyclonal activator *(638)*. In contrast to B cells from adults, peripheral blood lymphocytes (PBL) from cord blood did not differentiate into antibody forming cells upon culturing with type 4 pneumococcal polysaccharide *(639)*.

Because of ethical considerations, there is no information in human newborns and infants on antibody responses induced by immunization with foreign antigens, except the responses elicited by vaccines. This information will be presented and analyzed in Chapter 12.

4. ANTIBODY RESPONSE OF NEONATES ELICITED BY SOMATIC TRANSGENE IMMUNIZATION WITH PLASMIDS

Genetic immunization represents a new and appealing approach to induce antibody responses in newborns and infants. It based on two important findings: (a) the demonstration that a reporter gene (β-galactosidase) engineered into a plasmid is transcribed and translated in tissues at the site of injection *(640)*, and (b) injection of mice with a plasmid containing the *bovine growth factor hormone* gene resulted in the production of antihormone antibody *(641)*.

We first demonstrated that, in contrast to the inability of an inactivated influenza vaccine to induce a cytotoxic T lymphocyte (CTL) response in neonates, immunization of 1-d-old mice with a plasmid containing the influenza virus nucleoprotein (NP) gene (bearing epitopes recognized by T cells in association with MHC class I molecules) generated CTL activity comparable to that of adult mice injected with the same dose of plasmid. The cytotoxic activity was related to an expansion of CTL precursors as assessed by measuring pCTL frequency 1 mo after immunization *(642)*.

Our pioneering study stirred interest in the use of genetic immunization for the induction of humoral immune responses in newborns. Thus, it was shown that the immunization of mice after birth with a plasmid that encodes the full-length rabies virus glycoprotein (gP) under control of the SV40 promoter developed higher antibody responses compared to mice immunized with the empty plasmid. The majority of anti-gP antibodies were of the IgG2a isotype, indicating the participation of T cells known to be required for Ig class switching *(643)*. Induction of antibody responses in newborn mice induced by genetic immunization with a plasmid containing *influenza virus HA gene (pHA)* also was demonstrated.

Antibodies against HA and NA have been shown to confer protection against influenza virus. Anti-HA antibodies prevent the HA-mediated binding of the virus to the sialoprotein receptor of host cells and subsequent fusion of the virion with the plasma membrane. Meanwhile, anti-NA antibodies inhibit the enzymatic activity of NA, thereby preventing the cell-to-cell spread of virus.

HA-specific neutralizing antibodies are thought to play the major role in immunity to influenza virus. The induction of the HA-specific antibody response was studied in newborn Balb/c mice injected with an empty plasmid (pC) or with a plasmid containing the HA of influenza virus WSN strain (pHA). The antibody response was assessed by measuring the hemagglutination inhibition (HI) titer and by radioimmunoassay (RIA).

The majority of adult mice immunized with pHA displayed high HI titers at 1 and 3 mo after immunization and no detectable antibodies after 9 mo, corresponding to clearance of the plasmid from the site of injection.

In the case of mice immunized with pHA as newborns, high HI titers were observed in 75% of mice at 1 and 3 mo after immunization. Newborn mice immunized with pC and then challenged with WSN virus showed titers comparable to adult primary responses, whereas mice immunized with pHA exhibited titers characteristic of a secondary response (Table 23). These results demonstrated that, in contrast to adult mice immunized with WSN or with pHA that developed vigorous primary and secondary responses, mice immunized as neonates failed to mount an anti-HA antibody response after challenge with WSN virus. Strikingly, neonates immunized with pHA developed a weak primary response but exhibited a strong secondary response subsequent to challenge with virus *(644)*.

These findings suggest that the immunization of neonates with pHA primed the B cells and induced B-cell memory. This concept was supported by two additional groups of findings: (a) the isotype pattern of the secondary response of mice that were immunized as neonates and adults was quite similar and was characterized by the predominance of IgG2a and IgA antibodies, with the exception of an increased concentration of IgG1 anti-HA antibodies in mice that were immunized as neonates with pHA; and (b) the percentage of survival of mice immunized with pHA as neonates or adults and challenged with a lethal dose of live virus was similar *(644)*.

Analysis of the reactivity pattern of HA-specific clonotypes for six different strains of influenza (H1N1) that were obtained by spleen focus assay from mice immunized as neonates or adults with WSN virus or pHA showed very interesting results.

The immunization of adults with virus or pHA increased the frequency of B-cell clonotypes with a broad reactivity pattern. In sharp contrast, whereas the immunization of neonates with live virus induced a long-lasting unresponsiveness and the few clones stimulated in vitro produced only antibody specific for WSN, immunization with pHA led to the occurrence of clonotypes displaying an adult-like pattern of reactivity *(632,644)*.

The most striking observation comes from studies of neonatal DNA immunization and consists of an early shift of the neonatal repertoire toward the adult repertoire, as assessed by a broader reactivity pattern of B-cell clonotypes.

This is surprising, because it is known that the restricted neonatal B-cell repertoire results from position-dependent utilization of the J-proximal V_H gene family, exhibits shorter CDR3 length, lacks N-region diversity, and has a low rate of somatic mutation compared to adults. This may be related to increased receptor editing or revision. An antibody response was induced in newborn mice immunized with plasmids containing measles virus HA, Sendai virus NP, and tetanus toxoid C fragment *(645)*.

Monteil et al. have studied IgG-specific antibody responses following immunization of 1-d-old piglets with a plasmid containing the gP gene of pseudorabies virus followed by boosting on day 42 *(646)*. After the boost, the piglets developed medium levels of IgD-specific antibodies that exhibited virus-neutralizing activity in vitro. Furthermore, they developed an anamnestic response after challenge at day 115. However, in spite of the fact that the animals produced antibodies, no protection was observed after challenge. This may be related to the low expression of gP protein after intramuscular injection of plasmid.

Successful humoral responses were elicited by genetic immunization of newborn nonhuman primates. Thus, in chimpanzees immunized at birth with a plasmid containing the hepatitis B surface antigen, a transient increase of antibody titer was observed between d 12 and 20 after immunization. An increase in antibody titer, which was long lasting, was observed after challenge at 33 wk with 100 CID_{50} of Hepatitis B virus (HBV) *(647)*. From this study, it was concluded that DNA-based genetic immunization was able to induce a protective anti-HBV response in newborn chimpanzees. Significant levels of antibodies also were detected in chimpanzees immunized after birth with a plasmid containing the HIV gag/pol genes. Antibody responses were evident as early as 4 wk after intramuscular and intravaginal delivery of plasmid. It is noteworthy that the serum titers of antibodies in infant animals were comparable to the serum level of antibodies of adult animals immunized with the same construct *(648)*.

Similar results were obtained after neonatal immunization of baboons with a plasmid that encoded the type A influenza virus HA. HA-specific antibodies were detected by ELISA at 28 d after immunization, and by both ELISA and HI at 2 and 3 mo after immunization. It is important to note that the immunization of newborn baboons with 50μg UV-inactivated virus did not elicit antibody production *(649)*. The induction of memory cells was demonstrated by challenge of 18-mo-old baboons immunized with virus as neonates , resulting in an increased titer of IgG1 anti-HA antibodies. This finding demonstrated that genetic immunization of newborn baboons triggered long-lasting immune memory that persisted beyond infancy *(650)*.

These findings question the paradigm of neonatal tolerance because of the immaturity of B cells, which are more susceptible to antigen deletion or anergy.

Several factors may explain neonatal immune responsiveness to genetic immunization. First, transfected cells secrete small amounts of antigen. It is well known that the induction of peripheral tolerance in neonates requires large amounts of antigen ("high-dose tolerance") and that central tolerance (deletion) requires the recognition by B cells of antigen expressed at the surface of somatic cells, including the antigen-presenting cells. Second, genetic immunization results in the long persistence of antigen. This ensures the priming of newly emerging cells from the bone marrow and eventually the generation of memory cells, as illustrated by good anamnestic responses after challenge. Finally, neonatal immune responses may result from the intrinsic adjuvant activity of plasmids that are rich in CpG motifs. The binding of CpG-rich DNA to TollR9 may trigger signaling pathways, thereby circumventing the limiting number and immaturity of B cells. This also can increase the synthesis of GM-CSF, IL-12, and interferon types I and II, which have an adjuvant effect, and enhance the reactivity and maturation of B cells in neonates (reviewed in ref. *651*).

7

Effect of Maternal Antibodies on Neonatal B-Cell Response

1. INTRODUCTION

Mammalian embryos usually develop in a sterile environment because the placenta is impermeable to most macromolecules that are present in maternal blood. However, immunoglobulins (Igs), in particular the IgG fractions, are exceptional, because they can be transferred from mother to fetus through the placenta. After birth, IgGs along with secretory IgA (sIgA) and lactoferrin can be transferred to the nursing infant through breast milk.

Maternal antibodies transferred through these routes have three major effects on the neonatal immune system. First, they confer a naturally acquired passive immunity. This effect is beneficial during the earliest periods of life when, because of incomplete ontogenetic expression of certain B-cell clones, the immune system is not completely mature and antigen specificities are not completely developed. These maternal antibodies confer protection against those viruses and bacteria that previously had infected the mothers. Circumstantial evidence, such as the devastating effects of the mumps virus infection in an Eskimo population that was previously naïve to mumps, strongly supports the importance of maternal antibodies in the prevention of some infections. If the level of maternal transmitted antibodies decreases before the child's immune system is able to produce sufficient amounts of protective antibodies, then the susceptibility of such infants to infections will increase.

A second important effect of maternal antibodies is their ability to interfere with vaccinations aimed at inducing an immune response in infants. In animals, maternal antibodies were found to completely abrogate humoral responses, and in humans, maternal antibodies were shown to inhibit the induction of responses to both live vaccines, such as those for measles and poliomyelitis *(652,653)*, and inactivated vaccines, such as those for pertussis *(654)*, diphtheria, and tetanus toxoid *(655–657)*. These inhibitory effects of maternal antibodies result from formation of immune complexes between antibodies and

From: *Contemporary Immunology: Neonatal Immunity*
By: Constantin Bona © Humana Press Inc., Totowa, NJ

vaccine that are rapidly cleared from circulation by the reticuloendothelial system. The antigen in the immune complexes is degraded, and the B-cell-specific epitopes can no longer be recognized by B cells. However, the degradation of antigen in professional antigen-presenting cells (APCs) may generate peptides that can activate T cells. This explains how maternal antibodies can inhibit neonatal humoral responses without blocking T-cell-mediated responses.

Finally, maternal antibodies can exhibit a regulatory effect on the development of the B-cell lineage through either longlasting suppression or priming of B cells. In the following sections, these three major functions of maternal antibodies are more thoroughly described.

2. TRANSFER OF MATERNAL ANTIBODIES TO FETUS AND NEWBORN

Maternal antibodies are transferred through the placenta and milk to the fetus and the newborn infant. There are important differences among mammalian species in how such transfer occurs. In humans, guinea pigs, rabbits, and rodents, the maternal IgG are transferred to fetus through the placenta; meanwhile IgA and smaller amounts of IgG and IgM are transferred through colostrum and milk.

In humans, IgG1, IgG3, and IgG4 are transferred more efficiently than the IgG2 subclass. These transfers are active processes mediated by Fc receptors (FcRs) located on fetal syncytiotrophoblast cells, which bind to Fc fragments of IgG. Those FcRs that mediate placental transfer are called neonatal FcRs (FcRns) and are heterodimers composed of an α-chain homologous with HLA class I molecules that are associated with β2-microglobulin *(658)*. The FcRn recognizes isoleucine at position 253 and histidine at positions 310 and 435 at the interface of the CH2 and CH3 domains of the Fc fragment of IgG *(659)*. The FcRn binds IgG with relatively high affinity at an acidic pH but with low affinity at a neutral pH. This property is important in the mechanism of transcytosis of IgG from mother to fetus. Maternal IgG is taken up by the trophoblast through fluid-phase pinocytosis. Pinocytotic vacuoles move toward apical vesicles, which have an acidic pH that favors the binding of IgG to the FcRn. Because each IgG molecule binds to two FcRns, the vesicles contain dimers (IgG FcRn2). The vesicles then fuse with the basal membrane of the syncytiotrophoblast and are exposed to a neutral pH, which causes the dissociation of IgG from the FcRn, allowing IgG to enter the fetal circulation *(658)*. In the human fetus, the placental transfer of IgG becomes evident around the 24th wk of gestation and increases exponentially during the second half of pregnancy. At birth, the fetal blood level of IgG (15 g/dL) tends to exceed that in the mother (13 g/dL) *(660)*. After birth, maternal antibodies are transferred in colostrum and later in milk. The major subclass of milk Ig is represented by sIgA, whereas IgM and IgG are present in minute amounts. In adults, the majority of sIgAs are synthesized in the gut- and bronchus-associated lymphoid tissue systems. Thus, maternal antibodies transferred through milk protect against the pathogens found in gut flora such as *Escherichia coli, vibrio cholerae, Shigella, Camphylobacter*, and eventually against some parasites such as *Giardia*.

Milk sIgA is relatively resistant to enzymatic degradation, particularly during the colostrum feeding period when the gastrointestinal protease enzymatic system is not well developed. In human colostrum, IgA is the dominant subclass and sIgA represents over 90% of all the Ig that is present. In human milk, the level of sIgA is around 11 g/L, varying between 6 and 40 g/L, whereas the concentration of IgG is around 0.4 g/L and that of IgM is 0.3 g/L. In milk, the content of IgA decreases drastically to 0.5 g/L. The mechanistic details of sIgA transfer are poorly understood.

In addition to Ig, maternal lymphocytes can be transferred to newborn mice through milk. This was clearly demonstrated in a study using B-cell deficient mice. When foster-nursed on normal mothers, the B-cell deficient pups showed a partial reconstitution of the B-cell compartment in the spleen and bone marrow *(661)*.

In other mammalian species such as ruminants (e.g. cows, horses, sheep, and goats), maternal antibodies are not transferred via the placenta, and the offspring are born virtually without antibodies. In these species, the maternal antibodies are provided in the colostrum. Cows secrete colostrum for the first 7 d after delivery. Over 90% of colostral Ig are IgG, and the major subclass is IgG1. Similarly to humans, in pigs and horses, the transition from colostrum to milk-feeding of newborns is associated with a shift from IgG to sIgA.

Although IgG1 and IgG2 are present in equal concentration in ruminant blood, only the IgG1 subclass is transported from blood through mammary tissue to colostrum. IgG1 is transferred via alveolar epithelial cells. In sheep, this process is augmented 2–3 wk before parturition.

Apparently, the FcRn mediates the transfer of IgG1. The transcript of the α-chain of the FcRn was detected in the acinar and ductal epithelial cells of the mammary gland before parturition and for 1 to 5 d postpartum, corresponding to the time of secretion of colostrum *(662)*. The expression of a FcRn chain correlates with expression of the β2-microglobulin gene in rats *(663,664)*. These findings suggest that in ruminants, IgG1 may bind to the FcRn at the basal side of acinar epithelial cells and then is transferred to the luminal side for secretion into the colostrum and later into milk.

In newborns, the IgG from the ingested colostrum is transported across the intestinal wall and enters circulation. FcRns are expressed at high levels in intestinal epithelial cells of suckling mice, and this receptor is completely lost at the time of weaning *(665)*. It probably plays a role in the transport of IgG during the first 24 h after birth. For example, in newborn lambs the FcRn is expressed by intestinal crypt cells that contain IgG1 at their apical surfaces *(662)*. This observation suggests that in ruminants, the FcRn expressed on epithelial cells selectively binds IgG1 and transports it into the intestinal lumen. In other mammalian species, such as dogs, cats, and rats, the maternal antibodies are transferred through both the placenta and milk. In milk of these species, IgG is a major component of colostrum, whereas sIgA is a minor component.

3. THE EFFECT OF MATERNAL ANTIBODIES ON B-CELL DEVELOPMENT

The generation of mice with a targeted mutation of the μ gene provided an excellent tool to investigate the effect of maternal IgG on development of the B-cell lineage. Such studies were carried out on homozygous $\mu MT/\mu MT$ mice produced by mating of heterozygous $\mu MT/+$ females to $\mu MT/\mu MT$ or $\mu MT/+$ males. The F1 progeny originated from either Ig^+ or Ig^- mothers. As expected, F1 progeny born to Ig^+ mothers had detectable amounts of IgG until 42 d after birth, with a linear decay from d 21 to 25 corresponding to the 7-d half-life of IgG. These mice contained two- to threefold more bone marrow pre-B cells and B cells than did pups born of Ig^- mothers. F1 mice born of Ig^+ mothers also displayed a decreased number of IgM-producing plasma cells and lower serum levels of IgM *(666)*.

These observations suggest that maternal IgG has two different quantitative and qualitative effects on the development of B-cell lineage in newborns. First, there is an increased generation of pre-B cells (and subsequent mature B cells). Second, there is a decreased number of IgM-producing plasma cells, with lowered circulation of IgM. Because maternal IgG stimulates the expansion of pre-B cells that are devoid of a B-cell receptor (BCR), it appears that the IgG effect may result from interaction with the VpreB/λ5 protein complex. Maternal IgG does not affect the V_H gene family usage and has no effect on CDR3 diversity *(667)*, indicating that maternal IgG does not influence B-cell repertoire development of the offspring.

4. PROTECTIVE CAPACITY OF MATERNAL ANTIBODIES

Numerous experimental findings in animals and clinical observations in humans demonstrate clearly that the maternal antibodies provide protection against infectious agents after birth. This concept is best exemplified by the enhancement of natural passive immunity subsequent to maternal immunization against pathogens that cause life-threatening diseases during the first months of life. Indeed, immunization during pregnancy confers protection for women of childbearing age as well as their offspring. The protective capacity of maternal antibodies requires persistent high antibody titers, which may be transferred to the fetus through the placenta or to the newborn and infant through the colostrum or milk. Although maternal IgG and IgA antibodies that are elicited by T-dependent antigens protect newborns and infants, maternal IgM antibodies that are elicited by microbial polysaccharide T-independent antigens are not protective. IgM antibodies are not transferred through the placenta because the syncytiotrophoblast lacks an IgM receptor that could mediate transcytosis, and the IgM antibodies transferred in milk have a very short half-life of 1–2 d. This explains the high incidence of otitis, meningitis, and pulmonary infections in human infants caused by bacteria such as *Streptococcus pneumoniae*, *Neisseria meningitis*, or *Hemophilus influenzae*.

The protection conferred by maternal antibodies depends on their persistence in the fetus, newborn, and infant. Figure 34 shows the effect of transplacentally transmitted maternal antibodies on fetal survival subsequent to vertical transmission of infectious agents and the protection and/or attenuation of systemic and gut infection by antibodies transmitted to newborns or infants through milk. Thus, maternal immunological experience and memory is essential for the survival of vertebrate species during the early periods of life, when the immune system of the offspring is not completely developed and is unable to generate the T cells required for the production of long-lived neutralizing antibodies and protective responses.

Passive immunity acquired either transplacentally or through milk has been demonstrated in various animal models. For example, administration to pregnant mice of a rabbit antibody to Sip recombinant protein of group B streptococci or immunization with the purified Sip protein itself protected the newborns against a lethal challenge with group B streptococci. Detectable levels of Sip-specific antibodies were present 64 d after challenge in the sera of offspring born to dams that were immunized with recombinant Sip protein. This finding suggests that maternal antibodies generated after vaccination crossed the placenta and persisted long enough in the infant sera to confer protection *(668)*.

This result is important, because it suggests that maternal immunization may represent a method of prevention against infections caused by group B streptococci. These bacteria are the most frequent cause of fulminating sepsis and meningitis in the first 2 mo of life and of chorioamnionitis and urinary tract infections in pregnant women. There are also several observations demonstrating maternal antibody-mediated protection against viral infections. For example, the immunization of dams with rotavirus serotypes protected suckling mice against diarrhea caused by challenge with homotypic or heterotypic rotaviruses. The protection correlated with the titer of antibodies, which was elevated 15- to 80-fold by immunization of dams with virus and Freund's complete adjuvant (FCA) *(669)*.

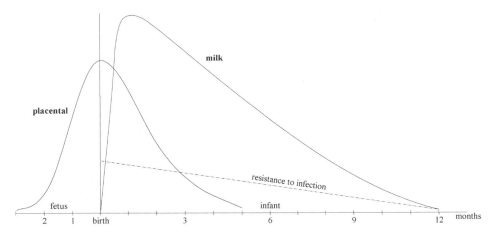

Fig. 34. Relationship between maternal antibodies transferred via the placenta or milk and the protection of offspring.

The infection of newborn mice with influenza virus is associated with severe morbidity manifested by pneumonia and high mortality occurring 2–8 d after infection. In mice, as in other species, antihemagglutinin (HA) antibodies that inhibit hemagglutination are protective. Protective anti-HA antibodies are transferred from mother to newborn mice by breastfeeding *(670)*. In mice born to dams immunized with influenza virus, these antibodies inhibit viral shedding from the nasal mucosa, block desquamation of the tracheal epithelium, and prevent development of pneumonia after challenge with virus.

Ferrets also are highly susceptible to influenza virus infection. Newborn ferrets infected with influenza virus die from severe obstruction of the airways and pneumonia. However, newborn ferrets were protected against infection with influenza virus by colostral- and milk-derived antibodies after suckling on mothers that had been immunized with either killed influenza virus vaccine *(671–673)* or a live vaccinia-influenza virus HA recombinant *(674)*. On the other hand, ferrets born to mothers immunized with vaccinia-influenza virus neuraminidase, polymerase, matrix protein, nucleoprotein, or nonstructural proteins were completely susceptible to viral infection, which means that only anti-HA antibodies are protective against lethal infections in newborn ferrets.

In mammalian species lacking transplacental transfer of antibodies, colostrum antibodies protect the newborn against microbial pathogens. In the case of newborn calves and pigs, the transfer of maternal antibodies via the colostrum within 12 to 24 h after birth is essential to survival. In these species, hyperimmunization of dams has proved to be efficient in protecting the newborns. For example, neonatal calves were protected against *Cryptosporidium parvum* by colostrum antibodies *(675)*; vaccination of pregnant sows protected newborn pigs against ETEC K88-induced diarrhea *(676)*; and vaccination of mares with inactivated rotavirus vaccine protected horse foals against rotavirus-associated diarrhea *(677)*.

There is a large body of evidence that immunization during pregnancy also provides protection to human newborns and infants. For example, vaccination of pregnant women with tetanus toxoid elicits IgG-specific antibodies, which cross the placenta and were detected at high concentrations in infant cord blood *(678)*. These antibodies protect both the neonates against tetanus neonatorum and the mothers against puerperal tetanus *(679)*. The role of colostrum antibodies in the protection of newborns and infants was clearly demonstrated in epidemiological studies, which showed that breast-fed infants had significantly less illness than bottle-fed babies during the first year of life *(680)*.

H. influenzae and *S. pneumoniae* are microbes that cause severe acute otitis, meningitis, and lower respiratory tract infections in early childhood. Maternal immunization with Hib vaccine protects children against these organisms because high amounts of antibodies are transferred across the placenta and—after birth—through the milk *(681)*. High titers of antibodies were found in infants delivered 2 wk or longer after maternal vaccination *(682)*. The incidence of *H. influenzae* in the throats of breast-fed babies is much lower than in bottle-fed infants. These observations explain why breast-fed children are protected against pneumonia during the first months of life.

The immunization of women in the third trimester of pregnancy with 23-polyvalent pneumococcal vaccine safely induces a modest increase of antibodies that could be transferred to the infant. Increased IgA-specific antibody concentrations in milk could significantly reduce serious infections during the first month of life. This was clearly shown in Papua, New Guinea, where maternal immunization reduced infant mortality caused by S. pneumoniae *(683)*. However, the acquisition of maternal antibodies does not reduce the overall frequency of carriers of bacterium.

Respiratory syncytial virus (RSV) causes serious respiratory disease in children and leads to serious morbidity in children with cystic fibrosis. Maternal antibodies may modify the severity of illnesses caused by RSV in the first month of life, especially in infants born to mothers with high levels of neutralizing anti-Fusion protein antibody *(684)*. Because 75% of infants with lower respiratory tract RSV infection are younger than age 5 mo, maternal immunization with a RSV vaccine may be more efficient than passive immunization with IgG anti-RSV antibodies.

Maternal antibodies may also protect against vertically transmitted infections. In the case of HIV, the rate of transmission from mother to child varies between 30 and 65%. Analysis of epitope specificity of maternal anti-HIV antibodies suggested that anti-gp120 and anti-gp41 antibodies correlated with the uninfected status of children born from seropositive mothers *(685,686)*. For example, in the case of gp120, antibodies specific for epitopes of the hypervariable loop of the PB1 region were exclusively found in the sera of mothers who gave birth to uninfected children *(685)*. It is well-known that the envelope glycoprotein gp120 plays a crucial role in the binding of virus to CD4 T cells and, therefore, in the mechanism of infectivity. The presence of maternal antibodies that are specific for epitopes of the hypervariable loop of gp120 in the sera of both HIV-infected mothers and their uninfected children suggests that such antibodies may block the spread of HIV from mother to fetus. Other maternal antibodies that were specific for a C-terminal epitope of gp41 protein also correlated with a lack of vertical transmission of HIV-1 *(686)*. The concentration of anti-HIV-1 maternal antibodies transferred to children showed an exponential decay. The half-life of passively transmitted anti-HIV-1 antibodies was 23.1 ± 4.2 d, with a median clearance of 13.3 mo *(687)*.

Cytomegalovirus (CMV) is the most common cause of congenital infection in humans, followed in some cases by permanent neurological sequelae. The infection of humans and other species with CMV can elicit neutralizing antibodies specific for viral glycoprotein B (gB). However, high levels of maternal anti-gB antibodies were found in infants with or without neurological sequelae; this indicates that the natural course of congenital infection is not modified by anti-CMV antibodies *(688)*. Also, in guinea pigs infected with guinea pig CMV (GPCMV), high titers of anti-gB antibodies developed, but these were unable to completely prevent maternal viremia, placental infection, and pregnancy loss *(689)*.

Taken together, the findings described in this section indicate that maternal immunization leading to transfer of antibodies from mother to fetus and newborn has a beneficial effect on the immune reaction against bacteria, viruses, and parasites during the first few months of life, when the immune system is not completely mature. The fundamental function of maternal antibodies is to prevent or attenuate infections and, based on the mother's immunological experience, represents a physiological, passive vaccination. The effect of maternal antibodies on vertically transmitted, congenital infections is variable, depending on the nature of the microbe and on the contribution of cellular immune responses to defense reactions. Figure 35 illustrates the protective effect of maternal antibodies on fetal and newborn defense reactions.

5. INFLUENCE OF MATERNAL ANTIBODIES ON THE IMMUNE RESPONSE INDUCED BY ACTIVE IMMUNIZATION OF NEWBORNS AND INFANTS

Although maternal antibodies play a crucial role by passively protecting newborns and infants against various microbes, the presence of maternal anti-

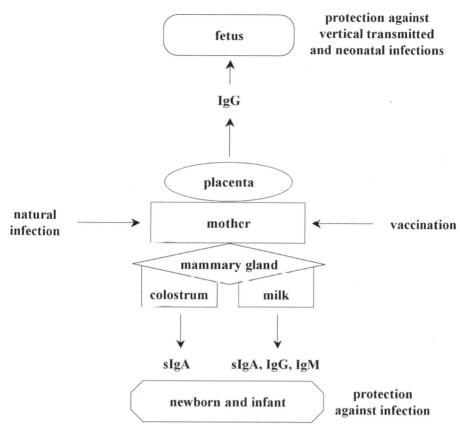

Fig. 35. Protective role of maternal antibodies transferred to fetus and newborn.

bodies may interfere with active immunization of infants by foreign antigens and vaccines *(690)*. The inhibitory effect of residual maternal antibodies at the time of immunization, coupled with their decline over time, may make infants more susceptible to bacterial, viral, or parasitic pathogens.

The inhibitory effect of maternal antibodies was initially related to prevention of the activation of B cells by antigens resulting from the formation of immune complexes, which are rapidly cleared and degraded by cells of the reticuloendothelial system *(691)*. This concept was supported by an experiment in adult rabbits that showed that passive administration of anti-Fab or anti-Fc antibodies 1 h and 7 d after injection of rabbit IgG had an immunosuppresive effect on antibodies specific for Fab and Fc determinants without affecting the response against unrelated antigens. These results also showed that the inhibition was at the level of antigenic determinants rather than the entire molecule *(692)*.

Table 24
Clonotype Reactivity Pattern Producing Anti-HA Antibody in Mice Immunized as Adults or Newborns With WSN Virus and a Plasmid Containing WSN Influenza Virus HA

Binding to influenza type A virus strains						Newborn			Adult Immunized with:			
WSN	PR8	CAM	WES	Den	BEL	WSN	pC	pHA	nil	WSN	pC	pHA
+						100[a]	70	47	76	64	55	40
	+						7.4				5	1.4
+	+							27	24	28	20	38
+		+										4.1
+			+					1.4				2
+		+	+					6.6			5	
+					+						10	
+	+							3.3				1.4
+	+	+										5.5
+	+		+		+		3.7	1.4		2.6		1.4
+	+	+	+	+			3.7					
+	+	+	+		+							
+	+	+	+	+	+			3.3		2.5		1.4
+	+	+	+	+	+		1.4					
+	+		+	+		14.8					5	1.4
+	+	+			+							
Frequency of HA-specific clonotype/10^6					0.13	0.34	0.3	0.15	0.32	0.16	0.9	

[a]Percentage of reacting clonotypes from the total number of clonotypes producing anti-HA antibodies.

Adapted from ref. 632.

Abbreviations: pC, control (empty) plasmid; pHA, plasmid containing HA gene of WSN strain; WSN, influenza virus strain WSN B2.

Table 25
Effect of Maternal Antibodies on Anti-HA Antibody Response, Virus Lung Titer, and Survival After Challenge of Offspring Born to Dams Immunized With WSN Virus or a Plasmid Containing Influenza Virus Hemagglutinin Gene (pHA)

Progeny from dams immunized with	Age at time of offspring immunization	HI[a] antibody titer Preimmunization	Challenge with 7 d after immunization	WSN virus Lung titer[b]	Survival
Saline	2 wk	<40	48±65	ND	ND
	3 mo	<40	213±92	3.7+/0.3	0/7
	3 mo[c]	60±20	613±384	ND	ND
pC[d]	2 wk	<40	356±229	ND	ND
	1 mo	<40	280±80	3.5±0.4	0/6
pHA	2 wk	106±41	53±20	1.6±2.0	8/9
	1 mo	<40	232±39	4.2±0.5	0/6
	3 mo	<40	1064±410	4.7±01	0/6
	6 mo	<40	3986±1943	4.9±0.4	0/7
UV-inactivated WSN virus	2 wk	864±453	618±76	0	5/5
	1 mo	340±129	100±40	1.8±0.1	0/7
	3 mo	<40	240+1-92	4.5±0.1	0/7
	6 mo	<40	845±536	4.3±0.4	0/7

[a]Hemagglutination titer expressed as mean ±SD of $\log_2$ dilution serum sample.
[c]This group of mice was immunized at age of 1 mo with UV-inactivated WSN virus.
[b]Data expressed as maen ± SD of $\log_{10}$ viral titer in $TCID_{50}$ units. Lungs were retrieved from each group at 7 d after infection with 3×10^7 $TCID_{50}$ WSN live virus, and virus titer was measured in standard MDCK assay.
[d]pC; empty, control plasmid
Adapted from ref. *708*.

The inhibitory effect of maternal antibodies was also observed in suckling mice. For example, the injection of IgG1 anti-hen egg lysozyme (HEL) monoclonal antibodies during the last days of pregnancy (–1 or –7) or 24 h after giving birth inhibited the HEL-specific antibody responses elicited by immunization with HEL that was emulsified in FCA in the offspring at ages varying from 2 d to adulthood *(693)*. The suppression of the anti-HEL response was not related to epitope specificity, dysregulation of the idiotype network, or Fc-mediated suppression. More likely, the suppressive effect in the offspring was related to a high interactive reaction with B-cell clones during sequential programmed development of the repertoire. Another example of the inhibitory effects of maternal antibodies on immune responsiveness was provided by an experiment carried out in 2-wk-old mice injected with serum from mothers that had been immunized with tetanus toxoid. Whereas immunization of control mice generated specific anti-tetanus toxoid antibodies, the immunization response of pups that had been previously injected with maternal antibodies was reduced, and the reduction was dependent on the titer of the maternal antibody *(694)*. Other studies showed low antibody responsiveness to immunization with rabies and Sendai viruses in offspring born to mothers that had been immunized against these pathogens (695). In this experiment, the failure to respond to viral immunization directly correlated to the amount of antibodies transferred from the mothers. This effect was longlasting, because offspring born to immunized mothers developed lower levels of antirabies antibodies even when challenged at age 6 mo, when maternal antibodies were no longer detectable.

These experimental findings demonstrate that the inhibition of the immune response to active immunization outlasts the period when maternal antibodies are present at protective concentrations in newborns or infants. An inhibitory effect of maternal antibodies was observed in 2-wk-old mice immunized with a fragment of the RSV-A G protein fused to an albumin-binding protein (694) or with acellular pertussis vaccine (696).

The effect of genetic immunization has been extensively investigated to determine whether it could circumvent the ability of maternal antibodies to inhibit active immunization of newborns. Experimental data indicate two reasons explaining why maternal antibodies fail to interfere with the genetic immunization of newborns. First, the persistence of plasmids as episomes in transfected cells may lead to a more rapid decline of maternal antibodies and the prolonged stimulation of newly emerging lymphocytes exported from bone marrow and the thymus. Second, the selective transfection in vivo of dendritic cells with plasmid (88–91) may facilitate the priming of lymphocytes, because dendritic cells are the most efficient APCs. There are several experimental reports indicating that maternal antibodies do not inhibit the humoral and cellular responses induced by genetic immunization.

For example, although newborn mice born to naïve mothers responded well to both inactivated herpes simplex virus (HSV)-1 vaccine and to a plasmid containing the full-length gB HSV-1 gene, newborn mice born to previously immune mothers only obtained effective immunity after immunization with the DNA complex (697). At 4 and 6 wk after immunization with gB DNA, mice born to HSV-immune mothers, when challenged with 10 LD_{50}, showed increased protection and exhibited increased blood levels of IgG1 and IgG2a. In addition, when lymphocytes from these mice were stimulated in vitro with HSV, these cells showed an increased production of interferon (IFN)-γ, interleukin (IL)-2, and IL-4 cytokines. Similarly, lambs that had high levels of antibodies acquired from mothers that had been immunized with bovine herpes virus gD responded to genetic immunization with gD DNA similarly to lambs born to naïve ewes (698). Also, when infant rhesus macaques were infused with measles-specific Ig and then immunized with a plasmid containing measles HA, fusion, and nucleoprotein genes, the animals developed a protective response after challenge at age 20 wk with pathogenic measles virus that had been grown in rhesus mononuclear blood cells. These infants exhibited high titers of neutralizing antibodies and reduced viremia, which generally correlates with the severity of measles and an increase in the number of cells producing Th1-type cytokines *(699)*. These findings are in agreement with those obtained in mice, which showed that the mice born to either naïve or measles-immunized mothers developed similar immune responses subsequent to immunization with a plasmid containing measles HA gene *(700)*.

In contrast, in mice experimentally infected with influenza virus, maternal antibodies inhibited the generation of protective anti-HA antibodies *(701,702)*. The data depicted in Table 25 show that the progeny from dams immunized with either the WSN virus or a plasmid containing the WSN *HA* gene, when challenged with UV-inactivated virus 2–4 wk after birth (when maternal antibodies were present in their serum), developed a poor anti-HA antibody response 7 d later. Two weeks after birth, offspring born to either WSN- or HA DNA-immunized mothers lacked neutralizing antibodies sufficient to protect them from a challenge with a LD_{100} dose of virus and to inhibit viral replication in the lung. However, maternal antibodies did not affect the induction of cell-mediated immune responses, in particular of CD8 cytotoxic T lymphocytes, after immunization with plasmids containing either influenza virus, the lymphocytic choriomeningitis virus *nucleoprotein* gene *(701,702)*, or the influenza virus *HA* gene *(703)*. These results strongly suggest that the genetic immunization of neonates may circumvent the inhibitory effect of maternal antibodies on humoral and cellular immune responses elicited by active immunization.

6. REGULATORY PROPERTIES OF MATERNAL ANTIBODIES

In addition to the ability of maternal antibodies to protect against infection and to inhibit active immunization in neonates, these antibodies can exert regulatory effects on the immune system. There is a little doubt that during fetal development of the immune system, the maternal antibodies interact with the BCR or T-cell receptor (TCR) of lymphocytes and that these interactions may be either suppressive or stimulatory.

6.1. Maternal Allotype Suppression

Allotypes are antigenic determinants of Igs and BCRs of B cells that are different in different groups of individuals or in inbred strains of the same species and are inherited in a Mendelian fashion. Allotype specificities were described in various mammalian species such as humans, rabbits, mice, rats, and birds within the IgG, IgM, and IgA subclasses. Allotypic specificities result from either a single or, at most, a few amino acid differences in the variable or constant regions of either the heavy or light chains of Igs *(704)*.

Dray first described allotype maternal suppression in 1962 in rabbits *(705)*. Newborn heterozygote rabbits, born to mothers that had been immunized against the males' *a* or *b* series allotype, failed to produce (or produced in an abnormally low proportion) B cells that expressed Igs containing the fathers' allotype. The suppression lasted for the entire life of the animal, and the suppressed offspring could not even produce antibodies subsequent to immunization with paternal allotype *(706)*. In the allotype-suppressed rabbits, there was an absence of B cells expressing the suppressed allotype on the BCR in peripheral blood and lymphoid tissues, including splenic lymph nodes and bone marrow. This was demonstrated by a lack of proliferation of B cells with antiallotype antibody *(707)* and a lack of binding of fluorescent- or isotope-labeled antiallotype antibodies in immunofluorescence or autoradiography *(708,709)*. This indicates that cells were either eliminated ("deleted") from the organs or that the synthesis of the paternally marked allotype was blocked ("anergy"). Our results favor the anergy mechanism, because we demonstrated that subsequent to in vitro stimulation with NWSM, a rabbit B-cell mitogen, the B cells from the spleen of an allotype-suppressed offspring were able to synthesize the paternally suppressed allotype *(710)*. The breaking down of longlasting allotype suppression by a polyclonal activator provides a strong argument for anergy rather than deletion as the mechanism that mediates allotype suppression. Maternal allotype suppression was also described in mice. In mice, naturally occurring T cells specific for the Ig allotype *(711)* mediate allotype suppression.

6.2. Maternal Idiotype Suppression

Idiotypes are phenotypic antigen markers of *V* genes that encode specific antibodies and, therefore, serve as clonal markers of BCRs expressed on those B cells that produce antibodies with single antigen specificity. Idiotypic determinants are expressed on the Fv fragment and, in particular, on the CDRs of either heavy or light chains; in rare cases, idiotypic determinants may be expressed on both chains. The Igs express either noninheritable, individual idiotypes that result from somatic mutations that occurred in a single clone, or there may be crossreactive idiotypes (IdX) expressed on all antibodies, with the same antigen specificity produced by all individuals of the same species and sometimes by individuals of different species (interspecies IdX). The IdX are markers of V germ line genes and are inherited in a Mendelian fashion. The expression of some IdX is allotype-linked.

The idiotype expressed on the BCR can bind anti-idiotype antibodies and can be recognized by T cells. Anti-idiotype antibodies produced by mothers and transferred to the fetus through the placenta and after birth during suckling may cause longlasting suppression of B cells that bear a BCR-expressing corresponding idiotype. This was demonstrated in several murine idiotype systems.

The T15 IdX is a clonal marker of antiphosphoryl choline (PC) antibodies. Maternal anti-T15 IdX antibodies transferred to offspring from Balb/c females that were immunized with T15 protein and mated with Balb/c males were unresponsive to immunization with PC when measured at ages 7 and 10 wk. At age 7 wk, the titer of anti-T15 IdX antibodies in the offspring was as high as that of adult mice immunized with T15 protein *(712)*. Clearly, maternal anti-IdX caused a longlasting suppression of B-cell clones expressing T15 IdX.

Anti-inulin antibodies express two major IdX forms: IdX G and IdX A. The expression of these forms of IdX is linked to an IgC_Ha allotype. CAL.20 females (congenic with Balb/c mice but carrying the VbH haplotype with C57Bl/6 mice) were immunized with an E109 myeloma protein bearing IdX G and IdX A and then mated to Balb/c mice. The offspring obtained were used at age 4 mo to study the anti-inulin plaque-forming cells (PFC) response and the expression of IdX G and IdX A. The data presented in Table 26 show complete suppression of the anti-inulin PFC response in offspring born to females immunized with E109 protein. However, offspring of mothers immunized with XRPC-24, a protein expressing the IdX of galactan-specific antibodies, showed no suppression of the anti-inulin PFC response. With respect to the expression of IdX, it was observed that whereas IdX G was completely suppressed, the expression of IdX A was not. Interestingly, the IdX A-bearing antibodies isolated from suppressed offspring were devoid of inulin-binding capacity. Isoelectrofocusing analysis of antibodies from suppressed offspring showed an absence of IgG binding to radiolabeled inulin–bovine serum albumin conjugate *(713)*. Interestingly, the inulin antibody response in Balb/c mice exhibits a substantial ontogenetic delay, and the inulin-specific B-cell precursors were detected several weeks after birth. This suggests that minute amounts of residual maternal antibodies, assuming that their half-life is about 1 wk, sufficed to induce the tolerance of inulin-specific B-cell precursors. Second, the dissociated suppression of the expression of IdX G and of IdX A antibodies that are devoid of inulin-binding specificity suggests that some B-cell clones expressing IdX A were actually stimulated by maternal antibodies. This explanation is supported by other studies that analyzed the effects of maternal anti-J558 IdX antibodies. J558 IdX is expressed on anti-α(1,3)-dextran antibodies. In one experiment, the anti-dextran antibody response elicited by immunization with dextran B1355 was studied in 112 offspring progeny. The progeny were generated from SJL females immunized with 3×10^7 Balb/c spleen cells expressing J558 IdX followed by a boost on day 18 of pregnancy with 1 mg of glutaraldehyde crosslinked J558 protein. Of 112 offspring tested, 111 were fully suppressed in their response to dextran B1355 up to age 12 wk, and half (56) failed to express J558 IdX by age 20 wk *(714)*. Similar results were obtained in offspring obtained from CAL.20 or A/J females that had been immunized with J558 protein and then mated with Balb/c males *(715)*. However, despite the fact that anti-α(1,3)-dextran was specifically inhibited *(see* Table 27), an impressive increase in the proportion of B

Table 26
Anti-Inulin Antibody Response and the Expression of IdX-G and IdX-A in 4-mo-old Maternal Idiotypically Suppressed C.B20x Balb/c F1 Mice

Mice	Anti-inulin PFC response per 10^6 spleen cells			Anti-inulin	Serum titer ($\log_2$)	
	Total	% IdX-G$^+$	% IdX-A$^+$	HA titer	IdX-G	IdX-A HI titer
C.B20xBalb/cF1	43±12	50	70	3±0	3±0.3	7.3±3
C.B20 anti E109xBalb/cF1[a]	0	ND	ND	0	0	5.8±0.4
C.B20 anti-XRPC24XBalb/cF1[b]	45±12	45	ND	3±1.1	3.5±0.7	6.8±1.8

[a]F1 born to dams immunized with inulin-binding E109 myeloma protein expressing IdX-G and IdX-A.
[b]F1 born to dams immunized with XRPC24 galactan-binding myeloma protein expressing X24 IdX.
All mice at age 4 mo were immunized with 10 μg bacterial levan, and antibody response was tested 5 d after immunization.
ND = not done.
Adapted from ref. 719.

Table 27
Anti-Dextran and TNP PFC Response and Frequency of B cells Expressing J558Id in 4-wk-old Maternally Suppressed CA1.20x Balb/c F1 (CAF1) Mice

Mice	Immunization	Dextran PFC	RIA(μg/mL) J558		% of B cells expressing J558	
			IdX	IdI	IdX	IdI
CAF1	Saline	0	<1	<1	ND	ND
CAF1	Dextran	2465±70	41±3	4±0.8	1.1	1.1
Suppressed CAF1	Dextran	9±1	<1	<1	1.9	4.0

Mice were immunized at age 12 wk with 100 μg dextran B1355, and the PFC response and the IdX+ antibodies were measured 7 d later. ND, not done.
Adapted from ref. *721*.

cells that bore the J558 Id was indicated by immunofluorescence staining. The staining was completely inhibited by preincubation of anti-idiotype antibody with J558 protein, and cocapping experiments showed comigration of J558$^+$ BCR with IgM and IgD. Some hybridomas obtained from these mice secreted J558 IdX-bearing antibodies that were devoid of dextran-binding activity *(715)*. These results resemble those obtained with maternal idiotype mice in the inulin system in which Igs expressing an IdX A that was devoid of inulin-binding activity were detected. Both observations strongly suggest that maternal anti-idiotype antibodies may display opposite effects: inhibition of antigen-specific clones that bear the corresponding dominant IdX and the activation of minor or silent clones producing antibodies that share the IdX but are devoid of antigen specificity.

7. TRANSFER OF MATERNAL IMMUNOLOGICAL EXPERIENCE TO THE OFFSPRING

The period of early development of B-cell clones is very sensitive to immunological imprinting by maternal antibodies. The development of the neonatal B- and T-cell repertoire may be considerably enhanced during this period. Animal experiments show that transfer of maternal anti-idiotype or idiotype antibodies resulted in a transgenerational priming effect, which guided the development of the neonatal primary repertoire. Thus, when female rabbits immunized with autoanti-idiotype antibodies specific for anti-*Micrococcus luteus* antibodies were crossed with naïve males, a significant proportion of offspring (40%) produced antibodies that were idiotypically crossreactive with maternal anti-*M. luteus* antibody. This finding clearly demonstrates that the maternal idiotype could strongly regulate development of the neonatal repertoire *(716)*.

Similar results were obtained in mice. In these experiments, female Balb/c mice were immunized with levan-binding UPC10 myeloma protein and then mated with naïve males. T cells from offspring were injected into irradiated Balb/c mice together with B cells from mice primed with TNP-Ova. Mice infused with T and B cells were immunized with Trinitrophenyl (TNP)-UPC10 conjugate, and the anti-TNP PFC response was measured 5 d later. In one set of experiments, T cells were treated with anti-CD4 or anti-CD8 antibodies and complement. The results of a PFC assay demonstrated that CD4$^+$ T cells from offspring born to mothers immunized with UPC10 mounted a significantly higher anti-TNP response after coinjection of B cells specific for TNP and immunization with TNP-UPC10 conjugate *(717)*. This result showed for the first time that maternal immunization with idiotypes might exhibit a regulatory effect not only directly on B-cell clones but also on neonatal T cells, which recognize idiopeptides and provide assistance to B cells. Similar findings showed that the activation of a silent levan-binding clone that expressed A48Id was activated

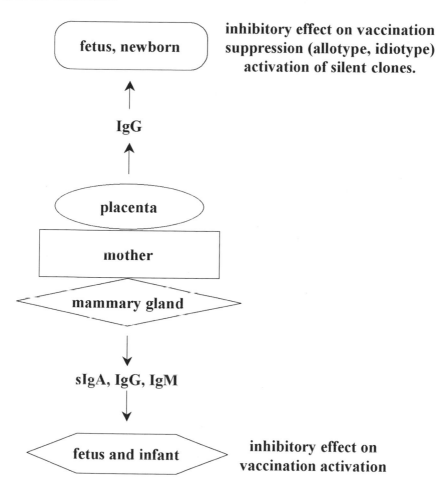

Fig. 36. Suppressive effect of maternal antibodies transferred to fetus and newborn.

subsequent to expansion of A48Id-specific CD4 T cells following injection after birth with idiotype *(718).*

Because maternal antibodies are mainly synthesized by B cells, which collaborate with T cells in response to T-dependent antigens, the development of the immune system reflects the entire immunological experience of the mother. Idiotype maternal experience is learned around the time of birth because idioype–anti-idiotype interactions, which contribute to selection of repertoire and have a long-term effect, appear to be limited to the fetal–neonatal stage of development. Learning of idiotype maternal experience by offspring is related to an exquisite property of idiotypic determinants, namely, their ability to be recognized by autologous T and B lymphocytes. Figure 36 illustrates the regulatory effect of maternal antibodies.

8. INHERITANCE OF MATERNAL IMMUNOLOGICAL EXPERIENCE

The maternal immunological experience transmitted to offspring through idiotype–anti-idiotype interaction is expected to be transient and to wane as the maternal antibodies disappear from the neonate. However, in the case of immunization with 2-phenyl-5 oxazolone (coupled with chicken serum albumin), maternal antibodies persisted in the offspring up to age 9 mo, depending on the level of titer of antibodies that were induced during a primary, secondary, or tertiary response. Interestingly, not only the F1 offspring but also F2 mice exhibited a prolonged increase of antioxazolone and anti-chicken albumin; 12 wk after challenge, they produced higher amounts of antibodies than those synthesized during a primary response. These findings suggest that maternal antibodies induced a state of memory that could be inherited, as illustrated by a faster and enhanced immune response in the F1 and F2 generations *(719)*.

Thus, in physiological terms, it is clearly an advantage for the offspring to learn and inherit the immunological experience of the mother, because this can result in the priming and expansion of precursors for a more vigorous defense reaction against the pathogens that prevail in a given species. This may explain the occurrence of epidemics in the human population after exposure to pathogens to which the previous generation had not been exposed. This is well-illustrated in the case of epidemics or pandemics that are caused by antigenic drift or a shift in type A influenza viruses.

Transmission of maternal experience to the offspring may represent a component of herd immunity that consists of equilibrium between susceptible and resistant individuals of a given species to infectious agents. Herd immunity depends on several factors, such as the natural genetic variation of the infectious agent, whether the infection was acute or persistent, the presence of animal reservoirs, and the level of immunity learned from maternal experience.

8

Neonatal Autoimmune Diseases Caused by Maternal Pathogenic Autoantibodies

1. INTRODUCTION

B cells exhibit the capacity to synthesize antibodies that are specific for both foreign and self-antigens. Active immunization with T-cell-dependent or -independent foreign antigens leads to production of antibodies with exquisite specificity for epitopes born by a large complement of foreign antigens. However, B cells can produce antibodies that display activity to self-antigens. Self-reactive antibodies are classified in three major categories:

   a. Natural, polyspecific autoantibodies. This subset constitutes a substantial fraction of the self-reactive repertoire. "Natural" serum antibodies are found in most species and are comprised of various Ig subclasses (IgM, IgG, IgA). They bind with moderate or low affinity to structurally dissimilar epitopes born by foreign and self-molecules *(720)*. In humans and mice, they are produced by CD5$^+$ B cells *(721)*, a subset that is enlarged in some animal strains prone to autoimmune disease *(722)*. Polyspecific autoantibodies can be found in increased concentrations in the blood of patients with autoimmune diseases, without induction of injury to normal tissue *(723)*.
   b. Autoantibodies with exquisite specificity for autoantigens. These autoantibodies exhibit high binding affinity to self-antigens and can be found at low levels in healthy humans and animals. Their concentration can be increased in some autoimmune diseases and may be used as a diagnostic criterion (e.g., antitopoisomerase I in scleroderma; anticentromere in calcinosis, Reynaud's phenomenon, esophageal motility disorders, *s* clerodactyly, and telangiectasia [CREST] syndrome; anti-transfer RNA (tRNA) synthetase or anti-Jo1 in polymyositis; and rheumatoid factor in rheumatoid arthritis). In certain conditions, autoantibodies can be pathogenic, as is the case of antithyroglobulin autoantibodies. Antithyroglobulin antibodies with similar epitope specificities are found in 50–70% of patients with autoimmune thyroiditis and 10–20% of normal subjects *(724,725)*.
   c. Pathogenic autoantibodies. These autoantibodies appear to facilitate the onset of autoimmune disease that causes injury to tissue bearing specific target autoantigens. Although they lack particular immunochemical properties, they exhibit distinct physiopathological properties. Production of pathogenic autoantibodies results either from breakdown of central or peripheral tolerance for self-

From: *Contemporary Immunology: Neonatal Immunity*
By: Constantin Bona © Humana Press Inc., Totowa, NJ

antigens or from immunization of mother with father antigens resulting from self-antigens displaying allelic polymorphism.

Based on tissue injury, the autoimmune diseases have been classified into two major categories: organ-specific and systemic. During the past few decades, intensive research aimed at understanding the effector mechanisms involved has led to further classification: autoimmune disease mediated by pathogenic T cells (such as multiple sclerosis, insulin-dependent diabetes mellitus [IDDM], uveitis, and Crohn's disease) and autoimmune disease mediated by pathogenic autoantibodies (such as myasthenia gravis, autoimmune thrombocytopenia, autoimmune hemolytic anemia, Graves' disease, and pemphigus).

Several criteria were proposed to define pathogenic autoantibodies to distinguish them from polyspecific antibodies or autoantibodies devoid of pathogenicity *(726–728)*. The most faithful criterion relies on the induction of damage and/or disease by passive transfer of autoantibodies. There are several examples of autoimmune diseases resulting from natural passive transfer of maternal pathogenic autoantibodies to a fetus from a mother afflicted by an autoimmune disease. Examples include transient myasthenia gravis, neonatal Graves' disease (a relatively rare condition resulting from transfer of maternal anti-thyroid-stimulating hormone receptor [TSHR] autoantibodies in normal or premature infants), neonatal lupus (caused by transfer of maternal anti-Ro and anti-La antibodies), and neonatal pemphigus (a rare condition related to transfer of antidesmoglin antibodies). Other neonatal autoimmune diseases are caused not by autoantibodies transferred from a mother affected by disease but by normal mothers that produce alloantibodies against the paternal antigen, as in the case of self-antigens displaying genetic polymorphism.

2. AUTOIMMUNE DISEASES CAUSED BY MATERNAL PATHOGENIC AUTOANTIBODIES

2.1. Neonatal Myasthenia Gravis

The neuromuscular transmission defect characterizing myasthenia gravis (MG) is mediated by autoantibodies specific for postsynaptic nicotinic AchR. The AchR is a pentameric glycoprotein composed of $\alpha2$-, β-, δ-, and α-chains in the adult and in $\alpha2$-, β-, γ-, and δ-chains in the fetus. Anti-AchR autoantibodies are produced by B cells lodged in peripheral lymph organs and in the thymus. The role of the thymus in the secretion of autoantibodies is well-documented by the presence in the medulla of a large number of B-cell clusters and germinal centers (GCs) that are indistinguishable from GCs found in the tonsils of healthy subjects. The majority of anti-AchR IgG autoantibodies in myasthenic patients are of high affinity and are produced by CD5$^-$ B cells.

Anti-AchR autoantibodies are directly pathogenic, because injecting AchR into normal mice, but not B-cell knockout mice, induces the production of autoantibodies that cause experimental diseases similar to human MG *(729)*. Similarly, the passive transplacental or milk maternal–fetus transfer of anti-AchR autoantibodies from a mother afflicted by disease can cause transient or chronic MG in a newborn or infant. Transient neonatal MG (NMG) occurs at high frequency (21%) in infants born to women with active disease and, less commonly, to women in disease remission *(730)*. In infants, disease correlates with the titer of antibodies specific for fetal rather than adult AchR receptor. Maternal anti-AchR is transferred mainly through the placenta during the second half of pregnancy and is found in both the serum and amniotic fluid of pregnant myasthenic women *(731)*. However, there is no explanation for antenatal myasthenic symptoms. Such disease suggests that maternal anti-AchR autoantibodies can be transferred through the milk. Brenner et al. *(732)* have studied the presence of autoantibodies in colostrum and milk. They found a high concentration of anti-AchR IgG autoantibodies in colostrum on d 1 and 4 postdelivery. This may explain the lack of antenatal symptoms and the occurrence of clinical disease in infants born to myasthenic mothers. Thus, breastfeeding may represent a source of maternal antibodies, which decay with time during postnatal life.

Study of the isotype of autoantibodies of seven mothers with myasthenia and their infants with NMG found anti-AchR IgG antibody in mothers and infants but no anti-AchR IgM antibody in infants *(733)*. This observation strongly suggests that disease is caused by maternal antibody transferred from the mother rather than those produced by the infant, because IgM is not transferred through the placenta.

The histopathological alterations of NMG have been studied by transferring maternal anti-AchR autoantibodies in rabbits. Ultrastructural observations of the intercostal muscles of rabbit neonates exhibiting an NMG-like syndrome showed degenerative alterations in the postsynaptic membrane. In addition, a morphometric analysis indicated the immaturity of postsynaptic membrane structures with underdeveloped secondary synaptic clefts *(734)*. Another rare yet dramatic neonatal disease produced by transfer of maternal antibodies manifests as arthrogryposis multiplex congenital syndrome, characterized by an irreversible contraction of muscles and neuropathies *(735)*.

2.2. Neonatal Liver Disease

Primary billiary cirrhosis (PBC) is an autoimmune disease, mainly of females, involving the liver and leading to cirrhosis and death from portal hypertension or liver failure. The hallmark of PBC is an antimitochondria antibody (anti-M2), which gives a characteristic immunofluorescence pattern in liver sections *(736)*. The autoantibodies are largely directed against the E2 subunit of the pyruvate dehyrogenase complex (PDC-E2) and tend to focus on the inner lipoyl domain, encompassing the lipoic acid attachment site at a specific lysine of the active site of E2 *(737)*. This autoimmune response may result from immunoregulatory defects. Direct evidence of an autoimmune origin for PBC is provided by the experimental transfer of autoantibodies or pathogenic T cells or by transplacental transfer of autoantibodies from mother to fetus. Hannam et al. *(738)* reported two cases of neonatal liver disease that were associated with transfer of maternal antimitochondria antibodies. Both children were born to a mother with high titers of antimitochodria antibodies, and both children presented clinical symptoms of cholestasis. The antimitochondria antibody in the children was of maternal origin because the IgG isotypes belonged mainly to IgG1 and IgG3 and exhibited identical epitope specificity. The pathogenesis of liver disease in the two infants remains speculative, because no finding provided direct evidence that antimitochondria antibodies caused their liver disease. However, the presence of perihepatocyte deposition of an IgG observed in liver biopsy is compatible with the idea that maternal antibodies mediated liver damage.

2.3. Fetal and Neonatal Thyroid Diseases

Transient neonatal thyroid diseases are relatively rare, occurring in 0.1–0.2% of pregnancies *(739)*. Such diseases result from transplacental transfer of maternal thyroid hormone receptor antibodies (TRAbs), which results in hyperthyroidism characteristic of Graves' disease, or from transfer of TSH-binding inhibiting antibodies (TBIAbs), which results in hypothyroidism *(740)*.

Graves' disease is a unique human autoimmune disorder characterized by diffuse goiter, with clinical and biochemical features of hyperthyroidism. In addition, 30 to 70% of cases exhibit ophthalmopathy. Graves' disease is mediated by autoantibodies specific for TSHR that stimulate cyclic adenosine monophosphate (cAMP) production, iodine uptake, increased synthesis of thyroglobulin and thyroid peroxidase, and increased growth and proliferation of thyroid cells. TSHR is a G protein-linked receptor comprised of two α- and β-subunits that uses cAMP and phosphoinositol pathways for signal transduction. Anti-TSHR autoantibodies are produced by B cells that accumulate within hypertrophied thyroid glands and can recognize both linear and conformational epitopes *(741)*. The pathogenicity of anti-TSHR autoantibodies was clearly demonstrated by human-to-human transfer of antibodies. Adams et al. *(742)* demonstrated thyroid stimulation in healthy subjects infused with serum from patients with Graves' disease.

Fetal and neonatal Graves' disease (NGD) observed in infants born to affected mothers results from transplacental transfer of antibodies that stimulate fetal thyroid cells. NGD is defined as the presence of tachycardia, goiter, hydrops, tremulousness, voracious appetite, ophthalmopathy, cardiomegaly and eventual congestive heart failure, and elevated thyroid hormone levels *(743)*. It can occur in successive offspring *(744)* and in infants born to mothers who have previously undergone near-total thyroidectomy resulting from Graves' disease. Appearance of NGD in infants born to mothers after surgical ablation of thyroid or radioiodine therapy is related to the persistence of TSHR antibodies in the mother *(745)*. Remission of NGD is most common by 20 wk and is nearly always seen by 48 wk after birth and correlates with the decay of the level of maternal antibodies. It is noteworthy that in some cases, NGD requires efficient therapy with antithyroid drugs, β-adrenergic receptor blocking agents, iodine, and, in some cases, glucocorticoids and digoxin *(746–748)*.

The induction of Grave's disease *in utero* is supported by clinical observations describing hyperthyroidism symptoms in premature infants born to mothers with poorly controlled disease. These patients demonstrated exophthalmos and marked goiter at birth and had maternal IgG anti-TSHR antibodies *(743,746)*. Fetal hyperthyroidism may be associated with intrauterine growth retardation, craniosynostosis, and intrauterine death *(747)*. The specificity of maternal autoantibodies that cause neonatal thyroid disease was studied by analyzing the specificity of monoclonal antibodies produced by hybridoma immortalized from mothers who gave birth to infants with NGD. Such monoclonal antibodies increased cAMP levels and iodine uptake in rat FRL-5 thyroid cells. Stimulating antibodies recognized a functional epitope on the *N*-terminus of the TSHR extracellular domain, requiring residues 90 to 165 for activity. In addition, blocking antibodies were produced that recognized three functional epitopes on TSHR *(749)*. Neonatal thyroidism with more persistent disease can result from a continuous production of anti-TSHR autoantibodies in patients with a mutation of the stimulatory G protein, as seen in McCune–Albright syndrome.

2.4. Neonatal Autoimmune Thrombocytopenia

Neonatal autoimmune thrombocytopenia (NAT) syndrome can occur in infants born to mothers affected by autoimmune thrombocytopenic purpura (AITP) through transplacental transfer of antithrombocyte antibodies or through subsequent allogenic immunization. AITP is an autoimmune disease characterized by persistent thrombocytopenia that results in bruising, purpura, and life-threatening bleeding. The pathogenicity of autoantibodies in AITP was demonstrated in a unique human-to-human transfer experiment. In this experiment, Harrington injected himself with plasma from a patient with idiopathic thrombocytopenia. Subsequent to injection, Harrington developed platelet depletion and a severe bleeding disorder *(750)*.

In AITP, the majority of autoantibodies are specific for various epitopes of integrin $\alpha_{IIb}\beta_3$ glycoprotein (GPIIbIIIa). A study of human monoclonal antibodies demonstrated binding to a peptide corresponding to amino acid residues 222–238 *(751)* and to a neoantigen of $\beta3$ *(752)*. In addition, it was found that 15–30% of antibodies from AITP patients bind to GPIb-IX, and 10–20% bind to GPV glycoproteins expressed on the surface of platelets *(753)*.

In NAT, fetal and newborn spleen cells may be the primary sites of platelet destruction. Macrophages bind to platelets covered with autoantibodies. This process is mediated by P-selectin (CD62P), which binds to the P-selectin glycoprotein ligand on macrophages. This interaction leads to upregulation of Fc receptors, mediating the phagocytosis of platelets. Studies in transgenic mice have implicated FcγRIIa in the immune destruction of platelets sensitized with antibodies.

NAT can also be caused by a maternal alloimmune response to fetal platelets. Five platelet glycoproteins exhibit polymorphism in Caucasian populations and are capable of eliciting maternal alloantibody responses that lead to NAT in the fetus and neonate. Thrombocytopenia results from antibodies specific for human platelet antigen (HPA)-1 in 78–89% of cases and for HPA-5b in 6–15% of cases.

A prospective study on more than 20,000 mothers and newborns found the incidence of NAT in newborns to be low (0.5%) *(754)*. The incidence of severe thrombocytopenia is 1 in 1100 infants. The number of asymptomatic cases of alloimmune NAT ranges from 10 to 25%; however, the long-term outcome in severe cases may be devastating. Intracerebral hemorrhage (7%) or resulting blindness, major physical disability, and neurological squeal (21%) manifest in severe cases. Cerebral hemorrhage occurs *in utero* usually between weeks 30 and 35 of gestation *(755)*.

2.5. Neonatal Pemphigus

Pemphigus is a group of heterogeneous autoimmune diseases characterized by blistering of skin mucous membranes and acantholysis resulting from epidermal cell–cell detachment. There are five major clinically distinct syndromes: pemphigus vulgaris (PV), pemphigus foliaceus (PF), pemphigus erythematosus, paraneoplastic pemphigus, and drug-induced pemphigus. PV and PF are autoimmune diseases caused by pathogenic autoantibodies. Autoantibodies target desmoglin-3 in the case of PV and desmoglin-1 in the case of PF. Both antigens belong to the cadherin family of calcium-dependent cell adhesion molecules.

It has been demonstrated that both antidesmoglin-1 and -3 autoantibodies are pathogenic. The following observations support the pathogenicity of autoantibodies:

a. PV autoantibodies are detected in the skin lesion *(756)*.
b. There is a good correlation between the titer of autoantibodies and the severity of the disease *(757)*.
c. Human IgG PV antibodies injected into newborn mice induce histopathological alterations similar to human disease *(758)*.

The concept of pathogenicity of PV antibodies also is supported by the existence of transient neonatal forms of pemphigus in infants born to mothers affected by PV or PF. In the case of neonatal PV, it was shown that skin involvement correlates with dermal histopathological alterations and the presence of autoantibodies detected by immunofluorescence staining *(759)*. Neonatal PF was described in two consecutive offspring born to a mother with classic PF lesions. High titers of IgG antidesmoglin-1 antibodies were detected in the serum of the mother and the cord blood of the newborns. The pathogenicity of the antibody in newborn cord blood was confirmed by induction of skin disease following antibody injection in newborn mice *(760)*. These observations demonstrate that neonatal pemphigus is caused by transplacental transfer of maternal antidesmoglin-1 and -3 autoantibodies.

2.6. Neonatal Lupus

Both human and animal models for systemic lupus erythematosus (SLE) are associated with autoantibodies that are specific for a multitude of antigens, such as ANA, single-stranded DNA, double-stranded DNA, Z-DNA, Ro, nRNP, Sm, Ku, La, P1/P2, laminin, human lymphocyte antigens (HLA) class I promoter-binding proteins, nucleolin, histones, and CD45 isoforms. Autoantibodies specific for these autoantigens also are associated with other autoimmune diseases (such as Sjogren's syndrome, mixed connective tissue disease [MCTD], rheumatoid arthritis [RA], and scleroderma) and may be found at low levels in healthy subjects. Among these, anti-Ro and anti-La autoantibodies fulfill the criteria of pathogenic autoantibodies, because they are responsible for neonatal lupus.

Neonatal lupus erythematosus (NLE) syndrome, first described by McCuistion and Schoch *(761)*, is a rare acquired autoimmune disease that is induced by maternal autoantibodies. It is characterized by cutaneous lupus lesions and congenital heart block (CHB) and, less commonly, by thrombocytopenia and cholestatic hepatitis *(762)*. The cutaneous lesions are annular erythematous plaques that develop 2–8 wk after birth. These skin alterations are transient and disappear by age 6 mo. Skin biopsy from lesions shows slight edema of the papillary dermis with dilated blood vessels, perivascular lymphocyte infiltration, and, in some cases, epidermal atrophy associated with lique-faction degeneration of the basal layer *(763)*. Maternal antibodies also target the heart *(764)*, leading to heart block syndrome. Heart block occurs in approx 50% of NLE infants, and despite early pacing, 10% of children die of heart failure during the first 12 mo *(765)*. With advances in fetal echocardiography, first and second degree heart block can be detected *in utero*.

NLE and cardiac injury observed in the fetus, which can progress postna-tally, result from maternal autoantibodies transferred to the fetus through the placenta. Therefore, NLE is not a spontaneous but an acquired disease result-ing from transfer of maternal autoantibodies. Four types of maternal autoanti-bodies have been implicated in the induction of NLE:

a. Anti-60-kd and anti-52-kd Ro/SSA—specific for 60-kd and 52-kd Ro/SSA zinc finger and RNA-binding proteins, both of which can interact with small cytoplas-mic RNA.
b. Anti-La/SSB antibodies—specific for a 48-kd protein that facilitates the matura-tion of RNA polymerase III transcripts and is required for 3'-endonucleolytic cleavage for tRNA maturation *(766)*.
c. Anti-α-fodrin antibodies—specific for human α-fodrin, a protein of 120 kd, rep-resenting an additional marker for the risk of NLE in anti-Ro/SSA-positive women *(767)*.
d. Anti-U1-RNP antibodies—present in NLE manifested with rash but without CHB *(768)*.

The appearance of anti-Ro and anti-La antibodies is more frequently associ-ated with Japanese women of the class II haplotypes DRB1*1101-DQA1*0501-DQB1*0301, DRB1*08032, and DQB1*0301. The mothers, who gave birth to NLE infants and exhibited both types of antibodies, were homozygous for DPB1*0501 *(769)*. This study suggested that major histocom-patibility complex class II association with NLE could vary depending on ma-ternal antibody profiles. Mothers with both anti-Ro and anti-La antibodies share many amino acids in the hypervariable regions of DRB1 and DQB1, which may bind the putative peptides that initiate or perpetuate autoantibody re-sponses. NLE caused by anti-Ro and anti-La autoantibodies can be associated with endocardial fibroelastosis. Collagen and elastin deposition, ventricular hypertrophy, and endocardial thickening characterize this condition. Endocar-dial fibroelastosis occurs in the presence of autoantibody-mediated CHB and has a very high mortality rate when developed pre- or postnatally *(770)*. The pathogenic role of maternal anti-Ro and anti-La autoantibodies in the induc-tion of CHB is supported by an interesting experiment showing that purified anti-Ro antibodies induce atrioventricular block in human fetal embryonic hearts and inhibit inward calcium flux through calcium channels in human fetal ventriculocytes *(771)*.

In vitro studies employing cardiac myocytes isolated from human fetal hearts provided evidence for a pathogenic link between autoantibodies and CHB and elucidated the mechanisms of injury caused by anti-Ro/anti-La autoantibodies. In apoptotic cardiocytes, the Ro and La antigens are translocated to the cardiocyte membrane, where they interact with maternal antibodies. Translocation of Ro and La antigens to the membrane is facilitated by apoptosis, as shown by inducing apoptosis with various agents in human fetal cardiocytes. In addition, apoptotic cells identified in fetal conducting tissue show redistribution of La antigen from the nucleus to the surface of apoptotic bodies and striking colocalization of human IgG with apoptotic cells in the atrium and atrioventricular (AV) node *(772)*.

Cells expressing surface La and Ro antigens become opsonized by maternal autoantibodies and are phagocytosed by activated macrophages, as illustrated by threefold increased expression of $\alpha_v\beta_3$ integrin and production of tumor necrosis factor (TNF)-α and transforming growth factor (TGF)-β cytokines *(773)*. TGF-β plays a crucial role in the fibrosis process. The supernatant of macrophages that are activated by incubation with apoptotic autoantibody-opsonized cardiocytes increases the proliferation of myofibroblasts, as assessed by the expression of α-smooth muscle actin. This effect was ablated by addition of anti-TGF-β antibodies. In addition, the activation of macrophages by apoptotic cardiocytes is associated with the phosphorylation and nuclear translocation of p44/p42 mitogen-activated protein kinase *(774)*. The involvement of activated macrophages is in agreement with cardiac alterations observed in a histopathological analysis of a biopsy from a 19-wk-old fetus with CHB. The alterations described consisted of dense lymphohistiocytic infiltrates and myocytic degeneration in the cardiac conduction system, including the AV node and bundle of His *(775)*.

These findings suggest that the apoptosis of fetal cardiocytes may lead to the expression of Ro and La antigens on the apoptotic blebs, which bind maternal antibodies, leading to phagocytosis by macrophages. This process activates macrophages that secrete cytokines, resulting in transdifferentiation of fibroblasts into proliferating myofibroblasts, as assessed by the presence of the myofibroblast marker α-smooth muscle actin in fetal cadiocytes. This process is associated with secretion of TGF-β, which in turn stimulates the growth of myofibroblasts. This leads to an entire spectrum of histopathological alterations consisting of the replacement of the AV node with fibrotic and fat tissue, the appearance of fibrous structures that contain crystalline structures in the conducting system, and the alteration of contractility of the myocardia secondary to myocardial fibroelastosis. Thus, these findings suggest that maternal anti-Ro and anti-La autoantibodies trigger an inflammatory cascade of events that results in major alterations of fibroblast function, ultimately leading to fibrosis of the conducting system, which is the histopathological signature of CHB.

2.7. Neonatal Autoimmune Neutropenia

Neonatal autoimmune neutropenia (NAN) related to antibody-mediated destruction of neutrophils has three major clinical entities:

a. NAN. This occurs in infants born to mothers affected with autoimmune neutropenia subsequent to maternal–fetus transfer of autoantibodies through the placenta.
b. Alloimmune neutropenia.This results from placental transfer of autoantibodies produced by women subsequent to immunization with alloneutrophil antigens obtained by blood transfusion or resulting from maternal–fetal incompatibility.
c. Autoimmune neutropenia of infancy. This is associated with parvovirus B19 infection and β-lactam antibiotics, probably related to crossreactive antibodies.

NAN is manifested with mild infection, predominantly of the skin and mucous membranes, that usually is caused by Gram-positive bacteria or otitis media. The diagnosis is based on the detection of neutropenia by laboratory tests such as granulocyte agglutination and granulocyte immunofluorescence. NAN should be distinguished from other infant diseases associated with neutropenia, such as infantile genetic agranulocytosis (Kostmann's syndrome), aplastic agranulocytosis, Lazy leukocyte syndrome, and myelokathexis. Infants with severe NAN respond well to hrG-CSF therapy. Life-threatening infections resulting in meningitis or pneumonia may occur in 5% of affected infants *(776)*. In addition to the direct cytotoxic effect on neutrophils, the autoantibodies may affect the metabolism of granulocytes, adhesion properties, the response to formyl chemotactic peptides, oxide radical production, phagocytosis, and cell motility (reviewed in ref. *776*).

Autoantibodies target human neutrophil antigen (HNA)-1a, -1b, -1c, Lan antigen, and SAR antigen located on FcγRII band; FcγRIIIb, HNA-4a, and HNA-5a located on β-integrin CD11b/CD18; and CR1, ND1, and NE1 antigens associated with the neutrophil membranes. All these antigens are polymorphic, explaining the alloimune responses. Antibodies bind and destroy mature neutrophils; this is reflected by increased numbers of metamyelocytes in the bone marrow. However, in some cases, the patients may display a maturation arrest at the myelocyte/metamyelocyte stage of differentiation. This may be related to a reduced frequency of $CD34^+/Kit^+$ $G\text{-}CSFR^+$ cells in patients with severe congenital neutropenia *(777)*. NAN was also reported in two premature twins, suggesting that the sensitization of neutrophils by autoantibodies can occur *in utero (778)*.

3. ALLOAUTOIMMUNE DISEASES

Hemolytic diseases of fetuses and newborns result from maternal antibodies specific for the parental blood group antigens that are transferred to the fetus through the placenta. The severity of this syndrome varies enormously and, in extreme cases, can lead to fetal or newborn death. The disease is generally associated with stillbirth, hydrops, jaundice, and kernicterus. It is caused by maternal alloantibodies against alloantigens inherited by the fetus from the father. These alloantibodies cause immune-mediated destruction of red blood cells or their progenitors. Alloantibodies occur because some blood group antigens exhibit genetic polymorphism. The likelihood of disease caused by each of the major human blood groups is as follows:

Anti-ABO	Usually mild disease
Anti-D (Rh), anti-KEL, and anti-Colton	Severe disease
Anti-Duffy and anti-Diego	Occasionally severe disease

4. EFFECT OF MATERNAL ANTIBODIES ON MURINE AUTOIMMUNE DISEASES

The study of pathogenesis of human autoimmune diseases is sometimes hampered by a lack of access to organs that are damaged by autoantibodies or pathogenic T cells. Animal models of autoimmune diseases facilitate the dissection of pathological events that lead to damage of organs. Recently, animal models of autoimmune diseases have been used to study the effect of maternal anutoantibodies.

Autoimmune ovarian disease (AOD) is the cause of premature ovarian failure *(779)*. In mice, this disease can be induced by a peptide of the zona pellucida 3 (ZP3) antigen corresponding to amino acid residues 330–342. This peptide contains a native B-cell epitope (amino acid residues 335–342) that overlaps with an epitope recognized by T cells (amino acid residues 330–342). This peptide elicits a strong antibody response to native ZP3 protein without concomitant T-cell activation. Setiady et al. *(780)* recently demonstrated that maternal autoantibody specific for a foreign peptide that mimics the ZP3 epitope induced AOD and premature ovarian failure when transferred to newborn mice 1–5 d after birth. In these animals, the autoantibody forms immune complexes with endogenous antigen and causes ovary inflammation and complete depletion of ovarian oocytes after 7–14 d. Apparently, the induction of AOD by maternal antibodies results from *de novo* induction of a pathogenic T-cell response mediating ovary inflammation. This concept is supported by the findings that (a) AOD did not occur in T-cell-deficient mice, and (b) CD4+ T cells from neonatal mice with AOD adaptively transferred ovary-specific inflammation to newborn mice *(780)*. Taken together, these results strongly suggest that maternal autoantibodies induce a T-cell-dependent autoimmunity that leads to neonatal AOD.

Juvenile IDDM is an autoimmune disease mediated by T cells. Nonobese diabetic (NOD) mice represent a murine model for human IDDM. IDDM in humans and NOD in mice are associated with islet-reactive autoantibodies, which have a predictive value for the predisposition and progression of disease. However, the pathogenicity of autoantibodies in diabetogenesis is extremely controversial. The role of maternal islet-specific autoantibodies was evaluated in newborn NOD mice born to B-cell-deficient NOD mothers and in progeny born to pseudopregnant mothers of a nondiabetic strain that were implanted with NOD embryos. The offspring from both animals were protected from spontaneous occurrence of IDDM *(781)*. These results highlight a potential pathogenic role for maternally transmitted autoantibodies in the development of IDDM and the eventual activation of diabetogenic T cells.

Maternal antibodies specific for the T-cell receptor (TCR) were studied in offspring born to mothers immunized with a chimeric TCR-IgG1 fusion protein. A TCR used for the construction of fusion protein was derived from a pancreatic islet-specific T-cell clone expressing a TCR encoded by Vα-2 and Vβ-8.2 genes. The immunization of SJL mice with this fusion protein induced the synthesis of TCR-specific antibodies, which specifically stained three T-cell lines expressing Vβ-8 family members. The SJLxAKR F1 born to SJL mothers that were immunized with fusion protein exhibited high titers of anti-TCR Vβ-8 antibodies, which persisted at least 3–4 wk in offspring. The 5- to 7-wk-old offspring lacked peripheral T cells stained with anti-Vβ-8.2 or anti-Vβ-8.3 antibodies, indicating that maternal anti-Vβ-8 antibodies depleted T cells that expressed a TCR encoded by Vβ-8 genes during the fetal and neonatal development of T cells. In the offspring, the recovery of T cells expressing Vβ-8.2 was surprisingly slow and occurred at age 28–30 wk. These results strongly suggest that maternal anti-Vβ-8 antibodies altered fetal and neonatal thymic maturation. This explanation is supported by findings that the T cells from offspring did not proliferate in vitro on exposure to the superantigen staphylococcal enterotoxin B, which selectively activates T cells using Vβ-3, -7, -8.1, -8.2, -8.3, and -17 gene segments; T cells also were not activated by pCA134-146 peptide, which specifically activates CD4 T cells using Vα-2 Vβ-8.2 pairs of TCR gene segments *(782)*. The information obtained from this interesting experimental study may provide new avenues for developing strategies to deplete autoreactive T cells that mediate autoimmune diseases such as IDDM, multiple sclerosis, uveitis, rheumatoid arthritis, and oophritis.

In summary, the findings reviewed in this chapter highlight the deleterious effects of some maternal antibodies. Maternal–fetal/newborn transfer of pathogenic autoantibodies can cause transient autoimmune diseases and, in some cases, severe clinical syndromes, which do not disappear after the decay of maternal antibodies. Some information presented in this chapter expands the information recently published in *Molecular Biology of B Cells* (T. Hondo, F.W. Alt, and M. Neuberger, eds., Elsevier Science, 2004).

9

Phenotypic Characteristics of Neonatal T Cells

1. INTRODUCTION

T cells act as the "chef d'orchestre" in the adaptive immune response. They cooperate with B cells in antibody production, are effectors of the antigen-specific cell-mediated immunity (CMI) response, and exhibit regulatory properties that modulate the function of antigen-presenting cells (APCs), B cells, and various subsets of T cells. By virtue of secretion of cytokines, T cells also modulate the function of nonlymphoid somatic cells.

T cells are divided into various subsets based on the structure of their receptor, the expression of cytodifferentiation antigens, and their functions. The defining marker of the T cell is the T-cell receptor (TCR).

Two distinct subsets of T cells have been characterized based on the structure of the TCR: TCR-α/β and TCR-γ/δ.

Based on cytodifferentiation antigens, T cells were classified into two subsets: CD4$^+$ and CD8$^+$. CD8$^+$ T cells are effectors of CMI responses. They are able to lyse autologous cells infected with microbes, allogeneic cells, or tumor cells. They recognize peptides derived from endogenous proteins bound to major histocompatibility complex (MHC) class I molecules. CD4$^+$ T cells recognize peptides derived from the processing of foreign or self-antigens. They recognize these peptides in association with MHC class II molecules.

The CD4$^+$ T cells have been divided into three subsets based on their functions: Th1 cells, which play a role in antimicrobial defense reactions and release cytokines with multiple pleiotropic properties; Th2 cells, which cooperate with B cells in the production of antibodies and secrete cytokines that exhibit various regulatory properties; and regulatory T cells. The regulatory T cells are divided in other minute subsets based on their pattern of cytokine expression or on the expression of cytodifferentiation antigens. Regulatory T cells producing mainly transforming growth factor (TGF)-β are called Th3; those producing mainly interleukin (IL)-10 are called Tr1; and those exerting their effect by contact with effector cells exhibit a defined phenotype: CD4$^+$ CD25^{high}. Table 28 illustrates phenotypic characteristics of subsets of CD4$^+$ T cells.

From: *Contemporary Immunology: Neonatal Immunity*
By: Constantin Bona © Humana Press Inc., Totowa, NJ

Table 28
Phenotypic Characteristics of Subsets of CD4 T Cells

Properties	Effector cells		Regulatory cells		
	Th1	Th2	Th3	Tr1	CD25^{high}
Cytokine production					
IL-2	+++	+	−	−	?
IL-3	++	+++	?	?	?
IL-4	−	+++	?	?	?
IL-5	−	+++	?	?	?
IL-6	+	+++	?	?	?
IL-10	+	+++	±	+++	?
IL-13	+	+++	?	?	?
IFN-γ	+++	−	?	?	?
TGF-β	+++	−	+++	±	?
Effect on B cells					
Activation of B cells	−	++	−	−	−
Class switching	IgG2a	IgG1, IgE	−	−	−
Autoimmunity					
Mediating autoimmune reaction	+	−	−	−	−
Preventing autoimmune reaction	−	++	+++	+++	+++

2. THE T-CELL ANTIGEN RECEPTOR: GENE REARRANGEMENT DURING THE ONTOGENY AND SIGNALING MECHANISMS

Like B cells, T cells are clonally distributed, because all the individuals of a clone share an identical TCR. The TCR is a heterodimer comprised of two chains (α and β or γ and δ), which are intimately associated with the CD3 complex. CD3 is comprised of five monomorphic polypeptides.

In humans, the TCR-α and -δ loci are localized on chromosome 14q11, the TCR-β locus on chromosome 7q35, and the TCR-γ locus on chromosome 7p15. The CD3 genes encoding γ, δ, and ε chains, which are structurally similar, are localized on chromosome11. CD3ζ 2 and CD3-ζ η are disulfide linked to CD3 and are important for signaling after the interaction of the TCR with MHC-peptide complex. The *TCR V* genes express clonotypic-idiotypic antigen markers, and some constant *TCR* genes express allotypic markers.

The TCR is encoded by three or four segments, which recombine during the development of T cells in the thymus. The organization of TCR-α and TCR(-γ genes is similar to that of genes encoding the immunoglobulin light chain, whereas the organization of TCR-β and TCR-δ genes is similar to that of genes encoding the heavy chain of immunoglobulin.

The TCR-α promoter located 5' to the V-α locus has two transcription sites: Pu, a purine-rich region, and GT, which is recognized by Sp transcription factors.

In humans, the TCR-α locus is composed of approx 50 V-α, more than 70 J-α gene segments, and one C-α. The enhancer is composed of four elements: (a) Tα1, which contains a DNA binding site for CRE;(b) Tα2, which contains sites for TCF-1 and Ets; (c) and Tα3, which contains sites for GATA, AP-2 and kE2 transcription factors. It is noteworthy that TCR V-δ locus is located between the TCR V-α and J-α loci. The transcription factors binding to Tα^4 are unknown.

The TCR V-γ locus is composed of 14 genes encoding variable chains (6 of which are pseudogenes) and two clusters of J-Cγ genes. The first cluster contains three Jγ1 and Cγ1 genes, and the second cluster contains two Jγ2 and one Cγ2 genes. The enhancer contains several segments: NFγ1, which binds GATA; NFγ2, which binds Ets; and NFγ3 and NFγ4, both of which bind CBF transcription factors.

The promoter of the TCR-β locus contains several potential binding sites for CP-1, Ap-1, poly designated as a polyoma virus enhancing element, two-conserved decamer, and one nonamer. In humans, there are about 60 V-β genes that can rearrange with one Dβ1, six J-β1, and one Cβ1 or with one Dβ2, seven Jβ2, and one Cβ2. V-β enhancer contains several regulatory regions.These include Tβ2, which binds GATA and Cre; Tβ3, which binds Ets; Tβ4, which binds CBF; and Tβ5, which can bind TCF/LEF-I transcription factors.

The TCR-δ locus is composed of three V genes encoding V-δ chains, which can recombine with three D-δ segments, three J-δ segments, and one C-δ segment. The enhancer of the TCR-δ/γ locus contains several segments that are able to bind transcription factors. Figure 37 illustrates the organization of human TCR loci.

The promoters of TCR-α and TCR-β loci are not lineage-specific and are active in various cells when coupled with various enhancers.

The rearrangement of various genes encoding TCRs follows the same rules as the rearrangement of gene segments encoding BCRs. This concept is supported by three groups of findings. First, the TCR-encoding genes have identical recombination signal sequences to those of V genes encoding the BCR. Second, TCR genes in embryonic conformation transfected into pre-B cells underwent rearrangements. Third, the immature T cells in the thymus express recombinant activating gene (RAG) enzymes. The rearrangement of genes encoding TCRs occurs in double-negative (DN) T cells in the thymus. RAG expression was found in immature CD4$^+$ CD8$^+$ CD3$^+$ T cells but not in the more mature single-positive (SP) thymic T cells. Thus, the coexpression of RAG1 and RAG2 in immature T cells in the cortical zone of the thymus mediates TCR rearrangement *(783)*. When productive rearrangement is achieved and the TCR-CD3 heterodimer is expressed on the surface, the expression of RAG may continue and allows for a secondary TCR-α recombination until the TCR is crosslinked during positive selection. RAG expression ceases in mature thymic T cells following TCR crosslinking and has never been detected in peripheral mature T cells in lymphoid organs.

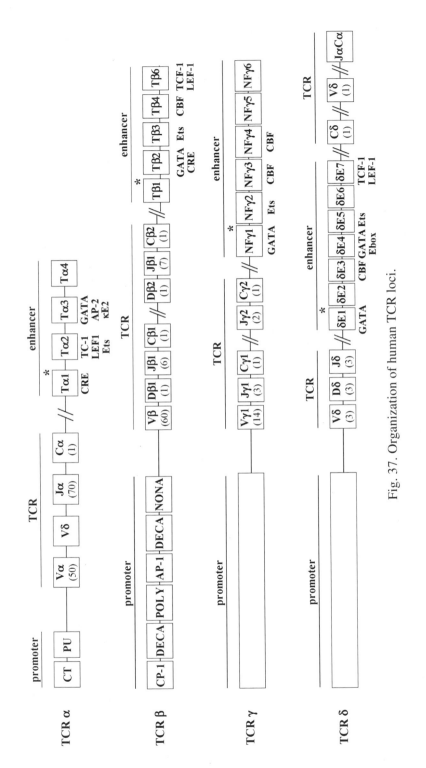

Fig. 37. Organization of human TCR loci.

In mice and humans, there is an order to the rearrangement of genes encoding TCR in the fetal thymus. In mice, the TCR-γ locus is transcriptionally active at d 14, reaches a peak at day 15, and rapidly decreases during gestation. The TCR-α and TCR-β loci are transcriptionally active by d 17 of gestation *(316)*. In humans, the TCR-δ locus is rearranged first, followed by TCR-γ, TCR-β and TCR-α loci *(336)*.

The expression of the TCR-CD3 complex is preceded by the expression of the pre-TCR complex in immature CD25$^+$ CD4$^-$ CD8$^-$ thymic cells. The pre-TCR was discovered in mice by von Bohemer and colleagues *(317)*. It is a heterodimer composed of pre-T-α, TCR-β, and CD3. The sequence of the pre-T-α gene revealed an opening reading frame of 618 nucleotides encoding a protein with a hydrophobic leader of 23 amino acids. The extracellular moiety consists of 130 residues, with two invariant cysteine residues that form interchain disulfide bonds like in Ig molecules. A third cysteine in position 119 could be used to form a disulfide bond between the pre-T-α and TCR-β chains. The extracellular domain has only 25% homology with TCR-α. The pre-T-α does not contain a J segment and ends at the Ig-like C domain. The intracytoplasmic region of 31 residues is proline-rich and contains an SH2 domain binding region and PPGHR motif also present in the tail of CD2, which is known to be involved in T-cell activation. The cytoplasmic tail of pre-T-α is longer than that of TCR-α and TCR-β chains. The pre-T-α–TCR-β complex is transported to the surface of immature T cells and is sufficient to promote T-cell development in the absence of other TCR chains. Intracellular signaling by the pre-TCR may be essential for the proliferation of immature thymic cells. During signaling via pre-TCR, the p56^{lck} may be recruited by the pre-T-α protein into the pre-TCR complex *(317)*. In humans, the pre-TCR complex is expressed in the CD4 immature SP stage of differentiation of thymocytes and is downregulated in immature double-positive (DP) T cells in which all loci are rearranged. CD4 immature SP thymic cells are defined as pre-T cells, which have lost the CD34 marker of hematopoietic stem cells (HSCs) and express CD1a, CD5, and CD4 but not CD8. The rearrangement of TCR loci is temporally coordinated with the expression of CD44, CD25, CD4, and CD8 antigens.

Engagement of the TCR by its natural ligand, the MHC-peptide complex, triggers impressive signaling machinery in T cells *(784,785)*. As the CD3-TCR complex lacks intrinsic enzymatic activity, its involvement in signal transduction is mediated by the interaction with nonreceptor protein tyrosine kinases (PTKs). The TCR recruits various signaling molecules by the conserved sequences on the cytoplasmic tails of the CD3-TCR complex, immunoreceptor tyrosine-based activating motifs (ITAMs) *(786–790)*. There are 10 tyrosine-containing ITAMs on the CD3-TCR complex (six from the ζ-homodimer, two from ε chains, and one each from γ and δ chains) *(791,792)*. Depending on the nature of TCR ligation, the tyrosine residues within the ITAMs can be differentially phosphorylated *(793)* and thus mediate the recruitment of particular signaling molecules, which in turn activate various biochemical cascades, leading to full T-cell activation, partial activation, or unresponsiveness *(794,795)*.

An early event following TCR ligation is the autophosphorylation of CD4-associated p56^{lck} *(796–800)*, an Src-family kinase expressed exclusively in lymphoid cells and especially in T cells *(801,802)*. The T cells that are deficient in p56^{lck} display a substantial reduction in TCR signaling capacity *(803,804)*. Animals deficient for this kinase exhibit a marked thymic atrophy associated with a significant decrease in the number of CD4$^+$ CD8$^+$, CD4$^+$ CD8$^-$, and CD4$^-$ CD8$^+$ thymocytes *(805)*. The p56^{lck} kinase phosphorylates the ITAMs of CD3 components (γ, δ, and ε) and the TCR ζ-chain *(786–789)*, generating docking sites for the SH2 domain of various PTKs and protein adaptors involved in TCR signaling (ZAP-70, phospholipase C [PLC]γ1, SLP-76, Vav, c-Cbl, Shc, and TRIM) *(806–813)* and in CD28 signaling (PI-3K and PI-4K) *(814,815)*. ZAP-70 kinase of the Syk-family *(816,817)* tyrosine phosphorylates LAT *(818)*, which is an adaptor for Grb-2 and PI-3K. The PI-3K kinase controls the inositol lipid metabolism *(819)*. The stimulatory capacity of the TCR alone on PI-3K is weak, but the combined signaling of the TCR and CD28 yields the optimal serine phosphorylation of the p110 subunit of PI-3K *(820)*.

Ligation of the TCR triggers activation of several other PTK substrates, including CD5 *(821)*, Erzin cytoskeletal proteins *(822)* vasolin-containing protein *(823)*, and PLCγ1 *(824)*. Recruitment of PLCγ1 to the TCR mediates events that control inositol lipid metabolism by generating inositol polyphosphates and phospholipids. These metabolites allow the TCR to regulate the intracellular calcium levels and the serine/threonine kinase family of protein kinase C (PKC) isoenzymes. The TCR can also activate the guanidine nucleotide binding protein p21^{ras} by a PTK-mediated mechanism independently of PLC-γ coupling to the TCR *(825)*. The p21^{ras} component is critical for the cytokine-mediated proliferation of T cells and is mainly regulated by the Shc/Grb-2/Sos complex *(826)*. The TCR triggers this pathway only in certain populations of T cells *(809,827)*. In activated T cells, ligation of the TCR involves another Grb-2-like protein, the Crk-C3G protein complex used to catalyze the guanidine nucleotide exchange on p21^{ras} *(828)*. Another PKC-sensitive Ras exchange protein that is activated by TCR signaling involved in the activation of T cells is the proto-oncogene Vav *(829)*, an exchange protein for Ras-related Rho/Rac proteins *(830)* that facilitates the intersection of TCR and CD28 signaling pathways *(831)*. The ERK1 and ERK2 of the mitogen-activated protein kinase (MAPK) cascade *(832)* mediate propagation of p21^{ras} signals to the nuclear transcription factors. In T cells, there are two signaling pathways for ERK2 regulation: one that involves Ras and another that involves PKC *(833)*. Activated p21^{ras} but not PKC couples the TCR to the MAPK cascade *(834)*. Another major function of p21^{ras} is to activate and recruit the serine/threonine kinase Raf-1 to the membrane *(835)*, which can trigger activation of ERK2. Lack of Raf-1 recruitment to the membrane was observed in some anergic T cells *(836)*. ERK2 kinase phosphorylates Elk1 *(837)*, a signaling molecule that associates in ternary complexes with a transcriptional activator serum factor that has roles in the regulation of Fos gene expression. Fos oncoproteins associate with the AP-1 transcription factor to induce activation of several cytokine genes. Two additional MAPK signaling cascades regulate JNK1 and JNK2 *(832)*. These two kinases integrate both TCR and CD28 signaling pathways with the Ca^{2+}/calmodulin system *(838)*. Regulation of JNK1 and JNK2 involves a kinase cascade similar to those of ERK1 and ERK 2. Ca^{2+}/calmodulin is another major signaling system activated by the TCR. The IP$_3$ inositol metabolite generated by PLC-γ binds to receptors in the endoplasmic reticulum to initiate release of intracellular Ca^{2+} stores. The rise of Ca^{2+} together with diacylglycerol (another PLC-γ-generated metabolite) activates PKC *(839)* and coincides with opening of CRAC channels that allow influx of extracellular Ca^{2+} into the cytoplasm *(840)*. Increased intracellular Ca^{2+} activates calcineurin (CaN), a ubiquitously expressed phosphatase with diverse functions*(825)*. CaN binds to NFAT transcription factors *(841)* and mediates its dephosphorylation-dependent translocation into the nucleus *(842,843)* in association with members of AP-1 family of transcriptional factors *(844,845)*. Increase of intracellular Ca^{2+} correlates with T-cell activation events *(846)*, whereas low- and noninducible calcium levels are characteristic for anergic T cells *(847,848)*.

These three major TCR signaling pathways (PKC, Ca^{2+}, and Ras) operate synergistically during the regulation of various transcriptional factors implicated in activation of the cytokine genes such as NFAT, NF-κB, and AP-1. Experiments involving dominant inhibitory mutants or specific inhibitors of these pathways suggest that the PKC system synergizes with the Ca^{2+} system in activating NFAT and AP-1. However, inhibition of PKC does not preclude activation of these transcriptional factors *(849)*. In contrast, the Ras signaling pathway is essential for the activation of NFAT *(850)* and can substitute for PKC signaling. A blockage of the Ras pathway, which is found in most of the anergic T-cell systems *(851)*, prevents the activation of ERK and JNK proteins *(852)* with subsequent downregulation of the AP-1 transcriptional activity. Activation of the Ca^{2+} signaling system can also suffice for transcription of the *IL-4* gene *(853)* but seems to be used mostly by the Th1 but not Th2 cells *(854)*. These observations revealed a branching nature of the TCR signaling machinery that is able to select particular biochemical pathways that ultimately lead to a specific T-cell effector function.

Tuning the TCR on T cells is the result of a fine balance between the PTKs and protein tyrosine phosphatases (PTPs).

3. EXPRESSION OF COSTIMULATORY RECEPTORS DURING THE DEVELOPMENT OF T CELLS

Numerous molecules are associated with the membrane of T cells (*see* Table 11). Some of these macromolecules function as coreceptors. Others represent markers of the T-cell lineage, activated T cells, or memory T cells.

3.1. CD4 and CD8 Coreceptors

CD4 and CD8 are markers that divide T cells into two main subpopulations. CD4 and CD8 display different functions and also function as coreceptors. CD4 is necessary for interaction with MHC class II molecules, which present peptides generated in the endosomal pathways, whereas CD8 interacts with MHC class I molecules, which present the peptides derived from the processing of endogenous proteins to the TCR.

CD8 is a heterodimer of 32 kDa made up of two chains, α and β, encoded by genes located on chromosome 2. CD8 binds to the α-3 domain of MHC class I molecules.

CD4 is a transmembrane glycoprotein of 55 kDa and is encoded by a single gene. The outermost domains of CD4 interact with MHC class II molecules, leaving the outer MHC domain that contains the peptide to interact with the TCR.

The interaction of the MHC class II-peptide complex with the TCR and CD4 is essential for the activation of T cells. This was clearly demonstrated by experiments in our laboratory. We prepared a chimeric, soluble, dimeric MHC class II molecule made up of a peptide that was derived from influenza virus hemagglutinin (HA) corresponding to110 to 120 amino acid residues, connected via a linker to the first exon of β chain of I-E^d and Fcγ2a. This chimeric molecule was coexpressed in a plasmid with the *I-E^d α-chain* gene, and after transfection, a dimeric soluble MHC class II-peptide chimeric molecule called DEF was obtained *(855)*. This soluble DEF molecule activated and induced the proliferation of T cells from transgenic (Tg) mice expressing the TCR that recognized HA110-120 peptide. The proliferation of HA-specific T cells was inhibited by both anticlonotypic and anti-CD4 monoclonal antibodies *(856)*. This finding indicates that the crosslinking of CD4 and TCR, and the resulting TCR-CD4 coaggregation, leads to stimulation of T cells as long as both TCR and CD4 molecules bind to the same ligand *(856)*.

Several observations suggest a functional integration of the CD4 and TCR signaling pathways in T cells: (a) CD4 associates physically with the TCR during T-cell activation *(857–859)*; (b) coaggregation of CD4 with CD3-TCR complex augments T-cell proliferation *(860)*; and (c) p56^{lck} coimmunoprecipitates with TCR phospho-ζ elements in activated T cells but not in resting or anergic T cells *(861)*.

The CD4 signaling pathways are not well defined. Several reports indicate that signaling of the CD4 coreceptor might affect the trend of TCR signaling cascades. Whereas some groups found that ligation of CD4 by antibodies induces T-cell activation independently of TCR signaling *(862)*, others found that anti-CD4 antibody induces production of tumor necrosis factor (TNF)-α and interferon (IFN)-γ but does not affect IL-2 or IL-4 production *(863)*, Ca^{2+} immobilization, tyrosine phosphorylation of Shc *(864,865)* or Ezrin protein *(866)*, or activation of p59^{fyn} *(867)*, AP-1 *(862)*, and NFAT *(864,867)*. Discrepancies among these studies may reflect experimental differences such as the CD4 epitopes recognized by various antibodies, the degree of crosslinking, and the differentiation status of the T cells analyzed. In other experimental systems, ligation of CD4 by antibodies or HIV-1 gp120 independently of TCR-CD3 signaling induced a long-term anergy *(868–870)*. Also, lack of CD4-MHC class II-peptide interaction leads to T-cell anergy *(871)*.

The CD4 coreceptor plays an important role in T-cell differentiation *(872–874)*. Lack of CD4 on T cells has been associated with poor differentiation of DN T cells into Th1 or Th2 effector cells *(875)*. It has been suggested that oligomerization of CD4 molecules with the TCR-CD3 complex is an important step for CD4-mediated signal transduction in T cells *(876)* by virtue of the intracellular crosslinking of CD4 with the TCR-CD3 complex via CD4-p56^{lck} kinase *(869–871,877,878)*. A Zn^{++}-based motif has been reported to mediate the noncovalent association of p56lck with the cytoplasmatic tail of CD4 antigen *(879,880)*.

3.2. CD28 and CTLA4 Coreceptors

Optimal activation of T cells requires two signals: one delivered by the TCR and another by CD28 superfamily coreceptors. According to the two-signal model, the lymphocytes fail to respond adequately in the absence of a CD28-induced signal.

The ligands of CD28 and CTLA-4 are CD80 and CD86, which are expressed on the surface of APCs.

CD28 is constitutively expressed on the surface of T cells, whereas CTLA-4 is rapidly expressed after the activation of T cells *(881)*. Binding of CD28 to CD80 and CD86 transmits a signal that synergizes with the TCR signal. The engagement of CD28 alone subsequent to exposure to anti-CD28 antibody does not activate the T cells in the absence of occupancy of the TCR by MHC-peptide complex. CD28 signaling regulates the threshold for T-cell activation and augments and sustains the T-cell response initiated by TCR signaling that favors T-cell proliferation, differentiation, and secretion of cytokines *(882)*. In contrast, the engagement of CTLA-4 subsequent to interaction with CD80 and CD86 delivers a negative signal that inhibits the signals delivered by the TCR, CD28, and CD4 or CD8. The signals delivered via CTLA-4 inhibit the synthesis of IL-2 and the proliferation of T cells and terminate T-cell responses *(883,884)*. Therefore, the magnitude of the T-cell response involves a balance of CD28-mediated activation and CTLA-4-mediated inhibition after interaction with CD80 and CD86 ligands.

In mice, CD28 is expressed very early in ontogeny in an 11- to 12-d-old embryoid body derived from CD45[+] HSCs. In contrast, CTLA-4 was not found in embryonic cells or embryonic bodies by staining with specific antibodies, or its transcript was not detected by polymerase chain reaction *(416)*.

Study of CD28 and CTLA-4 expression in human neonatal lymphocytes showed that cord blood resting lymphocytes expressed higher levels of CD28 than adults. The proportion of CD28[+] T cells declines throughout life and was noted predominantly in the CD8[+] subset. Following in vitro activation with PMA and ionomycine, the percentage of CD28[+] adult T cells increased to a level similar to that seen in neonatal T cells. In neonatal T cells, CD28 is functional because signaling via CD28 enhances proliferation and synthesis of cytokines by murine neonatal T cells stimulated in vitro with mitogens or anti-CD3 antibody. Higher expression of CD28 in neonatal T cells may allow increased crosslinking to provide signals required for the activation/proliferation of T cells in peripheral lymphoid organs. In contrast, CTLA-4 was not expressed in resting neonatal T cells even after the stimulation in vitro with anti-CD3 antibody. Interestingly, CTLA-4 was detected in the cytoplasm of neonatal T cells. This suggests that the translocation of CTLA-4 on the membrane of neonatal T cells may be differentially regulated relative to adult T cells, in which CTLA-4 is expressed on the membrane after activation *(417)*. Because the activation of resting T cells depends on the balance of the expression of CD28 and CTLA-4, these observations suggest that high expression of CD28 in neonatal lymphocytes represents an important factor in T-cell activation.

3.3. CD40 Ligand (CD154)

CD40 ligand (CD40L) expressed on T cells interacts with CD40 expressed on B cells. This interaction leads to activation of B cells and plays a crucial role in class switching. In contradistinction with adult T cells, the expression of CD40L in neonatal T cells is reduced or undetectable *(885–887)*. Neonatal T cells were induced to express CD40L by stimulation with anti-CD3 antibody *(887)*, PMA, and ionomycine *(419,886)*. The kinetics of CD154 expression subsequent to activation with anti-CD3 antibody was similar in neonatal and adult T cells. The expression of CD154 on activated neonatal T cells may be related to the observed differential regulation of CD154 transcripts by PMA and ionomycine *(419)*. The differences observed in the CD154 expression in young lymphocytes may be responsible for the predominant IgM secretion by B cells in postnatal life. The blocking of CD40L with CD40.G1 monoclonal antibodies, which bind to CD40L, prevented interaction with B-cell CD40 and inhibited the downstream switch reflected in inhibition of IgE and IgG4 antibody production *(887)*.

The expression of CD40L on T cells induced greater expression of CD86 on B cells *(887)* and also is able to induce the proliferation of thymic TCR-γ/δ cells and γ-mediated cytolytic activity and the secretion of IFN-γ and TNF-α *(888)*.

Thus, lack of expression of CD40L on neonatal T cells correlates with lack of class switching and the predominance of IgM production by neonatal B cells. However, T-cell activation by endogenous ligands leading to the expression of CD40L may favor class switching to IgE and IgG4 production during postnatal life.

3.4. CD2 (Lymphocyte Function-Associated Antigen [LFA]-2)

CD2 is expressed on all T cells. CD2 is an adhesion molecule of 55 kDa that interacts with CD48, CD58 (LFA-3), and CD59 expressed on different cells including APCs. The adhesion domain of human CD2 bears a single N-glycan at Asn65, which is required for adhesion to stabilize the polypeptide conformation *(889)*. The CD2–CD58 interaction, like anti-CD2 antibodies, induces the resting cells to be cycled and transduce an activating signal to the T cells. The interaction between CD2 and CD58 is facilitated by CD44, a glycoprotein of 80 kDa that functions as a homing receptor (reviewed in ref. *67*).

In humans, CD34+ common lymphocyte progenitors enter the thymus at wk 7–8 of gestation. These precursors can differentiate into T cells and natural killer (NK) cells. They do not express CD4, CD8 CD3, or TCRs and are termed triple-negative (TN) T-cell precursors. By d 8.5 of gestation, these precursors express CD2 antigen, and a few days later, CD3 ε-chain can be detected in their cytoplasm. This observation indicates a temporal sequence of expression of CD2 before CD3 ε-chain in the early phase of gestation within a relatively narrow window of time. At this stage, the CD2+ TN thymocytes can be stimulated to proliferate with anti-CD2 antibody and submitogenic amounts of IL-2 *(890)*.

Interaction of CD2 with CD58 increases cellular interaction and transduces activating signals to T cells. CD58 is expressed on thymic stromal cells. The binding of CD2 to endogenous ligand CD58 cannot trigger thymocyte activation alone but induces the expression of CD25 (IL-2R). Thus, CD2 expressed on a CD34+ TN T cell likely does not induce activation signal as in mature T cells but rather upregulates the expression of IL-4R and the CD2–CD58 interaction. In concert with small amounts of IL-4, these effects may drive the proliferation and subsequent differentiation into CD3+ DN T cells.

3.5. CD5

CD5 is a monomeric protein of 67 kDa that is expressed on T cells and a subset of B cells (B1). Its ligand is CD72, a C-type lectin expressed on B cells. CD5 has a long intracytoplasmic moiety, which is substrate for the tyrosine kinases *lck* and *fyn*. The intracellular fragment is in close association with CD3ζ-chain, and phosphorylation of CD5 occurs within seconds of binding the MHC-peptide complex to the TCR or after exposure to CD5 antibody. Stimulation via CD5 induces calcium mobilization, increase of cyclic guanosine monophosphate (cGMP), and the expression of CD25. Similarly to CD2, CD5 is expressed on CD34$^+$ TN immature thymocytes after wk 8–9 gestation.

3.6. CD34

CD34 is a cell-surface antigen of 120 kDa that is expressed on pluripotential HSCs and on the most primitive human T-cell precursors (TN thymocytes). CD34$^+$ TN thymocytes are present in the fetal thymus at wk 8.5 of gestation and differentiate into DN T cells. This concept is supported by several findings. First, thymic CD45$^+$ TN cells express the CD2 and CD5 antigens, which are expressed on all T cells *(891,892)*. Second, purified CD45$^+$ TN thymic cells dedifferentiate into DP T cells in fetal organic cultures using the fetal thymus from donors at wk 17–20 of gestation, whereas CD34$^-$ TN thymocytes lack this capacity *(893)*. CD34$^+$ TN thymic cells exhibit incomplete rearrangement of the TCR-δ locus displaying Dδ2–Dδ3 and Dδ2–Jδ2 rearrangements, whereas the TCR-γ, -β, and -α loci are in the embryonic germ line gene configuration.

In vitro culture of these cells with anti-CD2 antibody and recombinant IL (rIL)-4 for 2 d gives rise to TCR-δ^+ cells *(892)*.

The expression of CD34 decreases drastically during the thymic differentiation process at the stage of CD4$^+$ CD8α^+ β^- and ceases at the stage of DP T cells. These findings strongly suggest that CD34 is a marker of the most primitive T-cell precursors committed toward differentiation into T cells.

3.7. CD21 Receptor

CD21 receptor is a transmembrane molecule of 145 kDa. Its ligands are the C3b/C3g and C3d fragments of human C3, and it also has a low affinity for IgE, CD23, and Epstein–Barr virus (EBV) virus (reviewed in ref. *894*). CD21 is expressed on all stages of differentiation of the T-cell lineage but at the highest density level in the most immature CD34$^+$ TN thymocytes. On transition from the CD34$^-$ CD1$^+$ CD4^{low} CD8$^-$ stage to DN T cells, CD21 expression decreases, reaching the level of mature T cells. CD21 is shed from the membrane, and the levels of soluble CD21 increase with increasing gestation; however, reduced levels were detectable in cord blood *(894)*.

The function of the CD21 receptor during various stages of differentiation of the T-cell lineage is unclear *(895)*. One may speculate that it contributes to the selection of the T-cell repertoire by inhibiting recombination activating gene (RAG) activity and, therefore, TCR gene recombination. It is also thought to increase the susceptibility of immature T cells to EBV infection.

3.8. CD45

CD45 is present on all lymphocytes but exists in several isoforms that serve to distinguish various lymphocytes and are specifically expressed on various stages of T-cell development. The gene encoding CD45 is located on chromosome 1. Exons 4, 5, 6, and possibly 7 can be spliced in various ways, yielding eight isoforms that differ in extracellular domains. The CD45 is expressed in primitive T-cell precursors. CD45RA and CD45RB are expressed in naïve T cells, and CD45R0 interacting with CD22 is expressed in activated mature and memory T cells. In humans, the majority of T cells in cord blood express CD45RA, whereas those in adult peripheral blood express CD45R0.

CD45 can positively regulate the TCR signaling components by dephosphorylation of negative regulatory tyrosines on PTKs *(896,897)* such as Tyr505 of p56^{lck} *(898,899)*. Antigen stimulation in the absence of CD45 prevents T-cell proliferation and production of cytokines via hyperphosphorylation-mediated inactivation of p56^{lck} *(900,901)*. In contrast, antibody-mediated coaggregation of CD45 with the TCR can negatively regulate the TCR signaling machinery *(902)*, presumably by CD45 interference with TCR oligomerization-mediated signaling *(903)* or by excessive dephosphorylation of the positive regulatory tyrosines such as Tyr394 or p56^{lck} *(904)*. In general, the PTPs induce negative regulation of TCR signaling by dephosphorylation-mediated deactivation of PTKs. However, negative regulation of TCR signaling can be mediated not only by PTPs but also by some PTKs such as CsK tyrosine kinase *(905)*, which mediates phosphorylation of the inhibitory tyrosines of Src kinases (i.e., Tyr505 or p56^{lck}) *(906,907)*.

4. DEVELOPMENT OF THE T-CELL LINEAGE

During ontogeny, the development of T cells has been divided into three phases: the prethymic phase (which begins in the liver during gestation and continues in bone marrow during infancy and thereafter), the thymic phase, and the mature phase.

4.1. Prethymic Phase

In mice, the prethymic phase begins by d 14 of gestation in the fetal liver and continues in bone marrow during infancy and thereafter. Pluripotential HSCs present in the fetal liver or bone marrow differentiate into common lymphoid precursors and, thereafter, into T-cell precursors. Pluripotential HSCs express markers of both myeloid and lymphoid lineages such as Mac-1, Gr-1, Thy1, B220, Tae, 11, c-Kit, and Scal-1 *(156)*. From pluripotential HSCs arise bipotent T/NK-cell precursors identified as $CD117^+$, $CD44^+$, and $CD25^-$. The T/NK precursors reach the thymus through blood, enter into the cortical medullary junction by passing between endothelial cells of capillaries, and then migrate in the cortical zone *(908)*. Although the bone marrow HSCs and pluripotential HSCs exhibit the properties of fetal HSCs, they are phenotypically distinct because they express other markers, specifically $Thy1.1^-$, c-Kit^{bright}, and Rho^{high} *(909)*.

4.2. Thymic Phase

Upon entry into the thymus, bipotent T/NK precursors differentiate in the thymic cortex. This process is not autonomous and requires signals delivered after contact with various types of mesenchymal and thymic epithelial cells (TECs). The differentiation process of T-cell precursors is characterized by temporally coordinated expression of cell surface markers, the expression of RAG and TdT enzymes, and the rearrangement of genes encoding TCRs. The T-cell progenitors then enter into the thymus at the cortical medullary junction and migrate into the cortex. The most immature stages are characterized by the absence of the expression of CD4 and CD8 markers and are termed as DN.

In mice, DN cells undergo four major stages of differentiation. The phenotype of DN1 and DN2 thymocytes is $CD44^{++}$ $CD25^-$, and $CD44^+$ $CD25^{++}$, respectively. Both DN1 and DN2 thymocytes synthesize the pre-T-α-chain. The phenotype of DN3 cells is $CD44^-$ $CD25^+$, and these cells synthesize the TCR-β-chain. DN4 thymocytes do not express CD44; they express CD25 and pre-TCR encoded by pre-T-α and TCR-β. There is a subtle subset of DN4 in which no intracytoplasmic TCR-β protein has been detected. In that TCR-β^- subset, intracytoplasmic TCR-γ/δ was detected *(910)*. These cells may exhibit a low level of proliferation and may differentiate into TCR-γ/δ^+ cells in the cortex or medulla. Accompanying this maturation is a second round of expansion, which corresponds to the transition of DN3 toward DN4 thymocytes. The proliferation is mediated by pre-TCR, because the differentiation is arrested at the DN3 stage in pre-TCR knockout mice. In this mouse strain, no proliferation of DN3 thymocytes occurs *(911)*. DN3 and DN4 thymocytes express a newly characterized antigen, CD147 *(912)*. CD147 may play a role in cell cycling, because the fetal thymic organ cultures using thymuses removed at d 14–15 of gestation showed no DP thymocytes after incubation with the anti-CD147 antibody. These cultures showed a relative increase of DN1 and a drastic decrease of DN4 cells. This finding suggests a potential role of CD147 in the second phase of expansion of immature thymocytes.

In all differentiation stages, the DN thymocytes express CD2 and CD5 antigens, and the RAG enzymes are active. DN4 thymocytes differentiate into DP cells that express CD4, CD8, and TCRs. They lose the expression of CD44 and CD25, and RAG activity is absent or reduced to low levels sufficient for additional rearrangement of TCR-α genes (TCR editing).

DP T cells differentiate into SP T cells that express CD4 or CD8 and T cells that express TCR-γ/δ or TCR-α/β.

In humans, the pathway of T-cell development is similar to that described in mice, with the exception of the expression of different antigens. The T/NK-cell precursors are characterized by CD34$^+$, CD1a$^+$, and CD5$^+$. The DN cells display three phases of differentiation according to the model proposed by Blom et al. *(336)*. From pre-T cells CD34$^+$, CD1a$^+$, and CD5$^+$ arise the preTCD4 immature SPs CD34$^-$, CD1a$^+$, CD5$^+$, CD4$^+$, and CD8 . From these cells arise other types of DN cells called the EDP cells CD34$^-$, CD1a$^+$, CD5$^+$, CD4$^+$, and the CD8-α-chain. These cells differentiate into DP T cells exhibiting the phenotypes CD1a$^+$ CD5$^+$, CD4$^+$ CD8-α and -β$^+$ CD27$^-$, CD69$^-$, and TCR$^+$.

In the cortex, the majority (70%) of DP cells are not dividing cells; however, a small number (15%) are dividing cells that probably result from positive selection of DP cells. DP and SP T cells migrate from the cortex into the medulla. Kinetic analysis of DP and SP thymocytes suggests that the turnover time of DP and SP thymocytes in the medulla is significantly longer than that of DP in the cortex *(913)*. Once in the medulla, SP thymocytes are activated and express homing receptors. In the medulla, only 2–10.5 % divide, as assessed by a short-pulse labeling with BrdUrd *(913)*. In the medulla, SP T cells express HSA but not Qa2 antigen. The overall turnover time for medullar SP thymocytes is far greater than 1–2 d as was thought initially; it takes at least 6–9 d *(913)*. After residing in the medulla for several days, the SP T cells are exported to the periphery through veins and lymphatics. Their entrance into the vessels depends on expression of homing receptors, which are probably induced by cytokines in the medulla. Only the most mature SP thymocytes, which are HSA$^-$Qa2$^+$, leave the thymus.

The pathway of the differentiation process of murine and human T cells is illustrated in Fig. 38.

5. POSITIVE AND NEGATIVE SELECTION

Stochastic recombination of the gene segments encoding TCRs potentially create specificity for all peptides derived from the processing of foreign and self-antigens presented to T cells in association with MHC class I and II and CD1 molecules. The specificity of the T-cell repertoire is established during fetal development of the thymus.

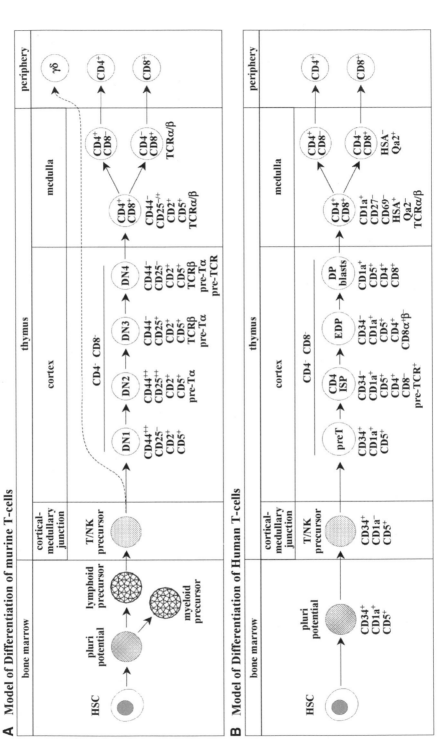

Fig. 38. Model of differentiation of murine and human T-cell lineage.

The major property of the immune system, including the T cells, is to discriminate between self and nonself. This implies a selection of the lymphocytes. T cells mediating the immune response against foreign antigens are positively selected, whereas a negative selection process deletes those that recognize self-antigen, which may cause autoimmune reactions.

Only T cells with a low affinity for MHC-peptide complex are positively selected, proliferate, and differentiate, whereas those exhibiting a TCR with high affinity for ligands are eliminated. This concept creates a paradox in which the signal induced by the ligand through the TCR results either in survival or death.

Positive selection is a multistage process involving interaction of T cells with the thymic environment and, in particular, with TECs expressing MHC molecules. TECs provide specialized accessory interactions that MHC$^+$ epithelial cells from other tissues do not. TECs and thymic stromal cells express other molecules such as BPM and TTS24, which could be essential in the positive selection process.

The most important question regarding the process of positive selection is: How does positive selection occur subsequent to interaction of TECs with thymocytes during fetal life, when the embryo is protected from exposure to foreign antigen that, with rare exceptions, cannot pass through placenta?

The paradigm of the positive selection process is that only cells that bear a TCR with low affinity/avidity for the self-derived MHC-peptide complex are positively selected. The positive selection process occurs in the thymus cortex at the most immature stage of differentiation of DP, large, dividing blast thymocytes that express a fully functional TCR and CD69, CD2, CD5, and Qa2 surface markers. Positively selected DP blast cells become small nondividing thymocytes located in the cortex. The interaction of the TCR with MHC-peptide complex is crucial for positive selection. This concept was supported by the study of TCRs in MHC knockout mice in which the differentiation of DP thymocytes was arrested (reviewed in ref. *914*). Positively selected DP thymocytes exhibit a new wave of expansion that appears to be MHC-independent and gives rise to SP thymocytes.

Positive selection is driven by binding the TCR to a single or mixture of self-peptides associated with MHC molecules on the surface of TECs. It is noteworthy that a few peptides derived from self-antigens have been identified. The majority of the peptides identified were not stimulatory for mature T cells, which require high-affinity interactions. Several transcription factors are critical for positive selection, such as Src and Syk family kinase proximally associated with the TCR, Ras, RasGRP, PLC-γ, ERK, helix–loop–helix family, Schnurri, and Egr1. The involvement of these factors in positive selection is supported by studies carried out in mice with targeted mutations in genes encoding these factors. In these mice, positive selection and the DN to DP transition processes are blocked (reviewed in ref. *915*).

Negative selection results from the high-affinity interaction of self-peptides with TCRs. This concept is supported by several findings demonstrating T-cell deletion by increased apoptosis. Pertinent findings include (a) deletion of T cells induced by endogenous antigens and by injection of high amounts of peptides in TCR Tg mice, (b) the increased expression of peptides in the thymuses of Tg mice, and (c) massive apoptosis caused by injection of anti-CD3 antibody.

Clonal deletion occurs early in T cell development at the stage of transition of DN cells to DP cells but also occurs late in the SP stage. In addition to TCR–MHC-peptide complex high-affinity interaction, the negative selection requires a second costimulatory signal delivered by CD28–B7 or CD40L–CD40 interactions. This concept is supported by the observations that CD28 knockout mice are resistant to anti-CD3 antibody or peptide-induced apoptosis *(916)* and that CD40-deficient mice do not exhibit the negative selection induced by endogenous super antigens *(917)*.

It was generally considered that the negative selection clonal deletion results from activation of apoptosis mediated by Fas ligand–Fas receptor and TNF-α–TNFR interactions. Most studies derived from mice with targeted genes for FasR, TNFR1, and TNFR2 revealed that FasL or TNF-α are not necessary for negative selection. Similarly, in the case of selection induced by endogenous peptides, it was shown that TNF signaling is dispensable for negative selection *(918)*. More recent evidence suggests that orphan steroid receptor factor Nur77, a downstream regulator of TCR involved in the apoptosis pathway, increases negative selection *(919,920)*. Studies in knockout mice suggest that Grb2 (an adaptor protein associated with the TCR) signaling is important for negative selection *(921)*. Also, p38, which is an activator of c-Jun, and MKK7, which is an upstream activator of JNK, increase negative selection. Clonal deletion requires both RNA and protein synthesis. These observations strongly demonstrate that negative T-cell selection is an active process.

6. TCR EDITING DURING T-CELL DEVELOPMENT

The process of BCR editing was first discovered in the case of immature B cells. There are some observations that the same process is active during the T-cell development. In the case of T cells, the editing process results from rearrangement of the TCR-α locus, which continues in the cortex DP cells and even in the medulla SP T cells. In one model, a rearranged Vα-Jα gene was introduced (knock-in) in embryonic stem cells and expressed in DP thymocytes with the *TCR*-β gene. Editing in these mice was induced by a superantigen and was associated with the internalization of one TCR-α *(922)*.

TCR editing also was described in a Tg mouse strain in which ovalbumin was expressed under the control of the human keratin 14 promoter, which drives the gene expression in TECs and skin, and tongue and esophagus keratinocytes but not in other tissues. In contrast to Ot-1 Tg mice that display a drastic reduction of DP thymocytes, in the K-14 OVA double-Tg mice, a significant proportion of DP thymocyte remained. These cells remained in the thymus because they expressed endogenous TCR-α; allelic exclusion of the TCR-α locus is not complete in mice. The DP thymocytes in these mice exhibited low expression of TCRs, CD4, and CD8 and an increased expression of CD69, indicating that they had encountered the antigen. Low expression of TCRs indicates that the autoreactive TCRs were internalized and that RAG expression was maintained in DP thymocytes of these mice. From these results, it was predicted that of the 10 to 27% of peripheral T cells expressing two functional *TCR*-α genes, some can express an autoreactive TCR *(923)*.

Taken together, these observations indicate that self-antigen presented by TECs can cause in DP thymocytes the internalization of TCRs and rearrangement of endogenous TCR-α, allowing for survival of DP T cells by a receptor editing process. Because these conclusions derive from studies carried out on Tg mice, it is difficult to determine the significance of the TCR editing process in vivo.

7. DEVELOPMENT OF T CELLS IN VERTEBRATES

CMI in T cells represents an important arm of defense reactions in all vertebrates. The thymus and T cells occurred 500 million yr ago, when jawed vertebrates diverged from other vertebrates. T-cell differentiation takes place in the thymus in all vertebrates. In all vertebrates, the TCR is the major marker of T cells, and the rearrangement of genes encoding the specificity of the TCR follow the same rules.

7.1. Ontogeny of T Cells in Fish

In all fish, T cells differentiate and mature within the thymus, which derives from the endoderm and the mesenchyme of pharyngeal pouches and the ectoderm of branchial clefts. The thymus anlage is the first lymphoid tissue that develops during ontogeny.

In fish, the pronephros is the organ that contains HSCs. From pronephros, the HSCs migrate into the thymus before the spleen.

Hansen and Zapata *(320)* divided thymic lymphopoiesis into four stages: (a) the occurrence of thymic primordium, (b) its colonization with precursors, (c) expansion and differentiation, and (d) the histological division of thymic tissue into the cortex and medulla.

In trout embryos, the thymic primordium is evident at 8 d prehatching. At hatching, the thymus consists of few layers of ETC, and at 1 d prehatching, lymphocytes become preponderant. One month after hatching the thymus is completely regionalized in the cortex and medullar areas. RAG activity was detected at d 10 postfertilization when neither pronephros nor thymus primordia were developed *(924,925)*. These findings suggest that thymic progenitors may rearrange the genes encoding the TCR before colonization of the thymus. V[D]J recombination was also described in the thymus anlage at d 15 postfertilization. At d 16–20 postfertilization, the rearranged TCR-βV2 do not exhibit N insertion despite the fact that TdT is expressed before hatching.

In catfish, the thymocyte population changes remarkably during the first 28 d posthatching. At d 1, the thymus consists of epithelial cells and only a few lymphocytes. By d 5, the number of thymocytes increases and by d 21 occurs in equal proportions throughout thymic parenchyma *(253)*.

In zebrafish, the formation of the thymic primordium occurs much faster: 60 h postfertilization. At 65 h, the thymus anlage contains small and large lymphocytes distributed throughout the meshwork of ETC, and at d 4 postfertilization the number of thymocytes increases considerably. RAG expression coincides with colonization of the thymus with lymphocytes at 65–70 h postfertilization *(926)*.

7.2. Development of T Cells in Amphibians

In Xenopus, the thymus primordia become evident at d 3 postfertilization and 1 d later are colonized with lymphocytes. The colonization of the thymus with precursors is characterized by several waves. The first wave takes place by d 4 postfertilization by progenitors from embryonic mesoderm. The second wave results from colonization of the thymus by precursors originating from dorsal lateral plates. Finally, the third wave, which takes place during metamorphosis, results from seeding of the thymus with precursors from the larval liver (reviewed in ref. *320*). After the first wave of entrance of progenitors, 20% of thymocytes express the T-cell-specific XTLA-1 antigen. The first CD8 antigen appears at d 12 postfertilization. By this time, the larval thymus exhibits clear demarcation of the cortex and medulla. Following the expression of XTLA-1 and CD8 markers, the vast majority of thymocytes after the second wave of colonization express the CD5 marker of T cells *(927)*. RAG expression was observed d 3.5 postfertilization, and 1 d later the transcripts of fully rearranged TCR loci were detected.

Later during metamorphosis, over 90% of thymocytes in the cortical area are deleted. This observation strongly suggests that there is a negative selection in frog thymuses.

7.3. T-Cell Lymphopoiesis in Birds

The TCR and major markers of T cells defined in mammals appear to be highly conserved in birds. Bird T cells express TCR-γ/δ and TCR-α/β, a pan-T-cell antigen recognized by the CT1 monoclonal antibody, and CD2, CD5, CD4, and CD8 *(928)*. Similarly to lower vertebrate species, in birds the thymus is seeded with precursors from blood in waves. Studies of T-cell development in the chick–quail chimera indicated that the thymus is the only site in which T cells expressing the TCR-CD3 complex are generated *(929)*. During T-cell development, the CD3 molecules were identified at d 9 of embryo development, and at d 11 about 20% of thymocytes expressed CD2 and then CT1 antigen. In the thymus there is a sequential differentiation of TCR-γ/δ and TCR-α/β subsets *(930)*. The thymocytes expressing TCR-γ/δ occur in the thymic cortex on d 12 of embryonic life, approx 5 d after HSCs enter the thymus and 3 d after the detection of CD3 molecules. By day 13 TCRs-γ/δ reach the medulla and their number increases, indicating that they enter into the cell cycle and proliferate. Intracytoplasmic TCR-β-chain was detected on d 12, and surface expression of the TCR-α/β-CD3 complex was detected in the cortex at d 14. The TCR-α/β subset quickly becomes predominant. The sequential development of thymocytes expressing TCR-γ/δ followed by those expressing TCR-α/β strongly suggests that in birds, these cells represent two different lineages. This concept is supported by an experiment that showed that the treatment of embryos with anti-TCR-δ monoclonal antibody prevented the development of TCR-γ/δ thymocytes without affecting the development of thymocytes expressing TCR-α/β. Similarly, treatment with anti-TCR-α/β antibodies prevented the development of TCR-α/β but not of TCR-γ/δ thymocytes *(931)*.

TCR-α/β thymocytes are DP and differentiate into SP T cells. They leave the thymus and occur in the spleen by day 19 and in the intestine by d 20 of embryonic life. It interesting that in birds, the majority of SP T cells in the periphery do not express CD2 *(928)*.

7.4. T-Cell Development in Lambs

As in other mammalian species, in lambs T lymphopoiesis takes place only in the thymus during the last trimester of pregnancy. Thymocytes and peripheral T cells expressing TCR-γ/δ occur before TCR-α/β. In the fetus during the last month of gestation, TCR-γ/δ represents 18% of total T cells, and their number increases in the cord blood to 60% *(932)*. Postnatal SP T-cell emigrants express CD11a/CD18, CD44, CD2, and CD58 antigens. Prior to export from the thymus, CD44 is upregulated on TCR-γ/δ cells, and both CD16 and CD58 are downregulated, suggesting that this process may be the final step of maturation of TCR-γ/δ cells. In contrast, there is a continuous upregulation of CD2 during thymic development as well as an upregulation of the expression of CD2 on both TCR-γ/δ and TCR-α/β T cells during postnatal life. Thus, it appears that the changes in the expression of costimulatory and adhesion molecules are the result of the maturation of thymocytes to a mature peripheral T cell *(933)*. The lifespan of thymocytes in the fetus is unknown. However, before parturition the fetal lamb develops a large pool of long-lived circulating T cells that is rapidly replaced by short-lived T cells during postnatal life, following exposure to environmental antigens (934).

7.5. Thymopoiesis in Pigs

In contrast to other mammalian species, the differentiation of T-cell lineage in pigs exhibits some particularities (329).

The first lymphocytes occur in the thymic rudiment at d 38 of gestation. The vast majority are DNT cells expressing the pan-lymphocytic marker CD45 and the promyelocyte-monocyte antigen SWC3a. Early T-cell progenitors (CD3-ε⁻, CD4⁻, and CD8⁻) have been identified only in the SWC3a⁻ population. From these cells arise immature thymocytes characterized by the expression of CD8 and the absence of CD3-ε and CD4 expression. These cells differentiate in DP CD3-ε⁻ thymocytes, which at day 40 express CD3-ε^{high} and CD25. The DP thymocytes have been identified in the fetal thymus at d 56–76 of gestation. All DP thymocytes are positive for CD5, CD2, and CD1 expression (935).

Thymocytes first differentiate into TCR-γ/δ CD3-ε^{high}. Until d 50 of gestation, TCR-δ thymocytes represent almost exclusively all CD3^{high} thymocytes. The number of TCR-δ thymocytes decreases, and by day 55 TCR-β cells become predominant. Thus, like in other mammalian species, the TCR-δ T-cell subset occurs earlier than the TCR-α/β subset (935).

Apparently, in pigs the thymus is colonized by at least two waves of HSCs; however, the influx of T-cell progenitors is discontinuous and decreases sharply between d 40 and 45 of gestation, when the frequency of CD45^{high} thymocytes increases significantly.

7.6. Ontogeny of Human T Cells

In humans, the thymus develops from the third branchial pouch at wk 6 of gestation. Originally, the majority are ETCs and the lymphocytes begin to appear at wk 8 to 9 of gestation. Gradually the thymus separates into the cortex and medulla, and eventually Hassall's corpuscles are evident, marking the full development of the thymus gland. In thymuses from fetuses at wk 15 to 26 of gestation, 50 to 96% of thymocytes express CD2 as assessed by the ability to rosette sheep erythrocytes (330). The immature thymic cells develop from CD34⁺ CD38⁻ fetal liver cells and, after birth, from CD 34⁺, CD10⁺ Lin⁻ c-Kit⁻ human bone marrow cells (894). From these, HSCs derive T/NK precursors, which differentiate into DN, DP, and then SP thymocytes expressing TCR-α/β. The TCR-α/β cells develop exclusively in the thymus.

By contrast, in humans TCR-γ/δ T cells can be identified before thymic development at wk 6–8 of gestation in fetal liver cells. These cells also have been identified in cord blood cells and expand in vitro vigorously upon culture for 14 d with rIL-2.

In conclusion, in all vertebrate species the T cells develop within the thymus with the exception of TCR-γ/δ cells, which may develop extrathymically. Development of T cells expressing TCR-γ/δ precedes the occurrence of TCR-α/β cells. During fetal life, the HSCs are harbored within fetal liver. The common lymphocyte progenitor and T/NK precursors are derived from HSCs. During postnatal life and thereafter HSCs are present within bone marrow. The T/NK precursor cells later enter into the thymus at the cortical medullary junction, from which they migrate into the cortex. There, they undergo various stages of differentiation (e.g., DN to DP to SP). In these stages of differentiation, they first express a pre-TCR, and at the stage of DP they express fully functional TCR-α/β.

8. FUNCTION OF NEONATAL T CELLS

Since the original observation of Billingham and Medawar *(607)* that mice neonates injected with allogeneic bone marrow cells were able to accept skin allogeneic graft, it has been believed that the poor CMI response in neonates is related to immaturity of T cell function and higher susceptibility to tolerance. However, tolerance by itself represents an active immune response because tolerant lymphocytes transferred into naïve mice conferred unresponsiveness to recipients. The concept of an active tolerance is supported by an experiment by Goldman et al. *(936)* showing that the activation of Th2 cells plays a role in the induction and maintenance of neonatal tolerance.

From a functional point of view, T cells are classified in three main subsets: (a) CD4 T cells, which were initially considered helper T cells; (b) CD8 T cells, which mediate cytotoxic reactions; and (c) regulatory T cells. CD4 T cells were divided in two additional functionally distinct subsets: (a) Th1 CD4 cells that produce IFN-γ and IL-2, which favor class switching to IgG2 and mediate the delayed hypersensitivity reaction and protection against intracellular microbes, and (b) Th2 CD4 cells that produce IL-4, IL-13, and IL-5, which participate in humoral responses and favor class switching to IgG1 and IgE.

Late studies from the 1970s that were carried out in mice challenged the concept of unresponsiveness of neonatal T cells. At first glance these studies were very crude in light of the progress made in T-cell immunobiology. However, these studies merit mention because they demonstrated that neonatal T cells are functional. Bosing-Schneider *(937)* measured the ability of neonatal T cells to secrete T-cell replacing factor (TRF), which is probably a mixture of cytokines secreted by Th2 cells. The study demonstrated that T cells from 1- to 2-d-old mice produce minute amounts of TRF; however, 1-wk-old mice had a sufficient number of T cells to produce as much of this factor as T cells from an adult. It was later shown that neonatal thymic cells are able to provide assistance to B cells producing IgM antibodies to TNP-BGG *(938)*.

Further studies carried out in mice demonstrated that neonatal CD4 T cells are functional and that Th2 responses dominate in neonates. Th1 responses are prevalent in adults. In vitro studies showed that although the frequency of neonatal murine Th2 cells in lymph nodes is similar to that observed in adult mice, virtually no IFN-γ-secreting Th1 cells were detected in neonatal spleens. The production of IL-4 by neonatal splenic Th2 was antigen-specific *(939)*. Thus, the neonatal naïve T cells are biased to secretion of IL-4, a Th2 cytokine, both under standard in vitro activation conditions *(939)* and after in vivo immunization of neonates with peptide delivered on an immunoglobulin platform that enhances the immunogenicity and provides adjuvant activity *(940,941)*.

Neonatal T cells rapidly lose the Th2 phenotype. By d 6 after birth, high production of IL-4 diminishes *(942,943)*. Nonetheless, the Th1 cells are also present in newborn lymphoid organs. This concept is supported by the following findings:

a. Upon in vitro culture of neonatal splenic cells in the presence of IL-6 or anti-CD28 antibodies, IL-2 production and proliferation of Th1 cells were enhanced, reaching the levels of adult T cells *(944)*.
b. In vivo administration of IL-12, a strong promoter of Th1 cell development, together with anergic cells induced the production of high levels of IFN-γ and IL-2, and these mice acquired the capacity to prevent the induction of neonatal tolerance *(945)*.
c. In vivo injection of anti-CD40 antibodies in neonates enhanced the alloantigen-specific Th1 response and prevented the induction of neonatal tolerance *(946)*.
d. Selective generation of neonatal Th1 responses were described with different modes of immunization such as immunization with hen egg lysozyme and Freund's incomplete adjuvant (FIA) *(947)* or subsequent to immunization with DNA vaccines. A robust Th1 response was described in newborn mice immunized with a plasmid containing influenza virus HA gene, as assessed by production of IFN-γ and IgG2a antibodies *(643)* or plasmids containing measles virus HA, C fragment of tetanus toxin, or Sendai virus nucleoprotein *(644)*.
e. Autoreactive Th1 cells develop soon after birth. This was clearly shown in two different animal models of autoimmune diseases. One model of juvenile insulin-dependent diabetes mellitus (IDDM) consists of double-Tg mice expressing influenza virus HA under rat insulin promoter in pancreatic β cells and a TCR specific for a dominant epitope of HA recognized by T cells in association with I-E^d MHC molecules. Five-day-old double-Tg mice developed periinsulitis, which coincided with an increased number of HA-specific diabetogenic T cells *(948)*. In a model for autoimmune ovarian disease (AOD), it was shown that immunization of females at d 2 and 5 after birth with pZP3 antigen in FIA led to development of AOD *(949)*. These observations clearly demonstrate that autoreactive Th1 cells, which mediate both IDDM and AOD, escape from tolerance and are present and functional after birth.

Under certain conditions, neonatal T cells mount a mixed Th1/Th2 response. This conclusion was strongly supported by an experiment in which mice immunized at birth with protein antigen *(950)* or DNA vaccines *(643,648,951)* were able to mount quantitatively and qualitatively indistinguishable mixed Th1/Th2 responses 1 wk after immunization.

Both in vivo and in vitro experiments demonstrate that exposure to antigen usually gives rise to a Th2-biased secondary response *(648,947)*. It is unclear whether the Th2 dominance resulted from lack of priming or from recall of neonatal Th1 cells. This question was particularly important because it was demonstrated that both neonatal Th1 and Th2 cells were able to mount a primary response *(648,950,951)*.

Recently, Li et al. *(952)* attempted to address this question using a model in which neonatal T cells from a Tg mouse strain expressing a TCR specific for an ovalbumin-derived peptide were transferred into normal newborn mice. In this system, priming with Ig-Ova induced both Th1 and Th2 responses; however, the recall with antigen induced only a Th2 response. Surprisingly, the Th1 response after recall was observed when IL-4 was neutralized by exogenous anti-IL-4 antibody. In addition, anti-IL-4 antibody prevented in vitro antigen-induced apoptosis of Th1, indicating that IL-4 and IL-13 may be involved in IL-4-mediated targeting of Th1 cells in vivo following the challenge with ovalbumin-derived peptide. Thus, it appears that IL-4 may exert its downregulatory effect on the secondary response of Th1, because IL-4R and IL-13R proteins are expressed on surface of Th1 cells *(952)*.

An apoptotic effect of IL-4 on neonatal Th1 cells is supported by results of microarray analysis of genes encoding antiapoptotic and proapoptotic factors. Neonatal Th1 exhibited upregulation of Lt-b, TNFR1, and TNFRSF11A, and Th2 showed an additional upregulation of myosin light chain (MLC)-1, an antiapoptotic factor. It should be noted that anti-IL-4 antibody inhibited the upregulation of TNFR1 and TNFRSF11A *(952)*. Therefore, the increased apoptosis observed during the secondary response of Th1 may be related to a defective expression of MLC-1.

Studies of in vitro maturation of cord blood lymphocytes also suggest a biased response of human neonatal CD4 T cells toward Th2 cells. Naïve neonatal T lymphocytes contain a subset characterized by CD4+ CD31- CD45RO- cells, which differentiate into IL-4-producing cells after long-term culture in IL-4 and IL-12 supplemented medium or stimulation with low doses of anti-CD28 antibodies *(953)*.

The biased development toward Th2 cells in newborns may be highly influenced by immune status during pregnancy. In mice, fetoplacental tissue is characterized by secretion of Th2 cytokines such as IL-4, IL-5, IL-10, PGE2, and progesterone, which downregulate the production of IL-12, promoting the development of Th1 cells (data reviewed in ref. *953*).

Overall, these studies indicate that neonatal T cells can respond to antigen stimulation in vitro and in vivo and that priming with antigen stimulates both

Th1 and Th2 responses. However, the secondary response of neonates is biased to Th2 responses. The biased neonatal Th2 response may be related to IL-2-induced apoptosis of Th1 cells in a recall response.

10

Expression of MHC Molecules in Neonates

1. INTRODUCTION

Whereas B cells recognize the epitopes on native antigens, T cells recognize only peptides derived from the processing of antigen by antigen-presenting cells (APCs) in association with major histocompatibility complex (MHC) molecules. Therefore, the expression of MHC molecules on APCs and the ability of APCs to process the antigens play a crucial role in the activation of T cells, which are the effectors of cell-mediated immunity (CMI).

In Chapter 9, we presented a multitude of evidence demonstrating that antigens can activate neonatal T cells. These results indicate that the low CMI response of neonatal T cells can not be attributed to T cell immaturity but rather to Th2 dominance. Other possible explanations for the low CMI response in neonates include poor (or absent) expression of MHC molecules and/or poor capacity to process the antigens *(954)*.

2. NEONATAL EXPRESSION OF MHC CLASS I MOLECULES

MHC class I genes encode highly polymorphic molecules expressed on the surface of somatic cells that present short peptides mainly to CD8 T cells. The peptides are derived from endogenous proteins degraded in the cytosol by the multicatalytic proteasome lmp2 and lmp7 subunits and are transported into endoplasmic reticulum by TAP molecules, which deliver the peptides to class I molecules. In all vertebrate species, class I MHC molecules are heterodimers composed of a heavy chain noncovalently linked to β-2 microglobulin *(955)*.

Few studies have examined the expression and the density of class I molecules at the surface of somatic cells. The majority of studies on the expression of class I molecules on the surface of APCs have examined how APCs present class I-peptide complexes to CD8 T cells. In low vertebrate species, the expression of class I molecules during ontogeny has been thoroughly investigated in amphibians. Therefore, the expression of class Ia (the equivalent of mammalian class I) and class Ib (the equivalent of CD1) molecules was studied by immunofluorescence with alloantisera. Transcript levels of class I genes were

From: *Contemporary Immunology: Neonatal Immunity*
By: Constantin Bona © Humana Press Inc., Totowa, NJ

also examined by polymerase chain reaction (PCR). Expression of lmp7, a component of proteasomes required for antigen processing, was also examined.

Immunofluorescence and immunoprecipitation studies detect class I molecules on Xenopus thymus epithelium but not in other tissues until the climax stage of the metamorphosis *(956)*. PCR studies of class I gene transcription indicate that the expression is not simultaneous in all tissues. Whereas class I transcripts are present in tadpole intestines, lungs, and gills, no class I transcripts can be detected in the thymus or spleen until after the metamorphic climax. The expression dramatically increases in all tissues after metamorphosis. In contrast, lmp7 was expressed at all stages of development *(957)*. Thus, in Xenopus, class I molecules are differentially expressed during ontogeny in concert with reorganization of many tissues at the metamorphosis stage.

In mice, class I molecules are expressed by inner cells at the late blastocyte stage but only at low levels on trophoblasts *(958)*. At d 12 of gestation, class I molecules appear in most embryonic tissues such as the gut, lung, limb bud, and heart; they appear in the kidney and gonads at d 15 of gestation *(959)*. The increased expression of class I molecules during embryonic life parallels the development of the immune system.

The expression of class I molecules on neonatal dendritic cells was studied by measuring their ability to prime cytotoxic T lymphocytes (CTL), which recognize peptides in association with class I molecules. Immature neonatal dendritic cells exhibited similar efficacy of uptake and processing of foreign antigen as their adult counterparts. In addition, dendritic cells from 7-d-old mice that were loaded with an L^d-restricted epitope 118 to 126 from the nucleoprotein of lympho choriomeningitis murine virus (LCMV) stimulated the activation of a CD8 T-cell hybridoma bearing a T-cell receptor (TCR) that is specific for this peptide. Furthermore, in vivo experiments demonstrated that neonatal dendritic cells were able to prime CD8 cells *(960)*. In these experiments, freshly purified neonatal CD11c$^+$ dendritic cells were pulsed with 118 to 126 peptide and then injected into adult syngeneic mice. Five days later, the CTL activity was measured. The magnitude of cytotoxic response in adult mice injected with neonatal peptide-pulsed dendritic cells was similar to that induced by the injection of adult dendritic cells *(961)*. These results demonstrate a high capacity of neonatal dendritic cells to induce a CTL response and strongly suggest that neonatal dendritic cells express sufficient class I molecules for efficient presentation of peptides to CD8 T cells.

There is little information regarding the expression of class I molecules during human fetal development. There is a report that very small numbers of MHC class I-positive fetal cells can be detected by FACS analysis at 6 to 8 wk of gestation *(961)*. Immunostaining with antimonomorphic antibodies indicates that class I molecules have widespread reactivity with both epithelial and hematopoietic cells during mid-trimester of gestation. The immunostaining results corroborate data from immunoprecipitation and PCR assays that indicate that HLA-A, -B, and -C class I proteins were not expressed in fetal livers, whereas nonclassical class I proteins such as HLA-F were expressed *(962)*. There is also compelling indirect evidence that MHC class I molecules are expressed in fetal life. First, maternal alloantibodies against the paternal class I antigens are detected in multiparous women. Such antibodies can be induced by the shed fetal class I molecules. Processing and presentation of peptides derived from fetal class I antigens would lead to activation of Th cells and production of antibodies against fetal MHC molecules *(963)*.

A second line of indirect evidence is the detection of adult-like CD8 T-cell responses in human fetuses with a congenital infection of *Trypanosoma cruzi*. The tremendous expansion of CD8 T cells was associated with major phenotypic changes, which were closely related to acquired effector functions by CD8 T cells, such as production of interferon (IFN)-γ and synthesis of high amounts of perforin *(964)*.

The *in utero* CD8 T-cell response of congenitally *T. cruzi*-infected newborns resembles the strong antigen-specific CD8 expansion observed in adults. This similarity indicates that this response results from the presence and presentation of antigens by class I molecules expressed in fetuses.

3. EXPRESSION OF MHC CLASS II MOLECULES DURING FETAL DEVELOPMENT IN NEONATAL ANTIGEN-PRESENTING CELLS

An MHC class II molecule is a heterodimer of two glycoproteins: α-chain of 34 kDa and β-chain of 29 kDa. Genes in the MHC locus encode both chains. Class II molecules are integral membrane proteins with intracellular and extracellular domains separated by a hydrophobic transmembrane fragment. The extracellular segment is composed of two domains. The outermost domain, encoded by α1 and β1 exons, has an immunoglobulin-like structure containing hypervariable residues that are responsible for allelic polymorphism and the binding of peptides. Class II molecules present the peptides that result from the processing of foreign antigen (reviewed in ref. *965*) and self-antigens (reviewed in ref. *966*) to CD4 T cells.

In contrast to class I molecules, which are expressed in all somatic cells, the class II molecules are constitutively expressed in professional APC, namely, macrophages, B cells, and dendritic cells. Figure 39 illustrates class II molecules on the surface of a rat macrophage detected with gold-labeled anti-class II antibodies. In certain conditions, other cell types, including myoblasts *(967)*, eosinophils *(55)*, epithelial cells of renal proximal tubule *(968)*, microglial cells *(969)*, astrocytes *(970)*, and intestinal epithelial cells *(971)*, can express class II molecules and present peptides.

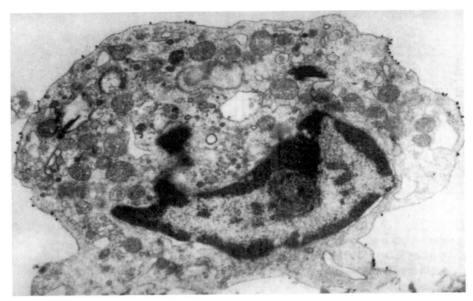

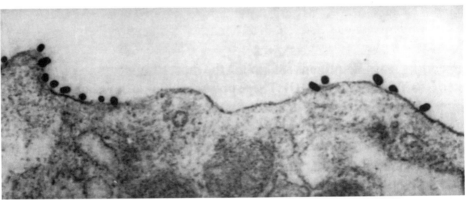

Fig. 39. Electron micrograph demonstrating the expression of MHC class II molecules on macrophages. Macrophages were incubated with gold-labeled anti-class II antibodies. Upper panel, gold particles appear as small black dots on the surface of an activated macrophage. Lower panel, higher magnification of a segment of the membrane. (From Bona C, Bonilla F. Textbook of Immunology. Harwood Academic Publ USA 1990, p. 225.)

There is a hierarchy in the ability of professional APCs to process and present antigens. In sum, the expression of class II molecules represents a potential important factor affecting the ability of APCs to generate peptides and present them to CD4 T cells.

3.1. Macrophages

Studies in mice demonstrate that both class II MHC expression and antigen presentation are defective in neonatal macrophages when compared to macrophages of adult mice *(972)*. Lu et al showed in various inbred murine strains that whereas 29% of peritoneal macrophages express class II molecules, only 2 to 9% of 7- to 10-d-old mice express class II antigens *(973)*. Low expression of class II antigens by neonatal macrophages correlated with an inability of those macrophages to stimulate Listeria-specific T lymphocytes when exposed to heat-killed Listeria. The macrophages obtained from 4-, 10-, and 15-d-old mice exhibited a reduction to 4.5, 8.4, and 11%, respectively, of the level of the proliferation of Listeria-specific T cells incubated with adult macrophages *(973)*. These results demonstrate that peritoneal macrophages from neonatal mice do not present antigen efficiently and that this is correlated with small numbers of macrophages bearing MHC class II molecules.

Similarly, rat neonatal alveolar macrophages fail to express class II antigens. It is well known that IFN-γ stimulation enhances the expression of class II molecules. The failure of rat neonatal alveolar macrophages was not related to weaker expression of IFN-γ-receptor but rather occurs at transcription level. The signaling events mediated by IFN-γ receptor in alveolar macrophages from 7-d-old rats showed a significant dose-dependent increase of interferon responsive factor (IRF)-1 and IRF-2 expression in response to IFN-γ stimulation. However, the expression of CITA, a transactivator of MHC class II and of invariant chain, was low or undetectable in neonatal alveolar macrophages stimulated with IFN-γ *(974)*.

These findings suggest that low expression of class II molecules in neonatal macrophages may be related to low activation of transcription factors controlling the expression of class II molecules and the synthesis of the invariant chain. The invariant chain is important in class II processing. It binds to nascent class II heterodimers in endoplasmic reticulum and mediates the translocation of class II molecules to endosomes.

3.2. B Cells

The major function of B cells is to synthesize antibodies. In addition, B cells have the capacity to take up antigens, process them, and present the peptides, in association with class II molecules, to CD4 T cells. There are three major mechanisms by which B cells internalize antigen. The first mechanism consists of fluid-phase pinocytosis. The antigen engulfed via fluid pinocytosis are localized within endocytic vacuoles, which fuse with lysosomes. The degradation of antigen takes place in low-density endosomes and lysosomal-dense compartments. The generation of peptides from antigen that are internalized via fluid pinocytosis is slow. It takes about 2 h for the peptides to be expressed on the membrane in association with class II molecules (reviewed in ref.*966*). The process of presentation of antigen taken up by fluid pinocytosis is enhanced by heat shock, which leads to the induction of Hsp70 protein. B cells incubated several hours at 42°C were able to present peptides from purified class II antigen more efficiently than B cells maintained at 37°C *(975)*. This may result from enhanced binding of peptides to MHC molecules mediated by Hsp70, which is a chaperone protein. Alternatively, the heat shock may affect the assembly of the processed Ag-class II complex rather than the quantity of peptide available for class II binding.

The second mechanism of the internalization of antigen within B cells occurs via immune complexes. This is a nonspecific mechanism mediated by the Fc and complement receptors (CRs). Both FcγR and CR2 are expressed by normal B cells. The formation of immune complexes promotes activation of the C classical pathway, which consists of fixation of C3dg onto antibody that interacted with the antigen, and the internalization of complex via CR2. The processing of antigen internalized as immune complexes via FCγR and CR2 leads to peptide-MHC complexes on the cell surface within 15 min after internalization. Thus, this pathway is more efficient than fluid-phase pinocytosis. The binding of immune complexes to both FcR and CR2 favors the expression of CD80, which is a costimulatory molecule required for T-cell activation *(976,977)*.

The third mechanism for antigen internalization is antigen-specific because the internalization is mediated by the B-cell receptor (BCR). The transmembrane region of the BCR is involved in both the internalization process and the intracellular trafficking of BCR-antigen complex *(978)*. The processing of antigen internalized via the BCR and fluid pinocytosis may be different, because the two antigen presentation pathways are differentially inhibited by emitin, a protein inhibitor, and by brefaldin A, which blocks protein export to endosomes from the endoplasmic reticulum. These observations suggest that the internalization of antigen by these different mechanisms targets the antigen to different cellular compartments with the result that they are then processed differently and presented with different efficacy.

Study of the expression of class II molecules on murine fetal cells from 16-d-old embryos showed that the B-cell progenitors, pre-B cells, and immature B cells lack MHC class II expression as assessed by flow cytometry and PCR *(979)*. This is in sharp contrast with pre-B cells from the bone marrow of adult mice, in which approx 90% express class II molecules *(980)*. Cell surface expression of class II molecules was measurable at birth and increases rapidly, reaching the level of adult by d 10 *(981)*. However, acquisition of the ability to process the antigen occurs later—at 18 d in the case of antigens internalized by fluid-phase pinocytosis and at 28 d in the case of antigens internalized via the BCR *(982)*.

The expression of class II molecules in neonatal B cells is increased by culturing the cells in presence of anti-IgM antibodies and interleukin (IL)-4 but not by anti-IgM antibodies alone *(983)*.

A cursory glance at the current evidence indicates that ability of neonatal B cells to process and present antigen is weaker than that of adult B cells. This was clearly shown in an experiment comparing the ability of young (3- to 28-d-old) and adult B cells to stimulate the proliferation of antigen-specific T cells *(984)*. The T-cell proliferation response using B cells from 3-d-old mice was less than 20% of the adult response, and adult-like presentation was not seen until the mice were 28 d *(984)*. It is still not clear whether the weaker capacity of neonatal B cells to present antigen is related to the fact that in immature B cells, class II molecules contain smaller amounts of peptides or that immature B cells do not develop class II transactivator CITA compared to adult B cells.

3.3. Dendritic Cells

Dendritic cells are the most potent class of professional APCs. In mice, dendritic cells are a heterogenous population characterized by two functionally different stages of differentiation. Immature dendritic cells are able to capture antigen but display poor capacity to stimulate naïve T cells. After the uptake of antigen and activation by microbial and inflammatory stimuli, the dendritic cells mature, a process associated with upregulation of the expression of class II and costimulatory molecules and ability to stimulate the proliferation of T cells.

Dendritic cells isolated from 3-d-old mice exhibit a similar morphology as those isolated from the spleen of adult mice, but fail to express the dendritic cell-specific marker CD11c *(984)*. In contrast, dendritic cells from 7-d-old mice express CD11c and similar levels of MHC class II and CD40, CD80 and CD86 costimulatory molecules as adult dendritic cell *(960)*. The plasmocytoid CD11c and $CD8\alpha^+$ are completely absent at birth and they gradually appear between 3 to 21 d of age (2 to 3% in 3 to 7-d old, 11 to 16% in 14-d and 21-d-old) reaching the level of adult mice (25%) at d 28 *(984)*. Following in vitro stimulation with lipopolysaccharide (LPS), neonatal dendritic cells mature rapidly like the adult dendritic cells with marked increase in surface expression of class II, CD40, CD80 and CD86 molecules *(960)*.

Neonatal and adult immature dendritic cell take up antigen with similar efficacy as assessed by the internalization of FITC-dextran. This demonstrates the efficient endocytic capacity of neonatal dendritic cells *(960)*.

Study of antigen presentation by neonatal dendritic cell was investigated by measuring the ability to stimulate T cells specific for foreign or alloantigens. These studies showed that dendritic cell isolated from mice which were less than 28 d old were less effective in stimulating the proliferation of T cells *(984)*. Similarly, human dendritic cells from cord blood are less effective than adult dendritic cells at supporting the proliferation of T cells in response to antigeneic or allogeneic stimulation. The mechanism responsible for poor stimulatory capacity of cord blood dendritic cells is unclear, however, it might result from reduced expression of class II molecules *(985)*.

Langerhans cells (LCs) represent a subset of dendritic cells located in the skin. LCs have been identified in fetal skin at d 19 of gestation by their expression of MHC class II molecules and cytological properties *(986)*. However, the Birbeck granules, a marker of maturation of LCs, are not detectable until d 4 postpartum *(987)*. Although LCs within neonatal epidermis from 3-d-old mice express MHC molecules at lower densities, they do not express the DEC205 molecule. DEC205 is first detected by d 7 after birth, and by age 14 d, both MHC class II and DEC205 expression are similar with adult skin. The expression of DEC205, which functions as an endocytic lectin-type receptor, correlates with antigen uptake of fluorescent haptens. Immaturity of neonatal LCs also correlated with a contact sensitivity response. Although the immune response of mice sensitized at age 14 d is not significantly different to that observed in adult mice, animals sensitized after birth or at age 7 d give significantly lower responses *(988)*.

These observations indicate that there is a sequential maturation of LCs after birth that is characterized by an initial expression of class II molecules, followed by occurrence of Bierbeck granules and the expression of DEC205 molecules, which correlates with a contact sensitivity response reaching the adult level by 14 d after birth. Taken together, these results suggest that there is a direct correlation between the expression of MHC class II molecules on neonatal APCs and their ability to function as efficient APCs. Neonatal dendritic cells rapidly acquire the phenotypic and functional properties of adult dendritic cells during postnatal life and are able initiate CMI responses.

11

Neonatal Cytokine Network

1. INTRODUCTION

The concept of network in physiology may be conceived abstractly as consisting of a set of cells or organs connected pairwise by one or more binary relations that determine the traffic of information between them. This concept resembles the semiotic supra structural phenomena in which the word represents the signal that transmits the message.

In semiotics, like in the physiological network, the structural message is composed of source → transmiter (signal) → receiver (interpreter) → message → destinee, which is an interpretant. In physiology, the networks could be divided into two categories: systemic and local.

There are numerous systemic networks. I would like to give as an example two familiar and vital physiological network systems.

The first example is the hypothalamus, pituitary gland, and corticoadrenal gland axis. The hypothalamus produces corticthrophin-releasing factor, which stimulates the production of ACTH by the anterior pituitary gland, which in turn induces the synthesis of corticoid hormones by the corticoadrenal gland. The corticoid hormones exert positive regulatory function on various somatic cells and negative feedback effects on both the hypothalamus and pituitary gland.

The immune network concept proposed by Jerne *(48)* represents a second good example. This concept envisions that the immune system in a steady state is based on the interaction of every member of the system with one or another member through a binary relation, leading to mutual regulation of their expression. In the immune network, the idiotype represents the signal. The idiotype signal is contained in an internal dictionary used by lymphocyte clones to communicate, or speak to each other.

In semiotics terms, the message in immune network is rather like a text, because it represents a set of signals (i.e., idiotypes) that connect the lymphocytes bearing receptors specific for the entire world of foreign and self-antigens. As in structural semiotics, in the immune network, the major characteristic

From: *Contemporary Immunology: Neonatal Immunity*
By: Constantin Bona © Humana Press Inc., Totowa, NJ

of the interpreter—namely, the lymphocyte—is that it is able to specifically select a definitive information input because of the specificity of its receptor, which is encoded by a genetic program performed during the development and contained in the structure of variable genes encoding the lymphocyte receptor *(989)*. The same interpreter-lymphocyte could develop a response to a specific signal; however, it could also develop a response to many other signals contained in a common text such as cross-reactive epitopes or idiotopes.

In contrast to the systemic network, the cytokine network is localized, consisting of a set of cells of one or several phenoytpes that communicate with each other by means of cytokines *(115)*.

The producer may secrete one or several cytokines, and the receiver cell sits in a milieu of a soup of cytokines. The cells are able to select the cytokine signal by virtue of the corresponding receptor that they are bearing. The cytokine receptor generally exhibits high affinity for a particular cytokine. The signal triggers in the receiver cell's specific pathways, leading to the activation of transcription factors, which may activate various genetic programs because of the ability of this factor to bind to the promoters of various structural genes.

In the cytosine network, a given cytosine could deliver multiple signals for other cells or possibly even autosignal genetic programs. It is noteworthy that the same cytosine signal may activate a genetic program in one cell and still exhibit inhibitory capacity in that cell or in a different cell *(990)*.

An important characteristic of the cytokine network consists of a high degree of redundancy and pleiotropy. Redundacy is explained by the fact that a given cytokine that binds to its private receptor can still bind to a public receptor used by other cytokines *(990)*. Pleiotropy of the cytokine network results from the capacity of a cytokine to trigger one or several signaling pathways, leading to activation and/or inhibition of different genes. Table 29 illustrates the complexity, redundancy, and pleiotropy of the cytokine network.

The cytokines produced by the fetus and placenta play an important role in the development of both innate and adaptive immunity and contribute to fetal protection against infections. During postnatal life, the cytokines represent the major link between innate and adaptive immunity.

It is well known that human neonates are markedly more susceptible to infections. Several hypotheses were proposed to explain increased susceptibility to infections, such as decreased phagocytic capacity of macrophages *(991)*, low complement levels *(992)*, immaturity and/or low number of memory CD45RO+ T cells *(993,994)*, and reduced capacity to produce cytokines.

Reduced production of inflammatory cytokines may represent a crucial element in neonatal bacterial sepsis and the high prevalence of complications secondary to infection, which could represent a major factor in neonatal morbidity and mortality *(995–997)*.

Therefore, investigation of the neonatal cytokine network may provide clues for understanding the increased susceptibility to infections of neonates.

2. CYTOKINES DURING FETAL DEVELOPMENT

Cytokines produced by the fetus and those produced at the maternal–fetal interface are of considerable interest for understanding the development of the immune system. In earlier phases of development, the fetus depends mostly on innate immunity; in later phases, the immune system develops, and the infant depends on adaptive immunity.

In humans, it is believed that Th2 cytokines are predominant at the maternal–fetal interface. More recent studies on the expression of cytokines in decidual macrophages and trophoblasts showed that the pattern of cytokine production is more complex.

The earliest form of fetal immune response is mediated by monocyte-macrophages, which play an important role in both embryonic remodeling processes and in fetal defense reactions. The CD14$^+$ decidual macrophages spontaneously produce more tumor necrosis factor (TNF)-α than blood macrophages as well as interleukin (IL)-10 amounts that are four times greater. The synthesis of both cytokines is increased upon in vitro exposure to lipopolysaccharide (LPS). The exposure of decidual macrophages to LPS upregulates the synthesis of IL-1β but not of transforming growth factor (TGF)-β. Because none of these cytokines have been detected in CD14$^-$ decidual cell preparation, it was concluded that they are produced by CD14$^+$ decidual macrophages *(997)*. IL-10 was also detected in human chorionic villi in the first trimester of gestation *(998)*. Transcripts of IL-2, IL-1β and IFN-γ were detected in first trimester decidua *(999)*, and transcripts of IL-4 and IL-13 were detected within placenta during wk 16–27 of gestation *(1000)*. These observations indicate that the balanced expression of both Th1 and Th2 cytokines is important for several reasons. First, it suggests that there is a bidirectional relationship between two sides of the fetoplacental unit that crosstalk via cytokines. Second, it indicates that the presence of Th1/Th2 cytokines may balance because the cytokines downregulate each other, and their expression depends on spatially and temporally different microenvironmental signals during various stages of development.

Fetal macrophages differentiate from common myeloid precursors without passing through the stage of promonocyte or monocyte. A significant proportion of them produce IL-8 at a higher level than adult macrophages. In vitro LPS stimulation increases the number of cells and the level of IL-8 synthesis. The addition to the cultures of IL-11 decreases the production of IL-8 *(1001)*. In contrast, a lower number of fetal macrophages and cord blood monocytes produces lower levels of IL-4 and TNF-α *(1001–1003)*.

Table 29
Structure of the Cytokine Network

Producer	Signal	Receiver (target cells)	Destinee (interpretant-function effect)
Monocytes, macrophages	IL-1	Thymocytes, endothelial cells, myocytes, adipocyte, liver, hypothalamus	Activation of lymphocytes, up regulation of cytokine synthesis, stimulates fibrinogen and CRP synthesis
CD4 T cells	IL-2	CD8 T cells, NK B cells stimulates Ig synthesis	Proliferation of T/NK/B cells, growth of CD8 T cells,
Macrophages, CD4 T cells	IL-3	Macrophages, B/T cells, eosinophils, basophils, HSC T/NK precursors, neural cells	Increases differentiation of HSCs, stimulates phagocytosis, degranulation of mast cells activation of macrophage/eosinophils
CD4T cells, mastocytes, NK T cells	IL-4	T/B cells, macrophages endothelial/LAK cells,	Activation of B cells, class switching, differentiation of mast cells, proliferation of T, and LAK cells, neutrophil activation, monocyte synthesis of IL-1/TNF-α, collagen synthesis
T cell	IL-5	B cells, eosinophils	B-cell differentiation, IgA synthesis, eosinophil development
T cell, monocytes, fibroblasts, hepatocytes, mastocytes, Endothelial cells	IL-6	B/T cells, hepatocytes macrophages	B-cell growth, Ig synthesis, proliferation of immature T cells macrophage activation

(continued)

	Source	Target	Function
IL-7	Stromal cells bone marrow, thymic epithelium	T/B-cell progenitors	Proliferation of T/B-cell precursors
IL-8	Monocyte-macrophages, endothelial cells, keratinocytes, fibroblasts, chondrocytes	T/NK cells, mastocytes monocytes, eosinophils, neutrophils	Chemotaxis, neutrophil degranulation, mastocyte histamin release
IL-9	Activated Th2 cells	T/B cells, mastocytes eosinophils, neuronal precursors myeloid precursors, megakariocytes	Proliferation of T cells, mastocytes, eosinophils, B cells, Ig production, differentiation myeloid precursors, differentiation of megakariocytes
IL-10	CD4 T cells, B cells, monocytes, placentas	T/B cell, NKs monocyte-macrophages mast cell precursors	B-cell proliferation, IgG and IgA synthesis, NK production of IFN-γ and TNF-α CD8 T-cell chemotaxis, T-cell activation, differentiation mast cell precursors
IL-11	Bone marrow stroma, osteoclas, alveolar cells	plasma cells, osteoclasts megakariocytes	Megacariocytopoiesis, plasma cell monocytopoiesis
IL-12	Monocyte-macrophages dendritic cells	Th1/CD8T/NK/LAK cells	Activation of CD8 T/NK, cells increases LAK activity, generation of Th1
IL-13	T cells	Monocytes, B cells fibroblast	Activation of B cells, IgG1, and IgE switching, monocyte production of cytokines, antigen presentation, ADCMC collagen synthesis

(continued)

Table 29 (*continued*)
Structure of the Cytokine Network

Producer	Signal	Receiver (target cells)	Destinee (interpretant-function effect)
T cells	IL-14	B cell	B-cell growth and activation, Ig secretion by plasma cells
Macrophages	IL-15	T/B/NK cells	B-cell Ig production, activation of T and NK cells
CD8 T cells bronchial epithelial cells eosinophils	IL-16	CD4 T cells monocytes, eosinophils	Growth of CD4 T cells chemoattractant of CD4 T/monocyte/eosinophils
CD4 T cells	IL-17	Stromal cells	Stimulates IL-6, and IL-8 production
Macrophages, dendritic cells, adrenal cells, osteoblablass condrocytes, keratinocytes, astrocytes, microglia	IL-18	CD4 T/NK cells	Differentiation of Th1 cells, NK cell activation, osteoclastogenesis
Th1/NK cells	IFN-γ	NK, macrophages endothelial cells	Activation of macrophages upregulation of class II anti-viral agents
Many tissues	IFNα/β	NK/B cells	NK activation, B-cell activation Ig synthesis, increases synthesis of dsRNA, antiviral activity, innate immunity
T cells, macrophages	TGF-β	T/B/NK/LAK cells, fibroblasts	Inhibits division of T/B cells, inhibits cytotoxic activity of T/NK cells LAK

Fetal T cells are unable to produce IL-2, IL-4, IFN-γ and TNF-α. Whereas TNF-α synthesis is increased subsequent to in vitro stimulation with PHA, no significant increased level of IL-2, IL-4, and IFN-γ was observed after stimulation with mitogen. In contrast, fetal T cells exhibited a spontaneous secretion of IL-10 and IL-6, which was enhanced by PHA stimulation *(1003)*. Spontaneous production of IL-13 was first observed in T cells from week 27 of gestation but was undetectable after week 37 of gestation *(1000)*. Thus, it appears that IL-6 and IL-8 proinflammtory cytokines that are involved in innate immune reactions are produced by fetal T cells before the synthesis of cytokines that are involved in adaptive immunity. In addition to inflammatory processes, the IL-6 is also an important cytokine that supports the expansion of myeloid cells during development. It is noteworthy that IL-6 and TNF-α are also synthesized by fetal macrophages *(1001,1002)*.

3. CYTOKINE SECRETION IN PRETERM INFANTS

Prematurity is a leading cause of perinatal morbidity and mortality. Preterm infants exhibit a 120-fold greater risk of death than term infants. The production of cytokine by mononuclear cells of preterm infants depends on two factors: the method of delivery (i.e., spontaneous vaginal delivery, elective cesarean section, emergency cesarean section) and neonatal bacterial infections. Extremely preterm infants may exhibit respiratory distress (apnea, bradycardia, and cyanosis), which can influence the pattern of cytokine production. In comparison with term infants, preterm infants are more frequently born after intrauterine infections. It is estimated that 20% of preterm infants are born to a mother with intra-amniotic infections associated with high levels of cytokines in amniotic fluid and umbilical cord blood *(1004)*.

Measuring the concentration of cytokines in serum of umbilical cord blood or in vitro stimulated cord blood mononuclear cells showed that premature neonates produce spontaneously similar levels of IL-1 but much less TNF-α. IL-6, and IL-8 proinflammatory cytokines compared to adults *(1005,1006)*. The synthesis of IL-6 and IL-8 and the stimulation of monocytes from both > or < 32 wk preterm infants is increased on in vitro LPS *(1006)*. This is in sharp contrast with the monocyte preterm infants with proven infection in which IL-6 and IL-8 serum concentration or cytokine production by monocytes was significantly higher compared to term infants. *(1006–1008)*. It is noteworthy that discordant results were reported concerning the levels of TNF-α in preterm infants with clinical sepsis. Although some investigators *(1009)* have found that the levels of TNF-α are normal, others have found higher concentrations in cord blood serum of pre1term infants with sepsis *(1009)*. Finally, McCloy et al. *(1010)* reported that IL-13 was undetectable in the serum of term infants but was detectable in low amounts in 70% of preterm infants and exhibited high levels in preterm infants with sepsis. Higher levels of IL-11 in preterm infants with sepsis may be important for understanding the defense reactions in these infants, because IL-11 is an important counterinflammatory cytokine. Increased concentration of IL-6 and IL-8 in amniotic fluid resulting from chorioamnionitis in the presence of acute deciduitis, chorionic vasculitis, and funisitis may have diagnostic value for fetal infections.

4. CYTOKINE PRODUCTION IN NEWBORNS WITH FETAL INFECTIONS

In utero exposures to antigens generally induce tolerance. However, there are numerous observations demonstrating that congenital infections stimulate fetal immune responses characterized by increased IgM synthesis and the number of CD45RO$^+$ T cells representing the memory cells. In fetal and newborn cord blood, CD45RA T cells are predominant. The presence of memory T cells exhibiting CD45R0 phenotype is considered a marker of congenital infections *(1011)*. The mechanism by which the fetus is exposed to bacterial or parasite antigens is uncertain but may be related to transplacental transfer.

In contrast to fetal T cells, which do not produce IFN-γ spontaneously or after in vitro stimulation with polyclonal activators, the fetal CD3$^+$ T cells of neonates born at 26–39 wk of gestation with neonatal infection produce higher levels of IFN-γ compared to uninfected newborns. The percentage of IFN-γ-producing CD3 T cells correlates with the duration of membrane rupture before the onset of labor *(1012)*.

IL-6 was also found to be increased in the cord blood of neonates with infections associated with morbidity *(1013)*. In contrast, any significant increase of IL-4 was detected in neonates with intrauterine infections *(1012)*

In utero exposure to helminthes and mycobacterial antigens also stimulates the production of IFN-γ, IL-5, and IL-10 cytokines, as assessed by studying in vitro production of cytokines by cord blood lymphocytes from newborn to mother infected with helminthes or *Mycobacteria* in endemic areas. An increased synthesis of IL-5, IL-10, and IFN-γ was noted after stimulation of cord blood lymphocytes with *Schisostoma hematobium* worm and *Brugia malayi* filarial antigens. In contrast, the stimulation with purified protein derivative (PPD) caused an increased production of IFN-γ only *(1014)*.

These findings demonstrate that human fetuses exposed to microbial antigens develop similar patterns of cytokine production as those observed in adults and that prenatal exposure does not lead to tolerance.

5. PRODUCTION OF CYTOKINES BY NEONATAL LYMPHOCYTES

The majority of studies of the production of cytokines in neonates was carried out using cord blood mononuclear cells.

Cord blood lymphocytes are prototypic recent emigrants from the thymus and bone marrow exhibiting some properties that make them different from adult lymphocytes. Thus, whereas in adults the memory T cells expressing CD45RO are predominant, in newborns, the T cells express CD45RA isoforms characteristic of naïve T cells. In addition, molecular studies have shown that the level of T-cell receptor (TCR) excision circles, which is a marker of recent TCR selection, is higher at birth and declines with age *(1015)*.

General strategy to study cytokine synthesis by cord blood lymphocytes consists of measuring the spontaneous production or enumerating the cells containing intracellular cytokines; production of cytokines after LPS stimulation of monocytes or of T cells with polyclonal activators such as anti-CD3 and/or CD28 antibodies; or stimulation with PHA or PBA polyclonal activators, allogeneic cells, or foreign antigen. The interpretation of the results of such studies is complex for several reasons.

First, the response to mitogens of neonatal lymphocytes is comparable to that of adults. In addition, more recent studies have shown that neonatal T cells develop proliferative responses upon stimulation with PPD, *Candida Chlamydia*, and environmental allergens, arguing for the presence of antigen primed T cells in neonates *(1016–1019)*. From this viewpoint, the study of cytokine production subsequent to allogeneic stimulation represents a cleaner tool, because the proliferative response in mixed lymphocyte culture does not require priming but does require antigen recognition similar to recognition of foreign antigen.

The second aspect of complexity of interpretation relates to the expression of cytokine receptors on cord blood mononuclear cells. The expression of cytokine receptors plays a crucial role in the cytokine networks that mediate crosstalking between cytokine-producing cells, because the activating or suppressing effects of a given cytokine depend of the expression of the corresponding receptor. Study of the expression of IL-2Rβ, IL-4Rα, IL-6R, IL-7R, TNF-αR, and IFN-γR on neonatal cord blood cells showed that their expression tended to be lower compared to adults *(1020–1022)*, whereas IL-2Rα and IL-2Rγ were similarly expressed in cord blood and adult lymphocytes *(1022)*. Thus, the level of the expression of cytokine receptors may influence the response to cytokines of cord blood mononuclear cells.

For the sake of simplicity, in this Subheading 5.1., we will present the available information regarding spontaneous or stimulated production of various cytokines by cord blood monocytes, dendritic cells, and lymphocytes.

5.1. Cytokines Synthesized By Neonatal Monocytes and Dendritic Cells

Monocyte-macrophages and dendritic cells exhibit several major functions in the immune response and defense reactions. Their role in adaptive immune response is related to their ability to capture, process, and present the antigen and to modulate the function of lymphocytes. Although the antigen processing process is independent of cytokine production, the immunoregulatory function is mediated by cytokines. Monocytes produce IL-12, IL-15, and IL-18, which induce the production of IFN-γ by Th1 and natural killer (NK) cells. The second function of macrophages is to promote inflammation, a crucial process in the defense reactions against microbes. This function is entirely dependent on production of acute phase and proinflammatory cytokines such as IL-1, IL-6, and TNF-α and on chemokines such as IL-8.

A comparative study of IL-1α and IL-1β production by LPS-stimulated monocytes showed that a lower proportion of cord blood monocytes produce these cytokines compared to adult monocytes (1022,1023).

There is conflicting information related to the production of TNF-α by cord blood monocytes. Recent studies showed that a reduced proportion of LPS- or PMA-stimulated cord blood monocytes produce TNF-α compared to adult monocytes (1022,1024). It is noteworthy that cord blood T cells also produce TNF-α. In contrast to adult T cells, in which TNF-α is produced mainly by CD45RO, CD4, and CD8 T cells, in newborns, it is produced mainly (81%) by CD4 CD45RA T cells (1024).

There is also conflicting information concerning the production of IL-6 by cord blood mononuclear cells. An early report indicated a lower IL-6 production by neonates when compared to adults (1025), whereas others found a normal production (1023,1026). A recent report showed that 3–7 h after in vitro stimulation with LPS, the percentage of IL-6-producing monocytes was much higher compared with adults (63 vs 51%, respectively). The synthesis of IL-6 by both neonatal and adult monocytes is inhibited by dexamethasone (1006).

Taken together, these results indicate that acute phase inflammatory, pyrogenic cytokines are produced by neonatal monocytes.

IL-8 belongs to the "CC" proinflammatory chemokine family, which exhibits chemotaxis properties and activating capacity of neutrophils. IL-8 was found in the cord blood of majority-term newborns (1008). Furthermore, it was reported that a higher number of IL-8 produced cord blood monocytes upon LPS (1006) or PMA (1027) stimulation (84% in neonates vs 70% in adults).

These observations strongly suggest that there is a spontaneous production of proinflammatory cytokines by neonatal monocytes that is enhanced upon in vitro stimulation with polyclonal activators such as LPS or PMA.

IL-12 and IL-18 are key Th1-trophic cytokines that promote IFN-γ synthesis. The production of IL-12p70 is markedly impaired at birth, and it matures slowly during childhood, reaching the adult level after age 12 yr *(1028)*. The production of IL-12 by cord blood mononuclear cells is diminished even after stimulation with LPS *(1029)*. Dendritic cells appear to be the main producer of IL-12 in cord blood. The relative inability of neonatal cells to synthesize IL-12 can be overcome by the provision of cytokines or stimuli that induce the maturation of dendritic cells such as granulocyte-macrophage colony-stimulating factor (GM-CSF) and IL-4 *(1028)*.

Because human neonates are susceptible to group B streptococcal infection, several investigators studied the IL-12 and IL-18 response of cord blood mononuclear cells to streptococcal antigen. Stimulation of cord blood cells with streptococcal antigen produced significantly less IL-12 and IL-18 compared to cells from adults *(1030)*. Less IL-12 production corroborated with less accumulation of IL-12 messenger RNA in neonatal cord blood cells *(1031)*. Inefficient or defective production of IL-12 and IL-18 may play an important role in poor IFN-γ production by cord blood lymphocytes.

5.2. Defective Production of Th1 Cytokines in Neonates

Th1 cells are functionally defined because they do not express a specific cytodifferentiation antigen. They mediate delayed-type hypersensitivity reactions (DTH) and are the effectors of autoimmune phenomena in some autoimmune diseases. The cytokines produced by Th1 play a role in defense reactions and in promoting the growth of other T-cell subsets. Thus, the IFN-γ activates the macrophages, allowing the killing of intracellular microbes, and IL-2 stimulates the growth of CD8 T cells.

It is generally accepted that neonatal Th1 cells are deficient with respect to their ability to produce IFN-γ. Neonatal T cells do not contain intracellular IFN-γ *(1032)* and produce low concentrations after stimulation with PMA (7% in cord blood compared to 39% in adult) *(1033)*, alloantigen stimulation *(1034)*, or stimulation with streptococcal antigen *(1031)*.

The mechanism of deficiency of Th1 to produce IFN-γ is not completely understood. It may be related to immaturity of APCs, which produce low levels of IL-12 and IL-18; the predominance of naïve CD45RA T cells, which may exhibit a different capacity to produce IFN-γ compared to CD45RA T cells from adults; and increased sensitivity to prostaglandins *(1035)*.

Human infants are more susceptible to infection than adults. This is related to both low levels of IFN-γ production and deficient IFN-γ receptor signaling in neonatal macrophages. Marodi *(1021)* has shown that whereas the expression of STAT-1 protein is comparable in cord blood and adult macrophages, the phosphorylation of STAT-1 in response to IFN-γ was significantly decreased in neonatal monocytes and macrophages.

In contrast to the deficient production of IFN-γ, the production and kinetics of IL-2 in stimulated cord blood is similar to activated adult T cells *(1033)* in spite of the fact that the proportion of cells expressing IL-2 was lower in cord blood lymphocytes *(1033)*.

5.3. The Pattern of Secretion of Th2 Cytokines in Neonates

Th2 cells produce multiple cytokines (IL-3, IL-4, IL-13, IL-5, IL-6, and IL-10). Studies carried out in mice show that neonates develop Th2-dominant responses (*see* Chapter 9).

Recent studies also suggest that human neonatal T cells exhibit Th2-polarized responses. In vitro IL-5 production subsequent to allogeneic and polyclonal stimulation with PHA or anti-CD3 antibodies was substantially elevated in neonates compared to adults *(1034)*. Similarly, the production of IL-4 subsequent to PHA or allogeneic stimulation did not significantly differ in neonatal lymphocytes compared to adults *(1035)*, although the number of IL-4-producing cells is lower in cord blood lymphocytes. The lower number of IL-4-producing cells is related to lower frequency of CD45RO T cells in cord blood *(1033)*. IL-13, another Th2 cytokine, is produced in higher amounts by neonatal naïve T cells stimulated with anti-CD3/CD28 antibodies and rIL-2 compared to adult T cells *(1036)*. It is noteworthy that CD8 T cells are the main producers of IL-13 in human cord blood and that they differentiate toward Tc2-like memory cells. High IL-13 production by neonatal CD8 T cells may be related to the intrinsic property of neonatal CD8 T cells to respond differently to microenvironmental stimuli *(1037)*. IL-10, like IL-4, is an anti-inflammatory cytokine. IL-10 is produced by monocytes, CD5+ B cells, and T cells.

Spontaneous or LPS-induced IL-10 production by macrophages was significantly lower in newborns than in adults *(1038,1039)*. However, neonatal CD4+ CD45RA+ T cells produce significantly more IL-10 than their adult counterparts subsequent to TCR ligation with anti-CD3 antibodies. The IL-10 production by cord blood T cells is regulated by other cytokines produced by macrophages. Thus, the addition of IL-1β to cord blood cells stimulated with anti-CD3 antibodies significantly inhibited the production of IL-10 *(1036)*.

5.4. Secretion of Cytokines by Neonatal NK Cells

NK cells mediate innate immune defense reactions against viral, bacterial, and parasitic intracellular pathogens and against tumor cells. In addition, through the ability to produce cytokines and growth factors, they participate in the regulation of hematopoiesis and adaptive immune responses. NK cells differentiate from a T/NK common precursor. A cytometric flow analysis of intracellular cytokines in cord blood and adult peripheral blood showed that there is no significant difference between the percentage of NK cells synthesizing IFN-γ and TNF-β but that those producing TNF-α were significantly lower in cord blood compared to adults *(1040)*. A minor subset of cord blood NK cells produce IL-13 *(1041)* and IL-5 *(1042)*. Cord blood contains NK cells in various stages of differentiation. The relatively immature stage (CD161$^+$ CD56$^-$) produces IL-13, TNF-α, and GM-CSF. The immature precursor in short-term cultures with IL-12 alone or IL-12 plus IL-2 differentiate into mature CD161$^+$ CD56$^+$ NK cells, acquiring the ability to produce IFN-γ without a concomitant decrease of the proportion of IL-5- and IL-13-producing cells *(1043)*.

Functional analysis of cord blood NK cells showed that they exhibit a distinctive response to IL-18 and IL-12 IFN-γ-inducing proinflammatory cytokines. In culture, cord blood and adult peripheral blood cells produced nearly the same level of IFN-γ, which was not augmented after addition of IL-12 alone. However, cord blood NK cells produced significantly higher amounts of IFN-γ subsequent to stimulation with IL-12 and IL-18. Increased IFN-γ production was paralleled by an enhanced expression of IL-18Rα and IL-18Rβ but not by an increased cytotoxic activity against K562 target cells *(1044)*. High response to IL-18 may compensate for the functional immaturity of cord blood NK cells, as it was determined through comparison of the ability of cord blood and adult peripheral NK cells to kill K562 cell lines, which do not express major histocompatibility complex (MHC) molecules *(1045,1046)*.

5.5. Cytokine Production by Neonatal NK T Cells

NK T cells are a subset of T cells that express a limited TCR repertoire encoded by an invariant TCR-α chain (Vα24-JαQ) and a few *TCR*-β genes. NK T cells recognize glycolipid antigens in association with nonpolymorphic MHC molecule CD1d. In adults, NK T cells produce large amounts of both IL-4 and IFN-γ subsequent to TCR ligation, indicating that they may exhibit immunomodulatory capacity *(110)*.

In humans, small numbers of NK T cells exist in cord blood, and their frequency is comparable to that found in adult blood mononuclear cells *(1047,1048)*. Neonatal NK T cells exhibit the memory phenotype CD45RO$^+$ CD45RA$^-$. They differ from adult NK T cells by the expression of CD25 and the lack of expression of adhesion molecules CD62L, CD69, and human lymphocyte antigen (HLA)-DR; however, they express the NK marker NKRP-1A at the same level as adult NK T cells *(1049)*. The fact that neonatal NK T cells express a phenotype characteristic to memory cells suggests that they develop during fetal life in the absence of exogenous stimuli and, given the selective expression of CD25 at birth, that they are activated by a self-ligand.

However, neonatal NK T cells do not produce cytokines after primary in vitro stimulation with a galactosyl ceramide, which is a ligand recognized in association with CD1 molecules. However, after secondary in vitro stimulation with PMA/ionomycin, a sizeable fraction of cord blood NK T cells were able to produce IFN-γ alone or IFN-γ and IL-4 *(1049)*. Lack of production of cytokines by neonatal NK T cells upon primary in vitro stimulation with CD1-glycolipid ligands suggests that they are not completely mature and need an additional second step to become fully mature effector cells of innate immunity.

Dendritic cells could modulate the synthesis of cytokine by NK T cells. Whereas the DC2 subset enhances production of IL-4, the DC1 subset polarizes the cytokine production toward synthesis of IFN-γ. It is noteworthy that whereas DC1 cells stimulate the differentiation of NK T cells subsequent to the ligation of TCRs to CD1d-antigen complex, the DC2 cells induce the differentiation of NK T cells in a TCR-independent manner *(1050)*. The induction of synthesis of different cytokines and the differentiation of different subsets of NK T cells probably results from the combination of various stimuli delivered by TCRs of NK T cells and costimulatory signals delivered by dendritic cells.

In summary, there are important differences in the pattern of cytokine production by fetal and neonatal mononuclear cells. Fetal macrophages produce mainly inflammatory cytokines such as IL-6, IL-8, and TNF-α. Fetal T cells do not produce Th1 cytokines but do produce IL-4, IL-3, IL-6, and IL-10 Th2 cytokines. Cord blood lymphocytes from preterm infants exhibit high synthesis of IL-1 and less production of TNF-α, IL-6, and IL-8; with intrauterine or congenital infection, they exhibit an enhanced production of acute phase cytokines and the synthesis of IFN-γ. This is in contrast with neonatal Th1 cells, which produce low amounts of IL-2 but not IFN-γ. In both humans and mice, the secretion of cytokines by neonatal T cells is biased toward a Th2 response *(1051)*.

12

Cell-Mediated Immune Responses in Neonates

1. INTRODUCTION

Cell-mediated immune (CMI) responses are mediated by T cells. T-cell subsets, such as Th1 and Th2, exhibit various functions. CD4 Th1 cells are the effectors of delayed-type hypersensitivity reactions, producing cytokines such as IFN-γ, which activates macrophage to kill obligatory intracellular pathogens, and interleukin (IL)-2, which promotes the growth of CD8 T cells. Th1 cells also promote class switching of IgM to IgG2. Th2 cells secrete cytokines to promote the B-cell activation and class switching of IgM to IgG1 and IgE. The CD8 cytotoxic T cells (CTLs) lyse cells infected with microbes (viruses, intracellular bacteria, and parasites) as well as cells expressing tumor-associated antigens. Therefore, CMI responses play an important role in immune defense reactions.

For a long time, it was generally believed that newborns exhibit an increased susceptibility to infection because of immaturity of neonatal lymphocytes, deficiency of antigen-presenting cell (APC) function, dominance of Th2 response, and the induction of tolerance. The concept of the immaturity of newborn T cells was supported by the observation that neonatal lymphocytes proliferate less than adult lymphocytes following stimulation of T-cell receptor with anti-CD3 antibodies *(151)*. The concept of high susceptibility to tolerance of neonatal T cells originated from the experiment by Billingham et al. *(607)* demonstrating that injection of newborn mice with allogenic cells prevents rejection of an allograft.

Fervent development of cellular, clinical, and molecular immunology during the past 50 yr has provided new findings leading to the revision of the concept that neonatal T cells can not mount cellular immune responses. These findings show that CMI responses in neonates could be induced in certain conditions by varying the dose of the immunogen, employing new antigen delivery systems, and using cytokines or costimulatory factors. Clinical studies also contributed by demonstrating that neonates and infants can mount efficient CMI responses following natural infections with bacteria or viruses and vaccinations with live-attenuated vaccines.

From: *Contemporary Immunology: Neonatal Immunity*
By: Constantin Bona © Humana Press Inc., Totowa, NJ

2. NEONATAL TOLERANCE TO ALLOANTIGENS IS NOT AN INTRINSIC PROPERTY OF NEWBORN LYMPHOCYTES

The CMI response to alloantigens is responsible for the rejection of allografts. CD8 T cells mediate graft rejection when the graft differs from the recipient only in major histocompatibility complex (MHC) class I alloantigen. Although CD4 T cells do not play a direct role in allograft destruction, they augment the CD8 T-cell activity by providing cytokines, such IL-2, that are necessary for the expansion of CD8 T cells. The CD8 T cells are expanded during graft rejection subsequent to recognition of peptides derived from processing of MHC class I molecules. In contrast, CD4 T cells may mediate the rejection of allografts bearing MHC class II antigens different from those of the recipient.

In the mouse, the precursors of alloantigen-specific CTLs were detected in the thymus of newborns and in the spleen of mice age 3–9 d *(1052,1053)*. It was believed that the precursors of alloantigen-specific CTLs exhibit an intrinsic tolerogenic property at birth, because injections of a high number of bone marrow allogenic cells prevented graft rejection of skin and consequently prevented a CTL response *(607)*. Ridge et al. *(1054)* analyzed CTL induction in female newborn B6 mice injected with male cells and tested the CTL response against male H-Y antigen. In this system, the in vitro H-Y-specific CTL response is completely dependent on in vivo immunization with alloantigen. Like in Billingam's experiment, tolerance was induced after injection of a high number of male cells (i.e., five male spleen cells to one female T cell). However, when females were injected at birth, not with male spleen cells but with male dendritic cells, a CTL response was observed. The CTL activity was detected 8 wk after injection, indicating that dendritic cells from adult males efficiently primed the precursors of H-Y CTLs at birth.

This finding demonstrates that mice receiving dendritic cells from an adult donor were resistant to tolerance induction and that the CTLs were primed to the same extent as adult female controls that were injected with male cells. In addition, this experiment showed that neonatal alloreactive T cells do not have an intrinsic property for tolerization but rather the immaturity of APCs controls induction of neonatal tolerance. It was shown that human cord blood dendritic cells have a poor capacity to stimulate naïve alloantigen-specific T cells compared to adult dendritic cells *(1055)*. The tolerance induced with bone marrow cells might be related to the high number of immature dendritic cells, which are unable to deliver costimulatory signals to alloantigen-specific naïve T cells in newborns. The requirement of costimulatory signals for neonatal naïve T cells to reach adult levels of function is supported by the in vivo requirement of multiple vaccine doses for infants *(1056)* and by the finding that CD40 binding prevents neonatal tolerance *(946)*.

3. NEONATAL T CELLS ARE ABLE TO MOUNT A TH1 RESPONSE IN CERTAIN CONDITIONS

Studies of neonatal T-cell function showed that the response to foreign antigen is skewed toward a Th2 dominant response in both mice and humans. In mice, immunization as early as the first week of life with vaccines such as tetanus toxoid, live-attenuated measles virus, or BCG-induced higher IgG2a antibody response, significantly higher IL-5 production, and lower IFN-γ synthesis by antigen-specific T cells. This pattern of response was maintained in adults, as assessed by measuring the response elicited by boosting with the corresponding vaccines *(645)*. However, recent studies have challenged this concept, demonstrating that under certain experimental conditions or during infection with certain microbes, Th1 responses might be induced in newborns, reaching into adulthood.

Several studies performed on newborn mice documented the ability to induce both Th1 and Th2 immunity. Injection of mice after birth with soluble hen egg lysozyme (HEL) protein induced tolerance; however, intraperitoneal immunization with HEL in incomplete adjuvant expanded cells that produce IFN-γ and IL-5 and favored the synthesis of both IgG1 and IgG2a anti-HEL antibodies *(945)*. The results of this study clearly showed that neonatal CD4 T cells are immunocompetent and that immunization with antigen and adjuvants elicits both Th1 and Th2 responses. A mixed Th1/Th2 response was also observed in mice immunized with a *Helicobacter pylori* extract in either complete or incomplete Freund's adjuvant. Although gastric diseases are typically manifested in adults, infection with *H. pylori*, which causes chronic gastric diseases, occurs in children under age 5 yr *(1057,1058)*. Newborn mice immunized with *H. pylori* lysates in adjuvant exhibit a protective immunity, as assessed by a decreased bacterial load in the stomach, a lower gastritis score, and a higher frequency of cells producing IFN-γ, IL-2, and IL-4 in recall assay *(1059)*.

The induction of neonatal Th1 responses by viruses depends on the replication capacity of virus in the host cells. This was clearly demonstrated in a study of protective immunity induced in neonatal mice by immunization with a single replicative cycle of herpes simplex virus (HSV) called disabled infectious single-cycle HSV variant (DISC). This variant lacks the gene that encodes glycoprotein H, which is essential for infection. Mice immunized 24 h after birth with DISC-HSV-1, but not with UV-inactivated HSV-1 virus, were protected from lethal HSV-1 infection, and the protection could be transferred to naïve recipients with both CD4 and CD8 T cells. The protective effect of CD4 T cells was related to Th1-mediated immune responses by IFN-dependent and -independent mechanisms. The protective function of transferred CD8 T cells might be caused directly by cytolytic activity or indirectly by secretion of IFN-γ cytokine *(1060)*. Similar results were obtained by immunizing newborn mice with a noninfectious strain of Sendai virus TR-5, a cleavage site mutant of F protein. This mutant is resistant to cleavage of functionally inactive F1 and F2 subunits by cellular trypsin-like proteases. Immunization with this mutant induced a mixed Th1/Th2 response, as demonstrated indirectly by production of IgG1 and IgG2a anti-Sendai virus antibodies *(1061)*.

Genetic immunization of neonates also induces a mixed Th1/Th2 response by circumventing deficient induction of Th1 cells during early life. We compared the cellular responses induced by immunization with a plasmid containing the influenza virus hemagglutinin (HA) gene in mice immunized as newborns or adults. DNA immunization protected both neonatal and adult mice from a challenge with a lethal dose of live influenza virus *(643)*. The immunization of adults elicited a Th1 response, whereas that of neonates elicited a mixed Th1/Th2 response. Similar results were obtained in newborn mice immunized with plasmids containing measles virus HA, Sendai virus nucleoprotein, or C fragment of tetanus toxin. In these experiments, the immunization of newborns with plasmids induced adult-like Th1 or mixed Th1/Th2 responses. These responses are characterized by production of IFN-γ by antigen-specific T cells. IgG2a was produced in mice immunized with measles virus HA plasmid, and both IgG1 and IgG2a was produced in mice immunized with a live recombinant canarypox vector expressing the same gene *(644)*.

The induction of Th1 responses by DNA immunization of neonates is related to CpG motifs contained in the plasmid. This was demonstrated by studying the response to hepatitis B virus in newborns. Mice immunized at 1, 3, 7, or 14 d after birth with hepatitis B surface antigen (HBsAg)-containing plasmid, HBsAg in combination with CpG oligonucleotide, or HBsAg in combination with CpG nucleotide and alum produced both IgG1 and IgG2a anti-hepatitis B virus antibodies. However, mice immunized with HBsAg and alum produced only IgG1 antibodies *(1062)*. These findings strongly suggest that the CpG motifs on plasmids that express various foreign genes may circumvent the biased Th2 response in neonates by stimulating the Th1 response. This effect is probably related to the activation of APCs following the binding of CpG to its corresponding Toll-like receptor. CpG binding to its receptor on APCs may trigger the IL-12 production that is required for the expansion of Th1 cells and the upregulation of costimulatory molecules such as CD40, CD80, and CD86. This concept is supported by data demonstrating that the immunization of newborn mice with plasmid that contains the antigen together with plasmid that bears IL-12 or IFN-γ genes enhanced the Th1 response *(1063)*.

In human newborns, the T-cell responses are also biased toward Th2, as illustrated by reduced IFN-γ production in cord blood lymphocytes stimulated with polyclonal activators *(1032,1064,1065)* that reach adult levels by age 12 mo *(1066)*. The defective Th1 response in neonates might be related to a lack of CD45R0 memory cells in the cord blood and/or immature dendritic cells. It is well known that dendritic cells are required for activating naïve T cells. The reduced capacity of cord blood dendritic cells to stimulate Th1 responses may be related to reduced expression of costimulatory molecules; autosecretion of IL-10; and failure to produce IL-12, an IFN-γ-inducing cytokine, even after stimulation with lipopolysaccharide (LPS), which induces dendritic cell maturation *(1055)*. In contrast to adult dendritic cells, cord blood dendritic cells fail to adopt a mature phenotype following in vitro LPS stimulation, as evidenced by lack of upregulation of MHC class II molecules, reduced expression of CD25 and CD83, and minimally increased expression of CD86 *(1055)*. Autocrine synthesis of IL-10 may be another limiting factor. This is illustrated by increased production of tumor necrosis factor (TNF)-α and IL-12 and the capacity to activate Th1 cells subsequent to treatment of dendritic cells with anti-IL-10 neutralizing antibodies *(1067)*. The most striking difference between adult dendritic cells and cord blood dendritic cells entails the inability of cord blood dendritic cells to produce IL-12 upon in vitro LPS stimulation *(1065)*.

Human neonatal T cells have the ability to mount a Th1 response in certain conditions. Yu et al. *(1068)* have shown that in vitro stimulation of cord blood mononuclear cells with *Dermatophagoides pteronyssinus* extract produced significantly increased amounts of IFNγ and equal amounts of IL-4 compared to adult peripheral blood cells. This is associated with the upregulation of the T-bet transcription factor required for gene activation of Th1 cells, followed by increased expression of GATA-3. This result suggests that stimulation of cord blood lymphocytes may trigger the activation of Th1 cells associated with changes in the kinetics of T-bet/GATA-3 expression.

In vivo studies also demonstrated that Th1 responses could be induced in newborns immunized with BCG or in young infants infected with *Bordetella pertussis*. In adults, immunization with BCG induced a Th1 immune response. Study of the cytokines produced by T cells in infants immunized with BCG after birth showed that subsequent to in vitro stimulation with pumped derived protein (PPD), smallpox antigen 85 complex *(1069)*, and 10 kDa antigen, the T cells proliferated and produced IFN-γ but not IL-5 and IL-13, which are produced by Th2 cells. This is in contrast to T cells stimulated with phytohemagglutinin (PHA), which produced IFN-γ, IL-5, and IL-13 *(1068)*. Similar results were obtained in another study that showed T cells from children immunized with BCG after birth produced IFN-γ after stimulation with PPD and exhibited an increased frequency of IFNγ-producing cells similar to that observed in BCG-vaccinated adults *(1070)*. These studies clearly showed that neonatal BCG vaccination induces adult-like Th1 immune responses.

Induction of Th1 immune responses was also reported in 2-mo-old infants infected with *B. pertussis*. An increased production of IFN-γ and an increased number of CD4 and CD8 IFN-γ-producing T cells were observed in lymphocytes obtained from acutely infected children following in vitro stimulation with *Bordetella* filamentous HA, pertussis toxin-specific antigens, or PHA *(1071)*. These results clearly show that lymphocytes from infants are mature and able to develop a Th1 response. The Th1 response induced by BCG and *Bordetella* is related to the activation of APCs by molecules of bacterial origin, such as peptidoglycan in the case of *Mycobacteria* or endotoxin in the case of *B. pertussis*, which bind to Toll-like receptors and activate the APC.

4. CTL RESPONSE IN NEONATES

CD8 CTLs play a major role in CMI responses against viruses and tumor cells. They recognize peptides derived from viral proteins and tumor-associated antigens presented by MHC class I molecules. It was long believed that, because of immaturity, neonatal T cells could not mount a CTL response against viruses, and, therefore, they could not kill infected cells or contribute to clearing the infected cells. Ensuing years have seen numerous findings that murine and human neonatal T cells can develop a CTL response in certain conditions.

We have studied the priming of CTLs in various stages of ontogeny with transfectoma cells that express a chimeric Ig heavy-chain gene bearing an influenza virus nucleoprotein (NP) peptide. The NP of influenza virus contains an epitope corresponding to amino acid residues 147-161 that is recognized by CD8 T cells in association with MHC class I K^d molecule. Through genetic engineering, we constructed a chimeric Ig molecule in which the CDR3 segment of the heavy chain was replaced with the NP147-161 peptide *(1072)*. The chimeric heavy-chain gene was transfected into SP/2 myeloma cells.

Study of CTL priming in adult mice showed that the NP-specific precursors can be expanded following immunization with NP peptide combined with Freund's complete adjuvant or with irradiated transfectoma cells bearing chimeric Ig heavy chain. Precursors could not be expanded with chimeric Ig-NP molecules or with SP/2 myeloma cells coated with NP peptide. In the same study, newborn mice were immunized on d 1, 3, and 5 after birth with 1 mg NP peptide, 150 µg Ig-NP, or 10^7 irradiated transfectoma cells. One month later, these mice were boosted with NP peptide in Freund's complete adjuvant, and 1 wk later, the lymphocytes were cultured with either NP peptide-coated or PR/8 influenza virus-infected cells. The CTL activity was then measured by using target cells coated with peptide. Our results showed that the immunization of neonates with the NP peptide or Ig-NP molecule failed to prime CTLs. In sharp contrast, mice injected at birth with transfectoma cells developed a cytotoxic response after in vitro secondary stimulation with NP peptide-coated spleen cells *(1073)*. These findings show that the generation of viral peptide from a

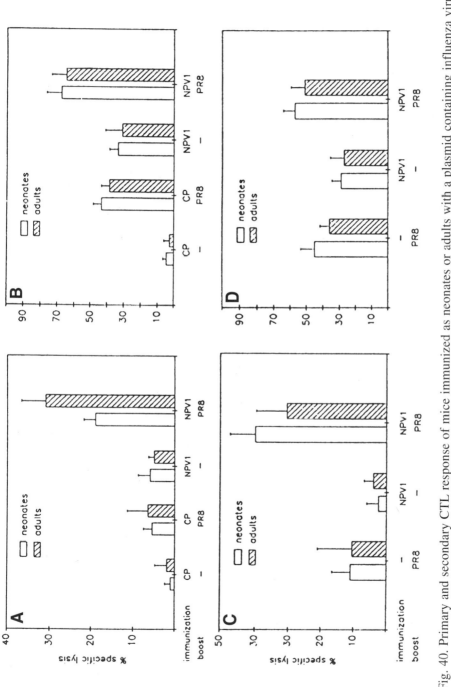

Fig. 40. Primary and secondary CTL response of mice immunized as neonates or adults with a plasmid containing influenza virus nucleoprotein gene. A and C are primary cytotoxic activity. B and D are secondary cytotoxic activity after immunization with empty plasmid (CP), plasmid containing nucleoprotein gene (NPVI), or PR8 influenza virus. (From Bot, et al. Dev Immunol 1998;5:197–210.)

chimeric gene in an endogenous processing pathway efficiently primes neonatal precursors of NP-specific CTLs. Meanwhile, the soluble NP peptide and Ig-NP molecule failed to prime CTLs in neonates, as in the case of adults.

The priming of murine neonatal CD8 CTLs was also induced by immunizing mice after birth with low doses (0.3 or 1 PFU) but not with high doses (1000 PFU) of murine leukemia virus. CTL activity was detected 10–15 d after infection and persisted for at least 28 wk. The inability of neonates to develop CTL responses subsequent to immunization with a high dose results from a polarized Th2 response, which induces humoral immunity. This was clearly demonstrated by measuring the synthesis of IL-4 and IFN-γ. Whereas mice immunized after birth with a low dose of virus produced IFN-γ and low amounts of IL-4, those immunized with a high dose produced IL-4 but failed to synthesized IFN-γ *(1074)*.

Expansion of CD8 CTLs was also reported in mice immunized after birth with polyoma virus, which is a potent oncogenic mouse pathogen. Polyoma virus induced tumors in newborns of an inbred strain resistant to the virus. In the resistant strain, the CTLs specific for MT389 peptide, which is derived from a polyoma viral protein, dramatically and rapidly expanded during acute infection of neonates, reaching adult levels and leading to virus clearance. Although capable of generating MT389-specific CTLs, neonatal mice susceptible to polyoma virus infection cleared the virus at a markedly lower rate *(1075)*.

Efficient CTL immune responses can be induced in neonates by delivering the antigen by naked DNA. Our laboratory first demonstrated that newborn mice immunized with a plasmid-expressing NP of influenza virus (NPV1) developed a significant cytotoxic immunity comparable to that of adult mice immunized with the same dose of plasmid *(641)*. Comparison of primary and secondary CTL activity of mice immunized with NPV1 plasmid as newborns or adults and boosted with PR/8 influenza virus showed significantly higher NP-specific primary CTL activity than that of mice immunized with plasmid or virus alone. In contrast, increased secondary CTL activity was observed in mice immunized with NPV1 plasmid that was a little lower than that of mice immunized with NPV1 plasmid and boosted with PR/8 virus (Fig. 40). Increased CTL activity of mice primed with NPV1 plasmid and boosted with PR/8 virus resulted from an increased frequency of NP-specific CTL precursors, as illustrated in Fig. 41.

The priming of CTLs by NPV1 plasmid was independently assessed by measuring IFN-γ production by T cells from immunized mice stimulated in vitro with NP-peptide in the presence of APCs. Significantly higher amounts of IFN-γ were detected in the culture of T cells from mice primed with NPV1 plasmid and boosted with PR/8 virus than in culture from mice immunized

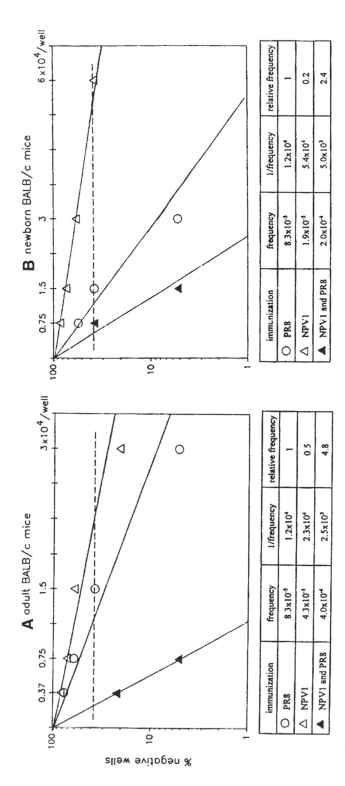

Fig. 41. Frequency of PR8 virus-specific pCTLs in spleens of mice immunized as adults (**A**) or neonates (**B**) with NPVI plasmid. The analysis of frequency of pCTL was carried out 4 wk after immunization with PR8 virus, NPVI plasmid, or both. (From Bot, et al. Dev Immunol 1998;5:197–210.)

A adult BALB/c mice

immunization	frequency	1/frequency	relative frequency
○ PR8	8.3×10^{-5}	1.2×10^{4}	1
△ NPV1	4.3×10^{-5}	2.3×10^{4}	0.5
▲ NPV1 and PR8	4.0×10^{-4}	2.5×10^{3}	4.8

B newborn BALB/c mice

immunization	frequency	1/frequency	relative frequency
○ PR8	8.3×10^{-5}	1.2×10^{4}	1
△ NPV1	1.9×10^{-5}	5.4×10^{4}	0.2
▲ NPV1 and PR8	2.0×10^{-4}	5.0×10^{3}	2.4

Table 30
Effect of Immunization With NPVI Plasmid on Pulmonary Virus Titer
and Survival After the Challenge With LD$_{100}$ Live Influenza Virus

Mice	Immunization	Pulmonary virus titer			Survival
		d 3	d 7	d 16	
Adult					
1 mo	Saline	4.6±0.5	3.8±0.1	NS	0%
after immunization	PR8 virus	0	0	ND	100%
	Control plasmid	4.8±0.1	3.7±0.5	NS	0%
	NPVI plasmid	4.0±0.3	0.9±1.5	0	80%
3 mo	NPVI plasmid	4.8±0.1	0.2±0.2	0	65%
after immunization					
Newborn					
1 mo	Control plasmid	5.9±0	4.6±0.2	NS	0%
after immunization	NPVI plasmid	4.5±1.2	1.2±2.1	0	30%
3 mo	NPVI plasmid	4.1±0.5	0.9±1.2	0	70%
after immunization					

Adult mice were immunized with 3 × 39 μg control or NPVI plasmid at 3-wk intervals in the anterior tibial muscle of the right leg. A group of adult mice were immunized i.p. with PR8 virus 7 d before challenge.

Newborn mice were immunized with 3 × 30 μg with control or NPVI plasmid 1, 3, and 6 d after birth in the right gluteal muscle.

Both groups of mice were challenged 1 or 3 mo after completion of immunization with aerosols containing a LD$_{100}$ dose (1.5 × 10^4 TCID$_{50}$) of PR8 influenza virus.

Pulmonary virus titer was measured by chicken red blood hemagglutination after 48 h incubation of MDCK cells with serial dilutions of lung homogenate. The results are expressed as mean ± SD of log$_{10}$ TCID$_{50}$ measured individually for each animal in a group of three mice.

NS, no survivors; ND, not done.

with virus alone or with empty plasmid (control). Decreased pulmonary viral titers and increased survival after challenge with live virus (LD$_{100}$) was observed in mice immunized as newborns or adults with NPV1 plasmid (Table 30). It is noteworthy that immunization with NPV1 plasmid induced CTL responses against two different influenza type A viruses. This effect might occur because influenza type A viruses that differ in the structure of the HA gene share an identical NP gene *(1076)*.

A robust adult-like CD8 CTL protective immunity was induced by the immunization of newborn mice with plasmid containing DNA clones of murine leukemia virus *(1077)*, NP gene of LCMV *(1078,1079)*, and HA of measles virus *(644)*. In all experiments, the CTL immunity induced by genetic immunization was long-lived and comparable to that induced in adults. These findings clearly demonstrate that DNA-based immunization of mice circumvents the ontogenic delay in development of CTL precursors and may prove an effective and safe strategy for the development of vaccines for infants.

Efficient induction of CD8 CTL immunity by genetic immunization may be related to in vivo transfection of dendritic cells by gene gun *(91)* or subcutaneous *(89)* immunization. Among various types of APCs, the dendritic cells are the most efficient in initiating the immune response of naïve T cells. Bot et al. *(89)* demonstrated that at the site of NPV1 plasmid injection, dendritic cells are transfected. Furthermore, adoptive transfer experiments showed that the expansion of NP-specific CTL precursors with class II$^+$ dendritic cell cells required 10 times less cells than with class II$^-$ cells.

It is known that generating memory CTL cells requires the presence of antigen *(1080)*. Long-lived responses induced by genetic immunization are probably related to the persistence of plasmid as episomes, allowing for continuous priming of newly emerged T cells from the thymus and for generation of memory cells during postnatal life. As an example, in humans, the expansion of HIV-1-specific CTLs was observed in an infant infected *in utero (1081)* and in infants born to seropositive mothers *(1082)*. The HIV-1-specific CTL activity was detected from age 3 mo to 5 yr in the infant infected *in utero* but only during late infancy in some children born to seropositive mothers with overt HIV-1 infection.

Secondary CTL responses were also observed in infants with acute respiratory syncytial virus (RSV) infections *(1083)* and in infants after natural infection or immunization with live influenza A virus *(1084)*. It is noteworthy that no influenza virus-specific CTL activity was detected in infants after immunization with cold-adapted or inactivated influenza vaccines. Failure to generate influenza virus-specific CTLs after immunization with inactivated vaccine is expected, because internalized killed virus is processed in the exogenous pathway, which does not generate peptide able to bind class I molecules. Lack of CTL activity in infants vaccinated with cold-adapted virus may be related to the lower replication rate of virus in vivo. In addition, limited replication in the nasal cavity but not in the lung might decrease the chances of activating CTLs by virus-infected pulmonary macrophages or epithelial cells.

In conclusion, the information presented in this chapter strongly supports the idea that the paradigm of unresponsive neonatal T cells has restricted validity. Neonatal lymphocytes can mount effector and memory cells in certain conditions related to antigen dose, delivery platform of the antigen, and the cytokine microenvironment, particularly the pattern of cytokines secreted by APCs induced by microbial agents. When adequate cytokines are present, the Th2 dominance of the neonatal response can be switched to Th1 responses, mediating defensive reactions against intracellular pathogens.

13
Fetal and Neonatal Tolerance

1. INTRODUCTION

The specificity of lymphocyte antigen receptors resulting from random recombination of several gene segments exhibits an extraordinary diversity that is able to recognize an entire complement of foreign and self-antigens estimated between 100 billion and 100 quadrillion different structures. However, in adult life the immune system does not struggle to distinguish between self- and non-self-antigens, because it learned this distinction during ontogeny. The ability to discriminate between self and nonself is a cardinal property of the vertebrate immune system.

At the beginning of the last century, Ehrlich was one of the first people to conceptualize this property by viewing the immune system as having two shoulders. One shoulder, bearing a light angel, recognizes the foreign antigens, whereas the other shoulder, bearing a dark angel, recognizes self-antigens. Although the response against the horde of aggressive foreign macromolecules of microbes is beneficial, the response against self-antigens is detrimental, leading to autoimmune diseases. Ehrlich coined the term "horror autotoxicus," or poisoning one's self, to define the detrimental immune response against self-antigens *(43)*. The concept of discrimination of self from nonself implied that the body is unresponsive to self-antigens and tolerates them throughout life under healthy, physiological conditions.

Ensuing years have seen numerous observations demonstrating that immune unresponsiveness might also be actively induced by self-, allo-, and foreign antigens. Clonal selection theory *(45)* provided a unifying framework for understanding the lack of response to self-antigens, proposing that the immune system is able to select and eliminate self-reactive clones during ontogeny. Therefore, the unresponsiveness and tolerance of self-antigens appears to be an active process in which some clones are eliminated or prevented from becoming functional. The concept that tolerance is an active process was supported by experiments demonstrating that unresponsiveness can be transferred from a tolerant animal to a lethally irradiated host with lymphocytes *(1085)*.

From. *Contemporary Immunology: Neonatal Immunity*
By: Constantin Bona © Humana Press Inc., Totowa, NJ

The two major types of unresponsiveness are (a) central tolerance and (b) peripheral tolerance. Central tolerance underlines the mechanisms of elimination-deletion of self-reactive clones in central lymphoid organs (such as bone marrow, which generates B cells, and the thymus, which produces T cells). Central tolerance is an active process that requires the recognition of antigens and the deletion of self-reactive clones in an activation-dependent cell death process.

Peripheral tolerance defines the unresponsiveness of clones in recognizing foreign and self-antigens as unable to become functional rather than being eliminated. Several mechanisms were proposed to explain this process.

Anergy is a process in which an antigen-specific clone becomes unresponsive because of an inadequate activation process *(1085)*. This can result from delivery of biochemical signals through an antigen receptor, which is different from those leading to activation or to lack of costimulatory signals. Costimulatory signals are necessary to activate lymphocytes, because this process requires two signals: one delivered by the lymphocyte receptor subsequent to binding of the antigen and the other delivered by molecules associated with lymphocyte or antigen-presenting cell (APC) membranes or by cytokines *(1086)*.

Clonal ignorance is another form of unresponsiveness in which self-reactive clones survive and are functional because not all self-antigens are expressed in the thymus. These cells migrate to the periphery but are harmless and remain ignorant until they are eventually exposed to self-antigens that are normally sequestered in so-called "privileged tissues." Such tissues include the brain, eye, and testes and are localized behind anatomic barriers that prevent the entry of lymphocytes. Following exposure to cryptic epitopes or foreign antigens that mimic sequestered self-antigens, self-reactive clones can be activated and may become pathogenic. Studies performed in transgenic (Tg) mice expressing glycoprotein (EP) or nucleoprotein (NP) of lymphochoriomeningitis virus *(1087,1088)* or hemagglutinin (HA) of influenza virus *(948)* in pancreatic β cells showed that T cells with potential self-reactivity appear to be ignorant to in vivo exposure to these antigens in some peripheral organs.

A third mechanism is mediated by regulatory suppressor T cells. Suppressor T cells have been found to be a major component in tolerance induced by low doses or extremely high doses of protein antigens. Tolerance induced in such conditions can be transferred to naïve recipients *(1089)*. There is increased evidence for the existence of regulatory cells and their role in the prevention of autoimmunity. Weiner and colleagues identified a new CD4[+]/CD45RB[low] T-cell subset (Th3) that secretes mainly transforming growth factor (TGF)-β *(1090)*. Murphy et al. described a regulatory type 1 (Tr1) CD4[+] T-cell receptor (TCR) α/β subset that secretes high amounts of interleukin (IL)-5 and IL-10 and low amounts of interferon (IFN)-γ and TGF-β *(1091)*. Th3 cells can induce a TGF-β-mediated suppression of Th1 autoreactive cells in the absence of CD8

T cells *(1090)*, and Tr1 cells can induce both TGF-β- and IL-10-mediated suppression of CD4 T cells *(1092–1096)*.

The regulatory/suppressor cells are primarily of the CD4 lineage. These cells are generated in the thymus, from which they migrate to peripheral lymphoid organs and expand. Most of these cells are CD62L⁺, a marker characteristic for cells with migratory abilities *(1097)*. Migration of regulatory T cells in periphery does not appear to be antigen-driven, although the presence of antigen in the target organ is instrumental for the suppressive functions of these cells *(1098)*.

Regulatory CD4 T cells (CD4⁺CD25⁺ and CD4⁺CD45RB^{low}) can be distinguished from the effector CD4 T cells based on their phenotype. Regulatory T cells are in an anergic/suppressive state; however, they can acquire markers of activation, such as CD69, in the target organ. In vitro, the regulatory cells can be activated upon polyclonal activation with ConA and IL-2 but not with ConA alone *(1098)*. Development of regulatory cells in the thymus greatly depends on IL-2. Interestingly, CD4⁺CD25⁺ T cells do not consume or use IL-2, however, they suppress IL-2 gene transcription in responder T cells . However, the presence of large amounts of IL-2 reverts their suppressogenic effect, making them autoreactive when transfused into nude mice *(1098)*.

The suppressive property of these cells was studied by reductionistic and subtractive approaches in animal models for human autoimmune diseases. Early depletion of regulatory cells from animals prone to autoimmune diseases led to acceleration of disease onset *(1096–1101)*. Alternatively, the adoptive transfer of regulatory cells into animals prone to or displaying autoimmune disease led to a significant delay or prevention of disease onset *(1097)*. It is typically believed, but not generally accepted, that the CD4⁺ CD25⁺ T cells exert downregulatory effects on autoreactive T cells by cell–cell contact rather than by releasing soluble suppressor factors *(1099)*. Unlike IL-10, the CD4⁺ CD25⁺ T cells do not act by downregulating the expression of costimulatory molecules on APCs and do not kill the responder T cells by the FAS-FASL mechanism *(1101)*.

There is a large body of evidence that both central and peripheral tolerance are induced in B- and T-cell subpopulations during fetal and neonatal life.

2. B-CELL TOLERANCE

The tolerance of B cells can be induced during fetal development and neonatal and adult life. The conditions required for the induction of tolerance in various stages of development and the mechanisms involved are quite different.

2.1. Self-Tolerance During Fetal Life

Central tolerance is the major mechanism operating during fetal development when B cells acquire surface IgM in the bone marrow and are able to interact with self-antigens. Among B cells newly emerged from the differentiation of the precursors, approx 75% are deleted in the bone marrow *(1102)*. Central tolerance can be induced in natural conditions during fetal life by self-antigens, maternal antibodies, or allo- and foreign antigens to which the immune system of the embryo might be exposed.

2.1.1. Central Tolerance in Antibody Tg Mice

For many years, it was difficult to demonstrate the deletion of self-reactive clones during fetal life because of the low frequency of clones recognizing self-antigens. This difficulty was overcome by developing Tg mice, in which the majority of B cells expressed rearranged V genes encoding antibody that is specific for a self-antigen. Because the transgenes can inhibit the further rearrangement of endogenous genes, the Tg mice have a large population of B cells that are specific for a self-antigen and, therefore, represent an excellent model to study self-tolerance. The knowledge acquired from studying self-tolerance in antibody Tg mice was particularly important because it recapitulated the events of tolerance induction, leading to the idea that developing lymphocytes pass through a tolerance-susceptible stage when the recognition of self-antigens causes the deletion.

In one model, Tg mice expressed V_H and V_L genes encoding specificity for major histocompatibility complex (MHC) class I ($H\text{-}2K_k$) molecules *(46)*, double-stranded (ds)-DNA *(529)* for an allelic form of the CD8 self-antigen *(451)*, or B cells producing rheumatoid factors (RF) that recognize self-IgG *(1103)*. In all these Tg mice strains, the B cells specific for these self-antigens were not present in the periphery, indicating that they were deleted in the bone marrow during the differentiation of pre-B cell (sIg^-) to immature B cell ($sIgM^+$) stages *(45,1104)*. When Tg mice expressing the rearranged genes of anti-MHC class I molecules were bred onto an H-2K or H-2B background, large numbers of B cells were detected in the bone marrow but not in the periphery, indicating self-reactive B cells were deleted in the bone marrow *(46)*. In the case of Tg mice expressing V genes with specificity for ds-DNA, the autoreactive B cells were deleted in bone marrow, and those that were not deleted matured in the periphery but lost the specificity for ds-DNA *(529)*. Similarly, high-affinity RF-producing B cells were also deleted in offspring generated from breeding the Tg mice with a mouse strain that produced the cognate self-antigen *(1103)*.

The second model involves double-Tg mice expressing the V genes that encode the specificity for hen egg lysozyme (HEL) and expressing HEL either as membrane multivalent antigen or as soluble oligovalent HEL (reviewed in ref. *1105*). These mice could be considered as a self-antigen model, because HEL was present in the bone marrow or in the fetal circulation. In the Tg mice expressing multivalent membrane-associated HEL, the extensive crosslinking of the B-cell receptor (BCR) on developing B cells resulted in the deletion of

HEL-specific B cells in bone marrow within 15 h. The deletion resulted from the strong antigen stimulation of immature B cells, and the absence of T cells related to immaturity of both T cells and APCs. In the double-Tg mice producing soluble HEL, the B cells were not deleted in bone marrow but were anergized in the periphery. The degree of B-cell tolerance was dependent on the amount of HEL. In a double-Tg strain producing low amounts of HEL, only 5% of BCRs were occupied, and B cells exhibited minimal BCR downregulation, normal function, and a lifespan of 4 to 5 wk. In sharp contrast, the B cells in another Tg strain producing high amounts of HEL, in which 45% of BCRs were occupied by antigen, the B cells were anergic, and the expression of surface IgM and costimulatory molecules was downregulated. Strikingly, the B cells in these mice had a much shorter lifespan (3–5 d) *(1005)*.

Studies conducted in antibody Tg mice strongly support the clonal theory that immature—but not mature—B cells are susceptible to tolerance. From the studies performed in Tg mice, two major conclusions were drawn. First, the recognition of membrane-associated multivalent antigens leads to central tolerance by deleting self-reactive B-cell clones, which could no longer be detected in the peripheral lymphoid organs. Second, the recognition of soluble, monovalent antigen leads to peripheral tolerance, namely anergy. The induction of anergy depends on the concentration of soluble antigen, the occupancy of BCRs, and the expression of costimulatory factors. Anergy is also mirrored in the lifespan of antigen-specific B cells. The expression of costimulatory molecules is particularly important for eliciting T-cell help in response to protein, with T-dependent antigen providing the second signal required for the activation of B cells *(1086)*.

2.1.2. Fetal Tolerance Induced By Maternal Antibodies

Dray *(705)* described the first study demonstrating the induction of a longlasting suppression by maternal antibodies as illustrated in maternal allotype suppression in rabbits. Allotypes are antigenic determinants of Ig and of the BCR of B cells that differ among distinct groups of individuals or inbred strains of the same species. The allotypes are inherited in a Mendelian fashion. Dray showed that in newborn heterozygote rabbits born to mothers immunized against the male's *a* or *b* series allotype, the B cells that produced Ig bearing the paternal allotype were entirely suppressed or expressed in an abnormally low proportion. The suppression lasts throughout the lifetime of the animal, and the suppressed offspring could make antibodies subsequent to immunization with paternal allotype *(706)*. This indicates that B cells producing the paternal allotype were either eliminated from the organs or the synthesis of the paternally marked allotype was blocked. Similarly, the offspring born to mothers producing anti-idiotype antibody exhibited a longlasting suppression of B cells that expressed the corresponding idiotype on their BCR (for details, *see* Chapter 6).

More recently, it was shown that maternal Ig is responsible for deleting B cells that produce RF in Tg mice expressing *V* genes that encode anti-IgG2a RFs. Wang and Shlomchik *(1106)* used a series of genetic crosses to show that maternal soluble Igs in RF-Tg mice are responsible for the induction of tolerance. This tolerance is maintained during postnatal life but remits 2–3 wk postweaning, and cells producing RF can be observed for weeks or months. This may be related to the production of low amounts of IgG2a in naïve mice, which prevents the deletion of newly emerging B cells in the bone marrow during postnatal life.

In contrast to maternal Igs, which induce a longlasting suppression of B cells producing antibodies specific for soluble monovalent antigens, the progeny derived from allophenic mothers preimmunized against an isoform of Thy antigen, which was expressed on the brain surface and on all T cells, failed to suppress the θ antigen in the offspring *(1107)*. This finding indicates that there are important differences between the tolerance induced by exposure to self-antigens and that induced by maternal antibodies during fetal development.

In both systems, fetal exposure to soluble monovalent antigen or to maternal Igs or antibodies induces anergy that is dependent on the concentration of antigen and the degree of occupation of BCRs. The anergy is evident in postnatal life; however, the autoreactive B cells remain thereafter. Meanwhile, *in utero* exposure to membrane-associated antigens induces central tolerance by deleting self-reactive cells, but the maternal antibodies specific for membrane antigens fail to induce tolerance. The mechanism of failure by maternal antibodies to induce tolerance that is specific for cell membrane-associated antigens remains poorly understood.

2.1.3. Fetal Tolerance to Alloantigens

The description of natural tolerance for alloantigens was a crucial finding that contributed to the formulation of clonal theory. The concept of tolerance to alloantigens originated from an "experiment in nature" observed by Owen *(1108)*, who studied blood groups in cattle. Owen noted that supposed monozygotic twins in cattle actually are dizygotic, because fetuses often exchange blood through anastomoses of placental blood vessels. Because of blood sharing by fetuses, each adult twin produces erythrocytes of each other without producing antibodies specific for blood groups. This observation brilliantly demonstrated that fetal exposure to blood groups allowed the twins to tolerate the alloantigen expressed on the red blood cells (RBCs) of twins.

Hasek repeated Owen's discovery under experimental conditions using chickens. In this experiment, synchorial parabiosis was performed between chicken embryos in the egg, allowing blood exchange. It was shown after hatching that the chicks were unable to produce antibodies to each other's erythrocytes *(1109)*. These findings clearly demonstrate that the chimerism established in different vertebrate species during fetal life leads to a longlasting central tolerance through the deletion of B cells exposed *in utero* to alloantigens.

2.1.4. Fetal Tolerance to Foreign Antigen

There are few studies concerning the induction of tolerance by fetal exposure to foreign antigens. Waters et al. *(1110)* reported the induction of tolerance following injection of pregnant mice with deaggregated human γ globulin. *In utero* exposure of offspring via maternal circulation of human γ globulin induced tolerance, which persisted until age 12 wk and then gradually disappeared. It is noteworthy that fetal tolerance induced by foreign Ig delivered by mother during pregnancy differs from classical tolerance induced in adults with high doses of deaggregated Ig, in which both B and T cells contribute to tolerance *(1111)*.

In human newborns of mothers chronically infected with hepatitis B virus (HBV), 22% of infants were unable to produce anti-HBV antibodies after vaccination with HBV vaccine *(1112)*. In the group of infants who were unresponsive to vaccine, HBV DNA was detected in peripheral blood lymphocytes by polymerase chain reaction (PCR). The unresponsiveness of the infants to HBV vaccination was specific, because the infants made an antibody response following vaccination with poliovirus types 1, 2, and 3 and immunization with tetanus toxoid or pneumococcal polysaccharide. This observation indicates that *in utero* exposure to low doses of HBV induced an immune tolerance.

Theoretically, congenital infection with microbes represents an ideal condition for the induction of central tolerance, because the fetal B cells may be exposed to microbial antigens, which under normal conditions do not cross the placenta. However, study of antibody responses in infants with congenital infections caused by mumps *(619)*, *Plasmodium falciparum (620)*, schistosomiasis *(622)*, rubella *(1113)*, cytomegalovirus *(1114)*, and leprosy *(1115)* demonstrated the propensity of human infants to make antibodies when exposed *in utero* to viral and parasitic infections. This may be explained by an acceleration of lymphocyte maturation in human embryos compared to other species.

3. NEONATAL B-CELL TOLERANCE

B cells are divided into two subsets: (a) B1 cells expressing CD5 antigen and producing multispecific antibodies and (b) B2 cells producing antibodies specific for foreign antigens and pathogenic autoantibodies. Both derive from Ig⁻ B-cell progenitors; however, there is a notable difference between the two subsets. Whereas B1 cells develop early in ontogeny and expand by self-replenishment, B2 cells develop continuously from Ig⁻ progenitors in bone marrow cells.

In mice, an important fraction of B1 cells in the peritoneal cavity and spleen produce antibodies specific for bromelain-treated RBCs. This antibody response is oligoclonal and encoded by restricted *V* genes (i.e., Vh11/Vk9 and Vh12/Vk4) *(448,449)*. B1 cells producing such antibodies are easily detected by anti-idiotype antibodies and by binding of liposomes containing phosphatidylcholine (PtC), a major component of RBC membranes.

Studies of the generation of B1 cells in the neonatal repertoire was performed in Tg mice expressing V_H12 and V_K4 transgenes. The development of B1 cells expressing transgenes that encode antibodies specific for PtC was studied in newborn livers and spleens in two Tg lines bearing a low or high copy number of transgenes. B1 cells producing autoantibodies were noted at birth. During the first 120 h of postnatal life, the number of PtC-specific B cells increased 20-fold compared to nontransgenic mice, indicating a strong clonal expansion and dominance of B1 cells in the peritoneal cavity *(1116)*. These B cells express IdX that is recognized by a rabbit anti-idiotype antibody. Kawaguchi *(1117)* showed that during d 4–10 after birth, the injection of anti-IdX antibodies markedly reduced B1 cells. The binding of anti-idiotype antibodies to the corresponding BCR of B1 cells probably delivers a negative signal to significantly inhibit the ability of B1 cells to expand or to produce autoantibodies after lipopolysaccharide (LPS) stimulation.

The induction of neonatal tolerance was described in early studies in which chronic administration of anti-IgM antibodies after birth eliminated immature IgM+ B cells from bone marrow and caused unresponsiveness to foreign antigens *(1118)*. In vitro studies showed that increased tolerance sensitivity of immature B cells did not result from apoptosis but from downregulation of the BCR, which could not be restored after culturing the same cells without anti-IgM antibodies *(462,1119)*.

In the case of B2-cell subsets, neonatal tolerance can be induced by both T-independent and -dependent antigens.

Bacterial polysaccharides are typically T-independent antigens (TI-1). Felton et al. *(1120)* observed that whereas small amounts of pneumococcal polysaccharide induced a protective immune response in mice, higher amounts (100 times more antigen) were unable to produce antibody and the mice died after challenge with a lethal dose of *Streptococcus pneumoniae*. The inhibition was specific, because the same mice were able to produce antibodies following immunization with SIII polysaccharide. The tolerance induced by polysaccharides was described for other antigens injected into neonates, such as dextran *(1121)* and levan *(713)*. The high-dose tolerance induced by T-independent polysaccharide antigen described by Felton was called "immune paralysis," because he considered it owing to persistence of polysaccharide antigens that could not be catabolized in mice. The persisting antigens eventually bind the antibodies and clear them from circulation while the antigen is present in the tissues.

Neonatal tolerance induced by foreign antigens requires smaller doses of antigen compared to those necessary to induce tolerance in adults. For example, the induction of tolerance against bovine serum albumin requires 0.5 mg/kg for newborn rabbits *(1122)* and 500 mg/kg in adult rabbits *(1123)*. The quantitative differences regarding the dose required for the induction of tolerance in neonates may be related to two factors. First, in mice, the number of lymphocytes in neonates is 220 times lower than in adults. The second, more plausible, mechanism is represented by the immaturity of neonatal B cells.

In vitro experiments showed a differential susceptibility of neonatal and adult murine spleen cells for the induction of B-cell tolerance. In this system, the induction of tolerance was studied using TNP17-human γ Ig conjugate. For a suppression rate of 50%, 10^3 more "tolerogen" were required in adult cells than in neonatal cells *(1124)*. Other studies support the concept that high susceptibility of neonatal B cells to tolerance depends on the maturation status of the B cells (reviewed in ref. *1125*). Analysis of neonatal clonotypes producing antibodies specific for haptens or viral proteins *(580–584)* indicated that clonotypes that arise early after birth exhibit a higher susceptibility to tolerogens than clonotypes that arise later in postnatal life. The induction of neonatal tolerance requires crosslinking of the BCR by the ligand *(1126)*. It is noteworthy that the requirement of crosslinking of the BCR by multivalent antigens was not anticipated by clonal selection theory.

Quantitative studies addressing the dose of tolerogen indicate that the amount of tolerogen must exceed a threshold of affinity. Therefore, only B cells that bear a BCR with high antigen affinity to a particular foreign antigen are deleted or anergized, leaving the B-cell repertoire intact for other antigens *(1125)*.

4. T-CELL TOLERANCE

T cells recognize peptides derived from the processing of foreign and self-antigens presented in association with MHC molecules. The T-cell repertoire is generated within the thymus during the process of differentiation of thymocytes from T/NK precursors. The differentiation of precursors into double-negative T cells (CD4⁻, CD8⁻) is associated with a stage of expansion and survival that is controlled by pre-TCR. The pre-TCR is composed of TCR-β and pre-T-α chains that associate with the CD3 molecule but not with proteins encoded by TCR genes of the TCR-α locus. TCR-α genes arrange later when the double-negative T cells progress to the double-positive (CD4⁺, CD8⁺) stage. Knocking out the pre-T-α or CD3 gene arrests the development of double-negative T cells at the stage of CD25⁺, CD44⁻ TCR-α/β⁻ *(1127)*.

The pre-T-α protein exhibits little homology with the TCR-α chain in its extracellular domain; however, the intracellular domain contains polar residues required for association with signal transducing CD3 molecule, which initiates signaling pathways by TCR ligation *(1128)*. This indicates that at the stage of double-negative cells, there is no selection of TCR-β genes, and the pre-TCR delivers signals required for the proliferation and survival of double-negative thymocytes. This leads to differentiation into double-positive (DP) cells, which express a functional and diverse TCR-α/β.

The double-negative thymocytes are the subject of positive and negative selection processes in which the thymus censors the self-reactive T cells. The censoring process leading to negative selection is responsible for central tolerance that is manifested by clonal deletion of self-reactive T cells. The positively selected cells differentiate further into single-positive CD4+ CD8− or CD4− CD8+ T cells that are able to interact with an entire repertoire of foreign antigens.

Apparently, the process of negative selection leading to central tolerance is related to the affinity of the TCR of DP thymocytes for MHC-protein complex. The T cells bearing a TCR with high affinity for peptides are deleted, whereas those with low affinity survive and differentiate into single-positive (SP) T cells, which thereafter migrate to peripheral lymphoid organs. However, a small number of DP T cells escape negative selection, possibly contributing to the initiation of autoimmune phenomena later in the life.

In the periphery, SP T cells may become unresponsive in certain conditions when exposed to low or high doses of antigen *(1129)*. The peripheral tolerance induced during neonatal or adult life results from anergy rather than from the deletion process in the peripheral lymphoid organs. The anergy is caused not only by the degree of the occupancy of the TCR but also by the lack of costimulatory molecules and/or cytokines. This concept is strongly supported by data demonstrating that in the absence of a second signal, T cells became anergic. Thus, T cells incubated with MHC peptide complex embedded in artificial membranes become unresponsive to recall stimuli *(1130)*; however, some cytokines, such as IL-2, can rescue T cells from anergy *(1131)*. The induction/ activation of regulatory T cells may also anergize T cells either by direct contact or via production of immunosuppressive cytokines, such as IL-10 and TGF-β. Furthermore, in vitro studies showed that murine or human CD4+ CD25high thymocytes and peripheral T cells *(1098)*, CD4+ T cells producing IL-10 *(1092–1096)*, or Th3 cells producing TGF-β induced by oral tolerance *(1090)* display immunosuppressive activity on self-reactive Th1 cells that mediate autoimmune diseases.

The neonatal environment favors the induction of peripheral tolerance, because APCs, in particular dendritic cells, express low levels of CD40 and B7 costimulatory molecules. Additionally, neonatal T cells secrete low levels of IL-2 because neonatal T cells are biased toward a Th2 response (reviewed in Chapter 9).

4.1. Tolerance of T Cells During Fetal Life

Clear evidence for clonal deletion to self-antigens has established that central tolerance is the major mechanism for maintaining self-tolerance. The first solid evidence of central tolerance came from pioneering studies reported by Marrack and Kapller *(1132)*, who showed that certain murine strains are tolerant to their own class II molecules. Murine T cells, which recognize class II I-E antigen, all use $V\beta17$ of the TCR-β family. In all strains expressing I-E molecules, the $V\beta17a^+$ T cells were deleted in the thymus and no $V\beta17a^+$ T cells were detected in the peripheral lymphoid organs. The fact that $V\beta17a^+$ T cells in these mice were detected in DP thymocytes but not in SP thymocytes indicates that the deletion occurs within the thymus at the stage of DP cells.

Other evidence came from studies of the TCR repertoire in mice that expressed a given minor lymphocyte stimulating (MLS) antigen haplotype. Originally, four MLS haplotypes were described in mice (MLS^a, MLS^b, MLS^c, and MLS^d), where MLS^b was not stimulatory *(1133)*. MLS antigens were unlike other alloantigens because their recognition by T cells, although dependent on class II molecules, was not MHC-restricted. Different alleles of class II molecules can be present in mixed lymphocyte cultures of the MLS antigen with the same T-cell clone *(1134)*. It was found that mice strains or recombinant inbred strains expressing MLS^a delete T cells from $V\beta6^+$ and $V\beta8.1^+$ gene families, whereas those expressing MLS^c delete $V\beta3^+$, $V\beta5^+$, and $V\beta11^+$ T cells.

Further studies showed that MLS antigens are superantigens, which cosegregate with endogenous mouse mammary tumor virus (Mtv) antigens (reviewed in ref. *1135*). The genetic segregation studies demonstrated that $V\beta11^+$ T cells were deleted by Mtv-8, Mtv-9, and Mtv-11; $V\beta3^+$ T cells were deleted with Mtv-1, Mtv-3, Mtv-6, Mtv-13, and Mtv-44; and $V\beta5^+$ T cells were deleted by Mtv-6 and Mtv-9. Partial deletion of $V\beta6$, $V\beta8.1$, and $V\beta9^+$ T cells was associated with Mtv-44, and Mtv-7 caused total deletion of T cells bearing a TCR encoding family members of these three $V\beta$ genes (reviewed in ref. *1136*). The Mtv antigens were found to be the product of the open reading frame present in the 3'-LTR of murine Mtv. Other studies demonstrated that induction of tolerance to MLS^a-encoded antigen results from intrathymic elimination of $V\beta6^+$ MLS^a-reactive T cells *(1137)* and requires dendritic cells and presentation of Mtv antigens by B cells in the thymus *(1138)*.

A second set of evidence for self-tolerance comes from studies using Tg mice. Pioneering studies were performed by von Boehmer using Tg mice that expressed a TCR encoding the H-Y antigen recognized in the context of class I molecules. All CD8$^+$ cytotoxic T lymphocytes (CTLs) were deleted within the thymus of male mice but were present in peripheral lymphoid organs of female mice, because the H-Y antigen is expressed only in male mice *(1130,1140)*.

The deletion of self-reactive T cells was reported in several Tg mice expressing peripheral tissue-specific proteins on thymic, stromal, or epithelial cells *(1141,1142)*. In one model, pancreas-specific elastase I was also expressed at low levels in the thymus, and it was shown to contribute to tolerance induction. This Tg mouse model, expressing SV40 T antigen in conjunction with elastase I under the control of the elastase I promoter in the pancreas, was crossed with a strain of Tg mice expressing a TCR that was specific for T antigen *(1142)*. The double-Tg mice obtained from this cross exhibited a reduced number of T-antigen-specific T cells in lymphoid organs and reduced Th1 activity with no decrease in Th2 and CTLs, as assessed by in vitro assays.

The induction of tolerance in fetal central and peripheral organs by self-peptides was demonstrated in a study in which a peptide of proteolipid protein (PLP)-encephalitogenic protein, recognized by CD4 T cells in association with I-A^s molecules, was delivered by an IgG2a chimeric molecule. The CDR3 of the V_H gene in the construct used in this experiment was replaced with PLP-derived peptide corresponding to amino acid residues 139–151. By virtue of IgG isotype, the chimeric molecule was transferred to the fetus via the placenta after it was injected into pregnant mothers. The resulting offspring were tolerized to experimental autoimmune encephalomyelitis (EAE), as illustrated by decreased disease severity or relapse when EAE was induced with free peptide in Freund's complete adjuvant (FCA). Interestingly, a chimeric IgG molecule carrying an altered peptide, in which four contacting amino acid residues required for TCR recognition were replaced, was unable to induce a tolerogenic effect *(1143)*.

We have shown that fetal tolerance can be induced by placental transfer of a peptide derived from influenza virus NP. The offspring born to mothers injected with 3 mg of peptide on d 15, 17, and 19 of pregnancy were not able to mount a CTL response 1 mo subsequent to the optimal schedule of the immunization with NP peptide. In contrast, those born to mothers immunized with 100 µg of peptide developed a significant CTL response subsequent to immunization with peptide 1 mo after birth *(1144)*. This result indicates that the quantity of peptide transferred from the mother during fetal development is critical for the induction of tolerance.

The induction of central tolerance is an active process, because the recognition of self-antigen in the context of MHC molecules is essential *(1145,1146)*. Several studies conducted on Tg mice expressing protein antigens within the thymus demonstrated that central tolerance results from apoptosis of DP T cells, mainly in the thymus medulla *(1141)*. These observations corroborate data that DP thymocytes migrate from the cortex to the medulla during thymic differentiation.

In summary, central tolerance within the thymus during development of the T-cell lineage results in deletion of self-reactive T lymphocytes. The deletion process targets DP thymocytes that display an increased density and diversity of TCRs. Deletion is an active process requiring the recognition of peptides in the context of MHC molecules, as in the case of mature SP T cells in the periphery.

4.2. Neonatal T-Cell Tolerance

Longlasting tolerance of T cells resulting from deletion occurs during fetal life within the thymus, which censors self-reactive T cells. However, there is a large body of evidence that not all self-reactive T cells are deleted. Self-reactive T cells that escape negative selection as well as T cells that are specific for alloantigens and foreign antigens can be rendered unresponsive, particularly during postnatal life. Like central tolerance, neonatal tolerance of T cells is MHC restricted, because it depends on recognition of peptides derived from the processing of foreign or self-molecules associated with MHC molecules.

4.2.1. Neonatal T-Cell Tolerance to Tissue Antigens

In vertebrates, the low frequency of T-cell precursors that are specific for a given antigen represents a major difficulty in determining the fate of T cells that are specific for self-antigens expressed in peripheral tissues. Advances in molecular biology have allowed the generation of Tg mice, which provide an excellent tool to address this issue. Such Tg mice were generated using constructs containing various genes expressed under the control of a cell-specific promoter.

Double-Tg mice were developed that expressed MHC K^b-specific TCR and K^b on hepatocytes *(1147)* or keratinocytes *(1148)* or viral antigens on pancreatic β-cells *(1082,1089,1149)*. Studies performed in double-Tg mice that simultaneously expressed K^b-specific TCRs and K^b on hepatocytes under the control of the liver-specific albumin promoter showed that the K^b-specific T cells were tolerant in vivo but could be activated in vitro subsequent to stimulation with spleen cells bearing K^b molecules *(1147)*. This phenomenon, called split tolerance, may result from downregulation of the TCR and CD8 coreceptor in anergized T cells. In double-Tg mice expressing K^b-specific TCRs and H-2^{bm1xka} mutant K^b molecules, CD8 T cells were deleted in the thymus, but $CD8^{low}$ T cells were present in the periphery. The $CD8^{low}$ T cells present in the periphery exhibited split tolerance, indicating that K^b-specific T cells that migrated to the liver after birth were deleted, whereas those migrating to the spleen were anergized.

In Tg mice strains, K^b-specific TCRs and K^b were simultaneously expressed in keratinocytes under the control of the keratin IV promoter. These mice exhibited peripheral tolerance, as demonstrated by the inability to reject K^b grafts. Tolerance induction to skin-expressed K^b antigen appeared to occur only during an early period after birth. This conclusion was supported by an experiment in which Tg mice were injected with anticlonotypic antibody. The animals that received antibody rejected K^b grafts as adults, whereas those that had not been subjected to antibody treatment accepted the grafts. This study established a time frame of 3 to 4 wk after birth during which T cells are sensitive to tolerance because the tolerance was not induced when the K^d antigen was expressed by mature peripheral tissue in the adult environment *(1148)*.

Intradermal trafficking of T cells in the newborn appears to be an important factor in the induction of neonatal tolerance. Treatment with anti-E and -P selectin antibodies during the first 15 d after birth reduced the homing of K^b-specific T cells in the skin and abolished tolerance, as assessed by allograft rejection *(1148)*. The results of this experiment indicate that the blockage of E and P selectins, known to function as skin-selective adhesion molecules, prevents contact with the antigen expressed in the skin and, therefore, prevents the induction of neonatal tolerance. The induction of tolerance by antigen expressed in peripheral tissues, namely the skin, is dependent on T-cell migration in the skin *(1148)*.

Studies conducted on Tg mice expressing the influenza virus HA gene in pancreatic β-cells under the control of the insulin promoter showed that peripheral tolerance occurs after activation of T cells through cross-presentation of the antigen by APCs. Cross-presentation is inefficient after birth, and tolerance is established only in 2- to 4-wk-old mice. This was clearly demonstrated by studying the occurrence of diabetes in Ins-HA Tg mice that were immunized with PR/8 influenza virus. Whereas 1-wk-old mice developed diabetes, 2- to 4-wk-old mice did not develop disease after immunization with PR/8 *(1154)*. This observation is consistent with observations made in Insulin (Ins)-HA/TCR-HA double-Tg mice showing that potential autoreactive T cells accumulate during the early neonatal period in the peripheral organ expressing the target antigen and that the induction of tolerance requires the maturation of APCs able to cross-present the antigen *(948)*.

4.2.2. Induction of Neonatal T-Cell Tolerance to Self-Antigens

Based on tissue injury, autoimmune diseases have been classified into two major categories: organ specific and systemic. In recent decades, intensive research aimed at understanding the effector mechanisms involved has led to further classification: autoimmune diseases mediated by antibodies and autoimmune diseases mediated by pathogenic T cells, such as multiple sclerosis, insulin-dependent diabetes mellitus (IDDM), uveitis, oophritis, Sjogren's syndrome, and inflammatory bowel diseases. Self-reactive T cells that recognize target antigens in brain, pancreas, eye, ovary, or intestinal cells escape deletion in the thymus and cause autoimmune disease under certain experimental conditions. In mice, parenteral administration of myelin basic protein (MBP) and proteolipid protein in FCA induces EAE (an experimental model for multiple sclerosis), *S*-antigen induces autoimmune uveitis, and zona pelucida protein 3 induces experimental ovarian autoimmune diseases (oophritis). The experimental autoimmune diseases are mediated by CD4 Th1 cells, which recognize the peptides derived from the processing of target self-antigens in the context of MHC class II molecules.

There are several reports demonstrating that the administration of peptides after birth induces tolerance and, in adults, prevents the occurrence of autoimmune diseases elicited by the administration of self-antigens in combination with other antigens. Thus, high doses of MBP and Freund's incomplete adjuvant (FIA), or of FIA and a peptide corresponding to immunodominant epitopes of MBP that is recognized by murine T cells in association with H-2^p or H-2^s, injected into newborn Lewis rats induced EAE resistance in adult animals. The tolerance induced during neonatal life lasts until adult life, as illustrated by failure to develop EAE after injection with MBP in FCA *(1150,1151)*. The requirement for FIA in the induction of neonatal tolerance can be circumvented by injecting newborn mice with a chimeric Ig bearing the peptide derived from PLP recognized by Th1 cells in the context of H-2^s molecules *(940)*. In this model, the induction of neonatal tolerance was caused by the deviation of the CD4 Th1 response to the Th2 response, producing IL-4. Exogenous IFN-γ and IL-12 rescued the anergic T cells, which exhibited in vitro proliferation in an antigen-specific manner.

Neonatal tolerance in a murine model preventing the development of primary Sjogren's syndrome was induced by intravenous injection of α-fodrin autoantigen *(1152)*. α-Fodrin is a candidate self-antigen in both animal models and humans with primary Sjogren's syndrome.

In summary, the findings described here demonstrate that neonatal tolerance induced by self-antigens, or the peptides derived from them, prevents the induction of autoimmune diseases in adults by anergizing Th1 cells producing IFN-γ and IL-12. Alternatively, disease is prevented by deviation of the immune response toward a Th2 response, which is dominant in the neonatal repertoire and can be propagated in postnatal life in mice that are tolerized after birth.

4.3. Neonatal T-Cell Tolerance to Alloantigens

Owen's *(1112)* description of dizygotic cattle twins, which are naturally "parabiosed" *in utero* as a result of placental fusion and are permanent chimeras unable to produce antibody against fraternal RBCs, represented the first example of central tolerance to alloantigens. Billingham et al. *(1153)* showed that a large proportion of dizygotic twins could accept skin grafts from the other twin. Later, Medawar et al. *(607)* performed experiments in mice demonstrating that injecting newborns with hematopoietic cells induced chimerism under experimental conditions. Indeed, such mice did not reject the skin of donor of hematopoietic cells when they reached maturity. This experiment demonstrated that exposure of the newborn immune system to alloantigens allowed tolerance to specific antigens as if it were self. The induction of neonatal tolerance to alloantigens was believed to result from the immaturity of neonatal immune cells, which are more susceptible to tolerogens. In neonatal tolerized mice, the donor cells were later detected by PCR *(1154)*, confirming the chimerism described by Billingham et al. *(607)*.

When these experiments were performed, little was known of the transplantation antigens or of the immune cells that mediate allograft rejection. Ensuing years have demonstrated that the target of allograft rejection and graft-vs-host reaction are major and minor MHC antigens and that the effector cells are CD8 and CD4 T cells (reviewed in ref. *67*). By virtue of their ability to lyse cells that bear alloantigens, CD8 T cells are the effectors of cell-mediated immunity against alloantigens. However, a subset of dendritic cells, natural killer (NK) T cells, and CD4 Th1 cells appear to be critical for tolerance.

In mice, the precursors of CTLs specific for alloantigens were detected in the thymus of newborns and in the spleen at age 3–9 d *(1052,1053)*. It was believed that the precursors of alloantigen-specific CTLs that were present at birth exhibited an intrinsic tolerogenic property, because injections of high numbers of allogeneic bone marrow cells prevented graft rejection of skin and a CTL response *(607)*.

Ridge et al. *(1054)* analyzed the induction of CTLs in newborn female B6 mice injected with male cells and tested the CTL response against the male H-Y antigen. In this system, the in vitro H-Y-specific CTL response is completely dependent on in vivo immunization with alloantigen. Tolerance is induced after injection of a high number of male cells (i.e., five male spleen cells for one female T cell). However, when females were injected at birth not with male spleen cells but with male dendritic cells, a CTL response was observed. The CTL activity was detected 8 wk after injection, indicating that dendritic cells from adult males efficiently primed the precursors of H-Y CTLs at birth.

This finding demonstrated that mice that received dendritic cells from an adult donor were resistant to tolerance induction and that the CTLs were primed to the same extent as adult female controls injected with male cells. This experiment also showed that neonatal alloreactive T cells did not have intrinsic properties for tolerization, but the induction of neonatal tolerance was related to the immaturity of APCs.

NK T cells represent a subset of lymphocytes that recognize glycolipid antigens in the context of CD1 molecules. Recently, it was found that a minute subset of NK T cells, representing 5% of NK T cells in the liver, exhibits a different phenotype, $CD8^+$ $NK.1.1^+$ $CD3^{int}$ TCR^{int}, and might recognize polymorphic MHC antigens such as allogeneic MHC class I molecules. This subset increased prominently to 16% in the livers of mice in which neonatal tolerance was induced subsequent to injection with allogeneic lymphocytes (i.e., BALBc/ c H-2^d lymphocytes infused into newborn C57BL/6 H-2^b mice). The CD8$^+$ NK T cells, which accumulated in the liver, migrated from the spleen, as demonstrated by a decreased number and loss of tolerance in mice splenectomized after injection of allogeneic lymphocytes. This result indicated that allogencic stimulation in the spleen was absolutely required for the expansion of CD8$^+$ NK T cells and the induction of neonatal tolerance. These findings strongly suggest that CD8$^+$ NK T cells stimulated with allogeneic lymphocytes suppress allospecific recipient lymphocytes, permitting unresponsiveness and establishing chimerism and allograft tolerance *(1155)*.

Neonatal tolerance is associated with a shift of Th1 to Th2 response and the expansion of Th2 memory cells. There are several observations strongly suggesting that prevention of the Th1 response is critical for induction of neonatal tolerance by alloantigens.

First, a 10- to 100-fold higher IL-4/IFN-γ ratio of cytokine production was observed in lymph nodes that drained tolerant grafts compared to lymph nodes that drained rejected allografts. Exogenous treatment with IFN-γ at the time of neonatal priming produced more IFN-γ and expanded more IFN-γ-producing CD4 and CD8 T cells, thereby rejecting the graft. This finding indicated that neonatal tolerance might depend on blockage of the Th1 response, which otherwise led to rejection *(1160)*.

Second, simultaneous injection of newborns with IL-12 and allogeneic cells prevented the Th2 alloimmune response. In vitro studies demonstrated that subsequent to this kind of immunization, the alloreactive T cells stimulated in mixed lymphocyte culture (MLC) produced high levels of IL-2 and IFN-γ and that the expansion of allogeneic-specific CTLs was increased. Thus, IL-12 inhibits the Th2 polarization of the newborn response to alloantigens and thereby prevents the induction of neonatal tolerance *(945)*.

Third, similar neonatal administration of anti-CD40 antibody and allogeneic cells resulted in increased IFN-γ production paralleled by enhanced CTL activity and decreased IL-4 synthesis *(946)*. Because newborn T cells express less CD40 ligand, the insufficiency of CD40–CD40L interactions might contribute to neonatal tolerance by blocking the IFN-γ/IL-12-dependent pathway after TCR–alloantigen interaction of Th1 cells *(1156)*.

5. NEONATAL T-CELL TOLERANCE TO FOREIGN ANTIGENS

Peripheral tolerance in adult animals can be induced with low or high doses of antigens. Neonatal T-cell tolerance results from inactivation of T cells after exposure to antigens during development and persisting into adulthood *(1157)*. The unresponsiveness of neonatal T cells may be related to deletion, anergy, or active suppression induced by antigens. The route of administration of antigens and the addition of adjuvants to immunogens represent important factors in the induction of neonatal tolerance.

The role of the administration route of antigens in neonatal tolerance is illustrated in an experiment describing tolerance in newborn mice that were induced with deaggregated human γ globulin (HGG). Newborns injected with the antigen after birth exhibited a defective antibody response and had anergic T cells when challenged with an immunogenic form of HGG/FCA in adulthood. However, the offspring born to mothers injected with 5 mg HGG after birth, in which the tolerogen was delivered via colostrum, were unable to produce antibodies, retained proliferating tolerogen-specific T cells, and were able to secrete IL-2 and IL-4 *(1158)*. From this study, it could be concluded that neonatal tolerance to HGG induced through lactation resulted in defective antibody responses but had no detectable effect on HGG-specific T-cell responses.

Neonatal T-cell tolerance was also induced experimentally with peptide corresponding to amino acid residues 93 to 103 of moth cytochrome c *(1159)*, amino acid residues 146 to 160 of acetylcholine receptor *(1160)*, or amino acid residues 139 to 151 of PLP *(940)*. In the last experimental model, anergic T cells failed to proliferate, produce IFN-γ, or express CD40L, leading to defective cooperation with APCs and a lack of IL-12 production. Impaired CD40 signaling in specialized dendritic cells called Langerhan's cells from murine neonatal lymph nodes was also described in neonatal cutaneous tolerance induced by 2,4-dinitrofluorobenzene *(1161)*. The role of a subset of $CD8\alpha^+$ dendritic cells in inducing neonatal tolerance also was shown in a different experimental system in which tolerance was induced by aggregated Ig-myelin oligodendrocyte glycoprotein *(1162)*.

The deviation of immune response toward Th2 type in neonatal T-cell tolerance has received considerable attention based on observations that administration of tolerogen with IL-12, IFN-γ, or anti-IL-4 antibodies rescues the anergic T cells. The development of the Th1 response is promoted by IL-12 and is dependent on the activation of STAT4. Meanwhile, Th2 cell development is stimulated by IL-4 and activated by STAT6.

Interestingly, studies on the induction of neonatal T-cell tolerance by postnatal injection with HEL in phosphate-buffered saline or in combination with IFA have shown that tolerance can be induced in wildtype as well as in STAT4- and STAT6-deficient newborn mice *(1163)*. This observation suggested that the T-cell populations that mediate neonatal tolerance are elusive and that STAT-6-independent Th2 cells may play a role in neonatal tolerance. Studies on neonatal induction of tolerance in rats injected with mercuric chloride, which induces an adult autoimmune glomerulonephritis mediated by Th2 cells, showed that tolerant animals exhibited activated $CD8^+$ T cells that produced IL-2 and IFN-γ but not IL-4 or IL-10. The results reported in this study suggest that the injection of mercuric chloride into tolerant rats preferentially activated Th1 cells that may be involved in induction and maintenance of tolerance to Th2-mediated dysregulation, leading to glomerulonephritis, increased IgE synthesis, and production of various autoantibodies *(1164)*.

These findings challenge the concept that neonatal tolerance is caused by inhibition of the Th1 response and subsequent deviation toward a Th2 response. The findings also indicate that understanding the mechanisms of this process requires further dissection of the components required for the establishment of neonatal T-cell tolerance.

14

Development of Efficient Prophylactic Vaccines and Theracines for Newborns and Infants

1. INTRODUCTION

Vaccines represent one of the most impressive successes of experimental medicine, allowing for the eradication of a causative infectious agent and extinction of diseases such as variola, which is caused by smallpox. The vaccine against variola was discovered by Jenner 200 yr ago based on the observation that the injection of a boy with cowpox was protected against two successive inoculations with the deadly smallpox virus. The global vaccination with vaccinia led to the almost total eradication of the smallpox virus. Classical vaccines developed later through discoveries pioneered by Pasteur and Ramon led to definition of a golden rule of vaccine preparation that consists of the principle of inactivation of the pathogenicity of a microbe or bacterial toxin without altering their immunogenicity—namely, the ability to induce a protective immune response. Fervent advancement in vaccinology established that an ideal vaccine should be endowed with the following properties: (a) The microbe used to prepare the vaccine should exhibit a constant antigen specificity without being the subject of genetic variation; (b) it should induce protective immunity; (c) the protection should be life-long, because it should induce immune memory, allowing a primed host to react rapidly to an infectious agent; and (d) it should be devoid of side effects.

The defense reaction of the host to infection comprises innate and adaptive arms of the immune system. Innate immunity component comprises cytokines, natural antibodies, phagocytes, and natural killer (NK) cells. The adaptive immunity component comprises B cells, which produce neutralizing antibodies, and T cells, which help B cells to produce antibodies or are effectors of cell-mediated immunity (CMI) responses.

Protective antibodies produced by B cells that are activated by vaccines act directly on the infectious agent, preventing the penetration of the viruses into permissive cells, covering the bacteria, and thereby facilitating the phagocyto-

From: *Contemporary Immunology: Neonatal Immunity*
By: Constantin Bona © Humana Press Inc., Totowa, NJ

sis or inactivating the microbial toxins. IgM and IgG antibodies protect against the microbes present in the blood, lymphoid organs, or tissues, whereas IgA protects against the microbes present on mucosal membranes.

T cells mediate CMI responses induced by vaccination. They are activated in the lymphoid organs but display the protective effects subsequent to migration into tissues at the site of multiplication of infectious agents. Their protective effect is indirect. Effector T cells, which mediate CMI response, either kill infected cells by a perforin-dependent cytotoxic ability or release cytokines, which activate macrophages and enable them to destroy the intracellular pathogens.

Life-long protective immune responses elicited by vaccination imply the induction of memory cells. Immunological memory correlates with increased frequency of antigen-specific lymphocytes and their quicker response to a second exposure to antigen. The induction of memory by vaccination is a very important point, because protective antibody titers usually decrease over time.

In the case of vaccines after one-dose immunization, the majority of antibodies produced during primary response are IgM secreted by plasma cells. Memory can not be sustained by plasma cells producing IgM antibodies, because the half-life of IgM is very short. The immune system overcame this problem through the ability to induce the differentiation of activated B cells not only in plasma cells but also in memory cells.

The maintenance of high titers of neutralizing antibodies can be related to the long persistence of antigen-antibody complexes on the surface of follicular dendritic cells; the long persistence of antigen, particularly in the case of latent virus infection; or the long persistence of bacterial polysaccharides, which are resistant to hydrolyses by mammalian enzymes.

The differentiation of memory cells in antibody-producing cells is related to re-exposure to antigen from an external source or from an antigen source in the host when bacteria or parasites are sequestered in granuloma.

Primed T cells last longer—about 3 wk after immunization or vaccination. Like B cells, primed T cells differentiate into effector and memory cells. Memory T cells are rapidly reactivated and become protective within the first 8–16 h subsequent to re-exposure to antigen in lymphoid organs *(1165)*. They can be continuously activated by persistent infections. Interesting examples of persistence of viral infections include HIV, herpes simplex virus, and hepatitis B virus (HBV) in humans and LCMV virus in mice. In humans, HBV persists at very low levels for decades after patient recovery and despite maintenance of an active cytotoxic T-lymphocyte (CTL) response *(1166)*.

For a long time, we were used to thinking of vaccines as a tool to prevent infectious diseases. The evolution of immunobiology in our understanding of both the beneficial and detrimental aspects of immune response has led to development of vaccines aimed at preventing or treating immune inflammatory diseases, including autoimmune and allergic diseases and tumors. Vaccines used in the treatment of diseases are termed therapeutic vaccines or theracines.

The infection of newborns and infants still represents a cause of high morbidity and mortality. The World Health Organization estimated that approx 3 million infants between ages 1 and 12 mo die annually of infection. Therefore, successful vaccination of newborns and young infants represents a global necessity. This represents a great challenge given the characteristics of the development of the neonatal immune system. There are several factors that limit the success of neonatal vaccination.

The first factor relates to the quality of neutralizing antibodies produced by neonates in response to vaccines. A typical feature of neonatal antibody response is the predominance of IgM. The ability to produce neutralizing IgG antibodies increases progressively during the first year of life. In addition, the antibody response elicited by administration of a single dose of vaccine is of short duration and thereby requires one or several booster doses in the following years. The Th2 dominance during early life has important implications on the class of IgG antibodies, because the switch of IgM leads to a strong predominance of IgG1 and IgG3 and low production of IgG2. The production of high-affinity antibodies also increases progressively because of the low rate of somatic mutation, which contributes to maturation of the affinity of antibody responses.

The second group of factors relates to Th2 dominance of the neonatal repertoire. The Th1 responses, which represent an important arm in defense reactions against the microbe, increase gradually during the first months of life. This leads to production of proinflammatory cytokines and the production of interleukin (IL)-2, which promotes the development of CD8 T cells. Proinflammatory cytokines and IL-2 are effectors of cytotoxic reactions, leading to clearance of infected cells.

Finally, the third group of limiting factors for the induction of protective CMI responses during early life is immaturity of antigen-presenting cells (APCs) that produce lower amounts of IL-12, which is required for the induction of interferon (IFN)-γ responses.

However, neonatal vaccination may result in efficient priming of lymphocytes, and this observation constituted the basis for the development of more efficient vaccines, new formulation for the administration of vaccines, and the optimal schedule of vaccination.

2. LIVE-ATTENUATED VACCINES

The preparation of live-attenuated vaccines was based on the principle established by Pasteur and Calmette, which states that culturing the microbe in special conditions leads to the loss of pathogenicity without altering the immunogenicity. In the case of viral vaccines, the discovery by Enders *(1167)* of a method of culturing in vitro in permissive cells with viruses also contributed to selection of temperature-sensitive mutants or naturally occurring mutants, which lose their pathogenic properties without damaging the ability to induce a protective immune response.

Live-attenuated vaccines induce humoral and cellular protective immune responses by their ability to replicate in permissive cells. The humoral immune response results from the interaction of B lymphocytes with CD4 T cells, which recognize peptides derived from the processing of microbes within APCs. These peptides are presented in association with major histocompatibility complex (MHC) class II molecules. The CMI response results from the processing of viral or bacterial proteins in the cells and the presentation of peptides in association with MHC class I molecules to CD8 T cells. Table 31 lists licensed live-attenuated vaccines.

The live-attenuated vaccines display two major advantages. First, they elicit a long-lasting immunity comparable to that induced by natural infection. The protective immune response can be induced by a single injection, followed or not followed by additional booster. Second, they induce both humoral and cellular immune responses and immunological memory. In spite of the fact that the vaccination with live-attenuated vaccines could not in all situations prevent viral replication and infection by infectious agent, their ability to induce a CMI response may lead to viral clearance.

A possible drawback of live-attenuated vaccines consists of the occurrence of reverse mutations.

With the exception of BCG and vaccinia, all infants vaccinated with live-attenuated vaccines require several boosts before age 6 mo because of the immaturity of the neonatal immune system and the progressive development of IgG antibody response during the first year of life.

2.1. Vaccinia Vaccination

During the past two centuries, the vaccination of infants with vaccinia has led to eradication of smallpox and variola. The immune response induced by vaccinia is mainly a Th1 response, as illustrated by the development of a delayed-type sensitivity reaction at the site of primary vaccination and revaccination. However, vaccinia vaccination induces neutralizing antibodies against the vaccinia virus. Neutralizing antibodies before vaccination were detected in 85% of subjects vaccinated at birth. After revaccination, a sharp increase of the titer of neutralizing antibodies was observed 14 d after boost. No significant decrease in antibody titer occurred in vaccinees within 3–20 yr following vaccination at birth and then at ages 8 and 18 yr *(1168)*. These observations strongly suggest that vaccina virus vaccination elicits a long-lasting immunity.

Table 31
Live Attenuated Vaccines

Vaccinia	Sabin poliovirus
Measles	Japanese encephalitis
Mumps	BCG
Rubella	Adenovirus
Varicella-zoster	Cold attenuated influenza virus

Abbreviations: BCG, Bacillus Calmette-Guèrin.

The majority of adverse reactions after smallpox vaccination are minor *(1169)*. They consist of atopic dermatitis and acute, chronic, or exfoliative skin conditions (eczema vaccinatum). In the case of immunocompromised infants, generalized vaccinia infection may occur. Progressive vaccinia is a rare, severe, and often fatal disease and requires aggressive therapy with immune immuno-globulin and cidofovir, an antiviral drug. Central nervous system complications, such as postvaccinal encephalopathy and encephalomyelitis occurring after vaccination, are the most common complications among infants age 12 mo or younger *(1169)*.

2.2. BCG Vaccine

BCG vaccination is generally carried out after birth in term and preterm newborns. BCG vaccination is compulsory in 64 countries and recommended in 118 countries. In 10 randomized trials conducted since 1930, it was shown that BCG neonatal vaccination afforded protection in 10–80% of cases, and in 80 to 100% of cases, it afforded protection against tuberculous meningitis *(1170)*. A Mantoux conversion rate of 81% was observed in both term and preterm neonates vaccinated at birth *(1171)*. A positive lymphocyte migration inhibition test, induration at the site of injection, a positive tuberculin test, pro-tein purified derivations (PPD)-induced proliferation, and the production of IL-2 indicate that BCG vaccination after birth induces a CMI response *(1170,1171)*.

BCG vaccination limits the multiplication and dissemination of bacillus rather than preventing the infection. In both mice and humans, the neonatal CMI response is characterized by Th2 dominance. However, the BCG vacci-nation after birth induces a strong Th1-type response that is necessary for the control of mycobacterial infection. Thus, it was shown that 2-mo-old infants vaccinated at birth displayed a strong proliferative response to PPD and high levels of production of IFN-γ. Interestingly, the level of IFN-γ synthesis by PPD- or phytohemagglutinin (PHA)-stimulated lymphocytes was higher in the infants vaccinated at birth than those vaccinated at age 2 mo age. In sharp contrast, no IL-4 reproduction by PPD-stimulated lymphocytes was observed in infants immunized at birth or at age 2 mo *(1069)*. The number of CD4 T cells producing IFN-γ after neonatal BCG vaccination was also increased *(1070)*. An analysis of cytokine produced by T-cell clones that were obtained from neonatal vaccinated infants showed that 9% of clones were specific for PPD. Among these clones, 41% were of Th1-type producing IFN-γ, and 59% were of Th0-type producing IFN-γ and IL-4 or IL-5 *(1070)*.

These observations strongly suggest that neonatal BCG vaccination deviates Th response from Th2 to Th1 response. Therefore, the early IFN-γ response in newborns plays a central role in their ability to control the infection with BCG and results in successful vaccination. The BCG-polarized Th1 response is likely dependent on the activation of APCs and, in particular, of dendritic cells involved in the priming of naïve T cells. It was shown that the infection of dendritic cells with BCG increases their ability to present antigen to T cells *(1172)*; the production of IL-12, which is a stimulator of IFN-γ production; and the expression of costimulatory molecules *(1173)*.

BCG neonatal vaccination induces long-lasting Th1 memory cells. This was clearly demonstrated by studying the Th1 response to PPD in a cohort of infants vaccinated with BCG at birth who were followed until age 1 yr. PPD-stimulated lymphocytes from this group of infants produced high levels of IFN-γ and only low levels of IL-5 and IL-13, which are Th2 prototype cytokines.

Neonatal BCG vaccination represents one of the first infectious agent encounters early in life and could have a strong impact on the development of the T-cell repertoire. This concept is supported by data demonstrating that infants vaccinated at birth with BCG and HeB or poliovirus vaccines exhibited increased anti-HeB and poliovirus type I antibodies at age 4.5 mo *(1174)*. The mechanism of enhancing the effect of the antibody response to unrelated vaccine by neonatal BCG vaccination may be related to the activation of s and the production of cytokines, because the lymphocytes from infants immunized with polio or HeB vaccines produce not only IFN-γ but also significant concentrations of IL-5 and IL-13.

2.3. Poliovirus Vaccines

Poliomyelitis is a paralytic disease of the motor neurons of the central nervous system, which is caused by polioviruses. There are three serotypes of poliovirus; each induces a specific immune response, as it was established by studies showing that infection with a serotype does not confer protection against the disease caused by other serotypes.

The development of live-attenuated vaccine by Sabin is based on the model of natural infection. It is considered that the poliovirus establishes infection on mucosal surfaces of the pharynx and intestinal tract. The virus then spreads from mucosa to the local lymph nodes, where it replicates and produces viremia, and then infects the central nervous system. Sabin-type vaccine was generated by selection of mutants of all three serotypes, which can replicate in the intestine subsequent to oral administration. Sabin-type vaccine induces local and systemic immunity, because the live-attenuated polioviruses multiply in the cells of the oropharynx and gastrointestinal tract and then spread to the lymph node like the wildtype viruses. It stimulates the production of protective IgA and IgG antibodies and provides a strong immunity that the natural infection would provide. Oral polio vaccine is given at birth as a single dose. If the vaccines respond to only one or two serotypes after a single dose, then multiple doses are given to elicit the production of antibodies against all three serotypes. Oral polio vaccination with Sabin-type vaccine may lead to elimination of wildtype poliovirus, and the progress toward this goal has been extraordinary. It is expected that in the next decade the eradication will be accomplished.

2.4. Influenza Virus Vaccine

Influenza types A and B are among the most common causes of respiratory tract infections in children. The annual incidence of influenza infection in children may exceed 30%. It is believed that children are an important factor in the spread of virus in the community. The inactivated vaccines are not very effective in infants. Live-attenuated cold-adapted trivalent vaccine administered intranasally is more efficient for the vaccination of children, because it replicates in the upper respiratory tract and induces local immunity.

The vaccine is updated annually by genetic reassortment techniques that substitute genes encoding the hemagglutinin (HA) and neuraminidase from contemporary influenza type A and B viruses.

A study carried out on a group of healthy children between the ages of 15 and 71 mo showed that the vaccine was highly immunogenic for the influenza A (H1N1 and H3N2) and B subtypes. After two doses of vaccine, 61% of initially seronegative children had neutralizing antibodies. The second dose of vaccine increased the antibody levels to influenza type A *(1175)*.

It is noteworthy that no influenza virus-specific CTL activity was detected in infants after immunization with live-attenuated cold-adapted vaccine *(1084)*. Lack of CTL activity in infants vaccinated with cold-adapted virus may be related to the lower replication rate of virus in vivo. In addition, limited replication in the nasal cavity but not in the lung might decrease the chance of activating CTLs by virus-infected pulmonary macrophages or epithelial cells.

2.5. Varicella Virus Vaccine

Varicella-zoster virus (VZV) causes varicella or chickenpox in children and herpes zoster in adults. Varicella results from primary infection with VZV. After infection, VZV becomes latent in the dorsal root ganglia and can be reactivated to cause shingles.

A live-attenuated VZV (Oka) vaccine was developed in Japan and was introduced to routine infant vaccination in various countries. Numerous clinical trials have shown that the vaccine is immunogenic and induces a protective immune response against infection with VZV *(1176)*.

VZV vaccination is recommended in children age 12 to 8 mo. VZV vaccination results in a significant rise of VZV-specific IgG antibodies and strong T-cell responses reflected in the expression of activation markers of both CD4 and CD8 T cells *(1177)*. Higher titers of antibody were uniformly associated with lower infection rates. In one study, children were followed 5 yr for the persistence of antibodies. Interestingly, the antibody levels increase over time after vaccination. The long-lasting immunity and increases of antibody levels could be associated with reactivation of Oka VZV as antibody titers decline or to stimulation of the immune system by wildtype VZV latent virus *(1178)*. Krause and Klinman *(1179)* recently showed that Oka VZV reactivates at a rate of 19% per year in children with low titers of antibodies. Surveillance of the effect of vaccination on the populations in California, Texas, and West Philadelphia from 1995 to 2000 showed the efficiency of vaccination, illustrated by a significant reduction in varicella cases *(1180)*.

2.6. Measles, Mumps, Rubella (MMR) Trivalent Vaccines

A combined live-attenuated measles, mumps, and rubella vaccine is used to immunize the infant population between ages 4 and 12 mo. The vaccine is safe and well-tolerated, and side effects are very mild, manifested sometimes with fever or rash *(1181)*. The global eradication of measles is a major aim, as measles still cause high morbidity and about 1 million deaths each year in developing countries *(1182)*.

CD46, a complement regulatory protein that binds C3b, is the cellular receptor for measles virus (MV) *(1183)*. Crosslinking of CD46 by MV inhibits IL-12 synthesis by monocytes and dendritic cells *(1184)*. IL-12 stimulates the production of IFN-γ by Th1 and NK cells and inhibits IL-4 production by Th2 cells, which dominates neonatal CD4 responses.

The major drawback in the induction of protective immunity against MV in infants includes Th2 dominance of neonatal response and maternal passive transfer of antibodies. Maternal antibodies can bind to MV and prevent its internalization within the cells. These considerations led to the recommendation of vaccination later after birth at age 6 to 9 mo, followed by two boosts at age, 4 to 6 and 11 to 12 yr. To reach the protective immunity of at least 95%, two doses are required *(1185)*. In Finland, where the two-dose strategy has been adopted since 1982, the elimination of measles has been achieved after 12 yr of vaccinations *(1186)*.

So far, the molecular mechanism of MV attenuation has not been identified. Live-attenuated MV vaccine is based on the Edmonton B strain of MV. It induces both humoral and cellular immunity. Cellular immunity represents the major arm of protection, a concept supported by the clinical observation that vaccinated agammaglobulenic children were resistant to repeated MV infections *(1187).*

The use of live-attenuated measles vaccine has led to a seroconversion rate of more than 95% and a very high protective efficacy. The production of anti-MV antibodies in infants vaccinated at ages 6, 9, and 12 mo was measured by enzyme-linked immunofluorescence assay (ELISA), plaque neutralization, and complement fixation assays. In seronegative children as in adolescents, the primary vaccination produced high seroconversion rates *(1188).* The seroconversion rate was 77% in 6-mo-old infants and 97% and 96% in 9- and 12-mo-old infants, respectively. Among the 6-mo-old infants who had residual passive-transmitted maternal antibodies, interference could not be distinguished from the age-matched infants who lacked passive antibodies at the time of vaccination *(1182).* There is a genetic association between humoral response levels after measles vaccine and HLA class IL genes. The HLA-DRB1*03 and HLA-DPA1*0201 alleles were significantly associated with seronegativity *(1189).*

Measles vaccination induced a strong CMI response with no age-related difference in 6-, 9-, and 12-mo-old infants with respect to in vitro proliferative T-cell response or cytokine production. No significant differences were found when the concentrations of IFN-γ and IL-12 were compared among the three infant groups. However, measles-specific IL-12 responses of infants were significantly lower than those of vaccinated adults *(1190).* A strong proliferative T-cell response is an indication that the vaccination induced memory CD4 T cells.

The immunization of 6- and 9-mo-old infants with live-attenuated MV induces changes in Vβ T-cell receptor (TCR) repertoire Thus, whereas the Vβ4 subset was depleted, the Vβ2 subset was increased 2 wk after vaccination before return to prevaccination levels at 3 mo. The increased expression of Vβ2 may reflect a clonally expanded T-cell subset, whereas the depletion of Vβ4 T cells may result from a superantigen present in MV vaccine *(1191).* The changes in the T-cell repertoire after MV vaccination differ from the changes observed in infants following natural infection. In this case, an increase of Vβ5 and Vβ8 T cells was noted *(1192).*

Live-attenuated mumps virus, a component of the MMR trivaccine, also induces both humoral and CMI responses. In children without maternal passive transmitted antibodies, the rate of seroconversion was 95% in 6- to 12-mo-old infants. The presence of passive antibodies did not result in lower titer of antimumps antibody after vaccination. Similarly, CMI response elicited by mumps vaccination did not differ among 6- to 12-mo-old infants with respect to proliferative response of T cells and in vitro production of IFN-γ in three groups of infants. It is noteworthy that after vaccination with MV vaccine, the production of IFN-γ in vaccinated children was lower compared to vaccinated adults *(1182)*.

Study of antirubella antibody response in children vaccinated with live-at-tenuated MMR vaccine showed seroconversion in 100% of infants *(1188)*.

Little is known on the priming of CTL response in children immunized with live-attenuated MMR vaccine. In the case of measles vaccination of 9-mo-old infants in Gambia, the magnitude of CTL response was found similar to that found in children or adults with acute measles infection *(1193)*.

3. INACTIVATED VACCINES

The generation of inactivated vaccines resulted from the development of methods to grow bacteria and to purify bacterial toxins. This allowed inactivation of the bacteria or toxins, which lost their pathogenicity but preserved the immunogenicity. The killing of bacteria was achieved by physical means, such as heating, or by chemical agents, such as treatment with formalin, which is a substance used to prepare inactivated Salk polio or influenza vaccines. Formalin is also used to convert the bacterial toxin in toxoid that is used for the preparation of vaccines against diphtheria or tetanus.

Inactivated vaccines can induce only humoral responses, namely, the production of protective antibody. The production of antibodies results from the activation of CD4 T cells subsequent to processing of vaccine by APCs and delivery of a second signal required for the activation of B cells, which recognize via BCR-relevant epitopes on the surface of vaccine antigens. The inactivated vaccines are very stable, do not exhibit reverse mutations, and induce the production of protective antibodies, or neutralizing antibodies in the case of vaccination with toxoids. Like live-attenuated vaccines, they can be administered as combined trivalent or quadrivalent vaccines. They exhibit some drawbacks. The major disadvantage is that they can not induce CTL responses and induce weak memory B cells, requiring several boosts to generate a response. Table 32 lists the licensed inactivated vaccines.

Among the inactivated vaccines, tetanus, diphtheria pretties trivaccine, Salk poliovirus, and influenza vaccines are used for the vaccination of children.

3.1. Poliovirus Inactivated Vaccine

Salk vaccine is used to vaccinate infants age 2 mo but often requires several boosts at ages 4, 6, 9, and 12 mo and 4 to 6 yr to induce high titers of protective neutralizing antibodies.

Table 32
Licensed Inactivated Vaccines

Rabies	Influenza virus formalin-inactivated
Salk formalin-inactivated poliovirus	Hepatitis A formalin-inactivated
Tetanus toxoid	Diphtheria toxoid
Bordetella pertussis heat-inactivated	*Vibrion cholerae*
Salmonella typhiod heat-inactivated	Japanese encephalitis virus

The persistence of neutralizing antibody was evaluated in groups of premature and mature born children with a follow-up 5 and 7 yr after primary vaccination. In the group of children in which the level of neutralizing antibodies was studied 5 yr after vaccination, the antibodies against poliovirus types 1 and 3 were generally high. No significant differences between preterm and full-term children were observed except for the concentration of antibodies against poliovirus type 3. A greater proportion of children and higher concentration of antibodies were observed in the group vaccinated four times at ages 2, 4, 6, and 13 mo than in those vaccinated at ages 3, 5, and 12 mo. A slight statistical difference between the two groups is of little clinical significance, because the immunity induced by killed poliovirus vaccine is considered similar to that induced by infection, which is longlasting and associated with immunological memory *(1194)*. No statistical differences were observed in the number of children with minimal protective titers in a group of children studied 7 yr after vaccination, with exception of lower titers against poliovirus type 3 *(1195)*.

3.2. Influenza Virus Inactivated Vaccine

The effectiveness of inactivated influenza vaccine in young children has been controversial. Inactivated influenza vaccine administered in young children induces high rates of seroconversion *(1196)* and a significantly lower prevalence of influenza-type virus infection in the vaccinated group than in the nonvaccinated group *(1197)*. However, in a randomized controlled trial, no significant difference was observed in the occurrence of acute otitis media in the vaccinated and placebo groups *(1196)*. Current influenza vaccination programs focus on children at high risk for influenza complications including infants with chronic cardiac and pulmonary diseases, type I diabetes, or with immunodeficiencies *(1198)*.

3.3. Diphtheria, Tetanus, Pertussis (DTP) Vaccine

Another important inactivated vaccine for children is DTP vaccine, which contains diphtheria, tetanus toxoids, and pertussis. Earlier, DTP vaccine consisted of toxoids and heat-killed or thimerosal-treated pertussis bacteria. The pertussis component of this DTP vaccine exhibited some side effects, causing local reaction in many infants and, on rare occasions, serious systemic toxic reactions including brain damage and death. Since 1981, heat-killed bacteria has been replaced with an acellular pertussis component, which contains formalin-treated pertussis toxin (toxoid), filamentous HA, and pertactin absorbed onto aluminum hydroxide. This vaccine appears to be effective and less toxic than the heat-killed vaccine. The current schedule for DTP vaccination of infants is the subject of debate regarding the timing and the frequency of dosing to induce the best memory response. The most common schedule of DTP vaccination is primary vaccination at ages 2, 4, and 6 mo and a booster dose at age 12 mo. This schedule of vaccination elicits high geometric mean titer (GMT) of antibodies for all three antigens in preterm and full-term children.

At the 5-yr follow-up, the concentration of antidiphtheria toxin antibodies was <0.01 IU/mL, the level generally accepted as the lowest level to give some degree of protection *(1194)*. At the 6- to 7-yr follow-ups, the GMT was lower in the preterm group than in full-term infants, with a minimum protective cutoff value of 0.10 IU/mL *(1195)*. The measurement of the avidity of IgG antidiphtheria antibodies in the 7-yr follow-up group showed that in both groups, the antibody had moderate to high avidity *(1195)*.

In the case of antitetanus toxin antibodies, all children in both preterm and full-term groups had titers above the minimum protective level, which is >0.01 IU/mL.

Antibody levels for pertussis toxin, filamentous HA, and pertactin did not differ between preterm and full-term children *(1195,1199)*. The high levels of antibodies to pertussis toxin, filamentous HA, and pertactin acquired after vaccination are associated with lower likelihood of acquiring disease caused by *Bordetella pertussis (1194)*.

The results of these studies clearly demonstrated the induction of immunologic memory after DTP vaccination *(1200)*. Of particular interest are the studies aimed at identifying CD4 T-cell cytokine response in the context of DTP vaccination, because it is generally accepted as an initial polarization toward the Th2 cytokine phenotype and the relatively poor development of the Th1 component during early infancy.

In a study of tetanus toxin-specific T-cell cytokine response, it was shown that at a 2-mo bleed prior to the vaccination, the tetanus toxin antigen induced IL-5, IL-13, IL-4, IL-9, and IFN-γ responses were infrequent or very low. The study of production of cytokines at four ages up to 12 mo showed that in spite of the large variation between individual infants, half of the group studied exhibited IL-4, IL-13, IL-9, and IFN-γ responses and one-third exhibited IL-5 responses. In contrast, the IFN-γ production level did not rise over the same period of time *(1201)*. These findings indicate a strong contribution of the Th2 cytokines to early vaccine response that corroborate to the presence and persistence of antitetanus toxin antibodies.

In other studies, the production of cytokines by pertussis-specific stimulated T cells was investigated in a group of DPT-vaccinated children. It has been shown that the recovery from pertussis and the immunization with heat-inactivated vaccine selectively induced a Th1 type of response *(1202,1203)*. By contrast, the vaccination with DT-acellular pertussis vaccine induces a type 2-dominated response characterized by production of IL-5 but not of IFN-γ by lymphocytes stimulated with pertussis toxin and filamentous HA. The Th2-type cytokine response was evident in full-term rather than in preterm infants *(1199)*.

Further studies are required to determine the importance of CMI responses elicited by DTP vaccination of infants.

3.4. Hepatitis A Virus Vaccine

Primarily, the fetal-oral route acquires hepatitis A virus (HAV) infection. The highest incidence rates occur among children ages 5–14 yr. Children likely play an important role in the transmission of HAV in the context of community outbreaks. Thus, the worldwide vaccination of children against HAV should lead to eradication of this virus. Both live-attenuated and inactivate HAV vaccines have been developed. A live-attenuated H2 strain HAV vaccine developed in China has been reported to be effective *(1204)*. However, the majority of other countries use an inactivated vaccine. The inactivated vaccine consists of formalin-inactivated HAV adsorbed on aluminum. HAV-licensed vaccine was approved for use in 2-yr-old children, however, recent studies indicate that a seroconversion rate of 100% could be achieved in infants vaccinated at ages 5 and 11 mo *(1205)*. A booster may be given 6–12 mo after the primary vaccination. The highest incidence dose is needed, and more than 97% of children vaccinated at age 2 yr develop a high level of protective antibodies *(1206,1207)*. Anamnestic antibody and CMI responses are lifelong, indicating that HAV vaccine elicits solid immunological memory. In spite of the fact that the level of antibodies decreases rapidly 1 yr after vaccination, it seems that the level of antibodies required for protection persists for at least 10 yr *(1207)*. There is an increased effort to develop inactivated HAV vaccines with enhanced immunogenicity. Such vaccines were prepared by incorporation of HAV antigen into influenza virosomes *(1208)* or into liposomes *(1209)*.

4. SUBUNIT VACCINES

Subunit vaccines represent a variant of inactivated vaccines produced by purification from bacteria of antigens that bear epitopes able to induce the synthesis of protective antibodies. Table 33 lists licensed subunit vaccines used for the vaccination of children.

The bacterial subunit vaccines consist of purified capsular polysaccharides (PSs). The PSs are type 2 T-independent antigens that are generally poor

Table 33
Subunit Licensed Vaccines

Haemophilus influenzae type b
Streptococus pneumoniae heptavalent vaccine
Neisseria meningitidis type A and C
Bordetella pertussis acellular vaccine

immunogens and induce the synthesis of low-affinity IgM antibodies, which exert their protective effect by opsonin-dependent phagocytosis mechanisms. PSs that exhibiting repetitive epitopes induce antibody synthesis subsequent to the crosslinking of BCRs. The anti-PS antibodies are produced by a subset of B cells that exhibits an ontogenic-delayed development; this explains the low efficacy of PS vaccines in young infants and the lack of response in infants with Wiskott–Aldrich syndrome who bear an X-linked gene that controls the development of the B-cell subset stimulated by PS. To increase the immunogenicity, a bacterial subunit vaccine is generally covalently linked to a protein carrier. The PS-protein conjugate vaccine displays an enhanced immune response related to the T-cell carrier effect.

A subunit vaccine is very stable, and the antibody response is restricted to a PS epitope. This is a real advantage compared to inactivate bacteria vaccines in which the antibody response to protective epitopes can be diluted by production of antibodies against numerous macromolecules present on the surface of a bacterium, which also bear nonprotective epitopes.

The major disadvantage of subunit vaccines is that antibody response is generally weak and requires several boosts. In addition, in the case of bacteria with multiple serotypes, the subunit vaccines should contain PS extracted from each serotype.

Polysaccharide-encapsulated bacteria such as *Streptococcus pneumoniae*, *Neisseria meningitidis*, and *Haemophilus influenzae* are among the most prevalent bacterial pathogens in humans and, in particular, a major cause of local and invasive infections in children. The protective antibodies against these bacteria are specific for capsular PS and prevent the infection by promoting opsonin-mediated phagocytosis and subsequent killing of bacteria by neutrophils and macrophages. The production of antibodies elicited by PS antigens does not require antigen processing and presentation of antigen by APCs to T cells. The role of T cells in the amplification of antibody synthesis elicited by T-independent type 2 antigens does not result from a physical contact with B cells but rather from secretion of cytokines into internal milieu where B cells are sitting. The role of T cells in class switching and affinity maturation of antibody response induced by T-independent type 2 antigen is often referred as noncognate T-cell help.

Early subunit vaccines containing the purified PS were so poorly immunogeneic that the need for more immunogeneic vaccine suitable for the induction of a protective response in children led to the development of a new generation of PS subunit vaccines. The new generation of PS vaccines exhibiting greater immunogenicity in infants is capable of eliciting immunological memory and stronger booster response. The new generation of PS vaccines was produced by coupling the PS with proteins. Various proteins such as diphtheria toxoid, tetanus toxoid, or meningoccocal outer membrane vesicle were used to prepare PS-protein conjugate vaccines.

The enhanced protective antibody response in young children results from carrier protein effect on the immunogenicity of PS in PS-protein vaccine. Protein carrier activates the CD4 T cells that secrete cytokines, which represent the second signal required for the activation of B cells subsequent to binding of PS antigen to specific BCRs. This concept is supported by a study carried out on infants ages 2, 4, and 6 mo who were vaccinated or not with tetanus toxoid at age 1 mo . The infants immunized with tetanus toxoid at age 1 mo had a higher geometric mean of anti-PS antibodies than infants who did not receive tetanus immunization. Therefore, this finding strongly suggested that the enhanced anti-PS response in children immunized with PS-protein conjugate vaccine resulted from the carrier priming effect of T cells

4.1. Haemophilus Influenzae Vaccine

Haemophilus influenzae are divided into six serotypes designated a, b, c, d, e, and f based on antigenic differences in their capsular material.

H. influenzae type b (Hib) was one the most common etiological agents of infantile bacterial infection. Even today, it continues to be a major cause of morbidity and mortality in developing countries. The virulence factor is the capsular PS consisting of high-molecular-mass repetitive units of 3-b-D-ribose(1-1) ribosyl-S-phosphate. The PS promotes survival of bacterium by inhibiting the phagocytosis and killing of bacteria. Whereas the neonates are protected by virtue of maternal antibodies, the infection rapidly increases, beginning after age 3 mo when the concentration of maternal antibodies waned and natural immunity elicited by nasopharyngeal colonization or infection by bacterium itself does not develop until about age 24 mo. These conditions explain why the incidence of infection peaks at age 6–12 mo and the vaccination is important in this age window. The incidence of infection declines and is rare in children older than age 5 yr. The subunit vaccine based on Hib-PS was poorly immunogenic in infants and failed to induce memory or a booster response. These drawbacks of earlier Hib-PS vaccine led to the development of more powerful vaccines that are able to induce a better response. The second generation of Hib-PS vaccines consists of chemical linkage of Hib-PS or oligosaccharide with a protein. The PS-protein conjugates have greater immunogenicity and are able to elicit recall responses because they elicit immunological memory.

Various companies produced several vaccines that consist of Hib-PS covalently linked to carrier proteins. All of them followed a similar rule, namely, to include in new formulation as carrier a protein from other vaccines known to display a priming effect in neonates. There are several Hib-PS conjugate vaccines that are currently licensed and used in various countries including the United States. They differ in the structure of PS moiety, the type of carrier protein, and the chemical nature of the covalent linkage of PS to protein.

The first conjugate vaccine licensed in the United States consisted of Hib-PS covalently linked to diphtheria. In one of the first trials carried out in Finland, it was shown that this vaccine conjugate is immunogenic and was 94% effective in the prevention of invasive disease after a schedule of three doses of vaccination in children at ages 3, 4, and 6 mo *(1210)*. Compared with other vaccine conjugate developed later, the Hib-PS diphtheria toxoid conjugate exhibits poorest immunogenicity and poor efficacy for the protection of a high-risk population. A more immunogenic vaccine that is able to elicit antibody with higher affinity was generated by covalent linkage of an oligosaccharide of 25 repetitive units derived from Hib-PS linked to CRM_{197}, a nontoxic protein fragment of diphtheria toxin. Furthermore, it was shown that the vaccines produced by conjugation of Hib-PS with tetanus toxoid or meningococcal outer membrane vesicles have also been immunogenic in infants after primary immunization at ages 2 and 4 mo or a single dose in infants as young as age 2 mo, respectively. It should be noted that the antibodies elicited by the vaccination with these two vaccine conjugates have lower avidity and lower bactericidal activity (reviewed in ref. *1211*).

Various clinical trials using these PS-conjugated vaccines alone, in combination with DTP, *(1200,1212)* or as pentavalent vaccines Hib-2-conjugated to tetanus toxoid, DTP, and poliovirus inactivated vaccines *(1194,1195)* showed that all children developed protective levels of anti-Hib-PS antibodies. In 5- or 7-yr follow-up studies of the vaccine response in preterm or full-term children vaccinated at ages 2, 4, and 6 mo *(1195)* or ages 3, 5, and 12 mo *(1194)*, it was shown that three priming doses induced higher geometric mean concentrations of antibodies with relative moderate avidity for all antigens contained in pentavalent vaccines. The positive correlation between the levels of antibody response specific for Hib-PS antigen and lack of correlation with antibodies against other antigens contained in pentavalent vaccines argues against carrier-induced epitope suppression operating through competition at the level of APCs that generate relevant peptides from the processing of vaccines. These vaccines may activate CD4 helper T cells required for the induction of an antibody response elicited by T-dependent antigens.

Studies aimed at characterizing immunochemical and molecular properties of anti-Hib-PS antibodies have advanced our knowledge on the development of immunity against Hib-PS. These studies strongly suggest that like murine anti-PS antibody response *(606)*, in humans anti-Hib-PS antibody response is oligopauciclonal. This concept is supported by several findings.

First, isoelectrofocusing analysis of affinity-purified anti-PS antibodies from various individuals showed the presence of only one to four clonotypes, which persisted even for prolonged periods after the secondary immunization *(1213)*.

Second, anti-Hib-PS antibodies express crossreactive idiotypes that are encoded by V gemline genes. The presence of a few crossreactive idiotypes in an inbred population is strong evidence that the response is oligoclonal, because the crossreactive idiotypes are encoded by V gemline genes. Two major crossreactive idiotypes—Hibld-1 expressed on the V_KII-A2 allele and Hibd-2 marker of $V\lambda$-VII—are preferentially expressed on specific anti-Hib-PS antibodies *(1214)*. In Hib1d-1 antibodies, the V_KII-A2 chain pairs most frequently with members from the V_HIII gene family. It is interesting to mention that the V_KII-A2 gene rearranged preferentially with J_K2 segments has a conserved arginine residue at position 95 at the V_K-J_K junction *(1215)*. The conservation of invariant arginine residue at position 95 in the CDR3 of the V_KII gene may play an important role in the binding of the Hib-PS antigen. This is supported by an experiment by Lucas et al. *(1216)*, who made various V_KII-A2 mutants with different amino acid residues at position 95. V_K with a junctional arginine or lysine at position 95 exhibited the highest affinity, whereas those having threonine, glycine, tyrosine, alanine, leucine, or serine displayed low affinity. Interestingly, a construct made of canonical V_KII-A2 containing arginine at position 95 but recombined with J_K3 instead of J_K1 had a very low affinity for Hib-PS antigen. Sequencing of V_H and $V\lambda$ genes expressed in monoclonal antibodies that were produced by hybridomas obtained from adults vaccinated with all four types of Hib vaccines showed a biased use of members of V_HIII. There was particular use of $V_HIII.23$ paired with V_KII-A2 and of V_H 3–15 paired with various $V\Lambda$ ($V\lambda II$, $V\lambda III$, $V\lambda VII$) and rarely with V_KII-A2, indicating again the pauciclonality of the response. Most Hib-PS antibodies exhibit somatic mutation, and approx 60% of nucleotide differences resulted in amino acid replacements. Some human anti-Hib-PS antibodies exhibit multispecific binding properties to self-antigens, such as DNA, cardiolipin, or myosin, or crossreactivity with *Escherichia coli* K100 PS. It is noteworthy that antibodies exhibiting crossreactivity are not encoded by canonical V3-15 or -23 with V_KII-A2, however, most frequent various V3 members pair with other V_K or V_L genes (e.g., V_K1 or V_K3) (reviewed in ref. *1211*).

Study of the expression of major crossreactive idiotypes and avidity of anti-PS antibodies of children vaccinated at ages 2, 4, and 6 mo with Hib-PS conjugate showed variations with the type of vaccine used. For example, HibId-1 idiotype is expressed on 46–68% of antibodies from children vaccinated with PS linked to tetanus toxoid or with oligosaccharide linked to CRM_{197} protein, whereas it is expressed on only 47% of antibodies from those vaccinated with PS-meningococcal outer membrane protein formulation. Based on the antigen-binding property, in particular to Hib-PS and other antigens and to the ability of PS to inhibit the binding of anti-idiotype antibodies, infant anti-PS antibodies were classified into two categories: (a) high affinity, antigen inhibitable and (b) low affinity, non-Hib-PS inhibitable *(1214)*.

The sequencing of a few monoclonal antibodies obtained from vaccinated children showed 100% homology with germ line genes in the case of V3-23 gene and V_KII. They also have an arginine at the $V_KII–J_K3$ junction that is typically found in the adult Hib-PS repertoire. Low-affinity monoclonal antibodies expressing noninhibitable idiotypes of infants are encoded by multiple genes belonging to the V_H3 family (V3-7, V3-21, V3-23, V3-30) and a V_H4 family member. Eight different V_K and Vλ segments, including the V_KII-A2 gene, were paired with V_H genes. The nucleic acid homology of V_H and Vλ genes encoding infant non-PS inhibitable antibodies that display low affinity exhibited 96–100% homology with the corresponding germ line genes and had low frequency of replacement mutations *(1211)*.

The analysis of binding properties, the affinity, the usage of the V gene family, and the rate of somatic mutation of infant PS-specific antibodies suggest that the Hib-PS repertoire of infants is more diverse than that of adults vaccinated with Hib-PS conjugates. Thus, it is possible that more restricted pauciclonal adult repertoires derive from memory cells expressing a BCR with high affinity in the infant repertoire.

Antibodies elicited by vaccination represent an important defense mechanism in young children. Whereas neonates are rarely affected because of the presence of maternal antibodies, the incidence of infection rapidly increases beginning at about age 3 mo and peaks at age 6–12 mo. The infection declines in older children because the vaccination induces memory cells that can be stimulated repetitively in older children and adults by Hib, which is found in the upper respiratory tract of approx 30% of individuals.

4.2. Streptococcus Pneumoniae Vaccine

The pneumococci are divided into more than 80 serotypes on the basis of the structural differences in their PS capsules. Antibodies against PS are protective. The pneumococcal cell wall also contains a C carbohydrate analogous to the Lancefield antigen and an M protein that is similar to group streptococci. Unlike group streptococci M protein, the pneumococcal M protein is not antiphagocytic and anti-M protein antibodies are not protective.

S. pneumoniae is the causative agent of pneumonia, meningitis, and acute otitis media in children. Antipneumococcal vaccine is a subunit vaccine containing PS from seven different serotypes.

The heptavalent PS vaccine is recommended for children with recurrent or severe otitis and to prevent invasive pneumococcal disease. Plain PS pneumoccocal vaccine is poorly immunogeneic in infants. In the new pneumococcal vaccine, the PS is covalently linked to CRM_{197} protein. The PS-protein conjugate vaccine caused an impressive reduction in invasive pneumococcal disease over a period of 1 yr in 1-, 2-, and 5-yr-old children. The vaccine may be protecting against otitis media as well as against 98% of antibiotic-resistant isolates *(1217)*. The vaccine has also been highly effective in preterm infants. A recent trial aimed to evaluate the efficacy of the vaccine in the prevention of otitis media in older children who have had previous episodes of acute otitis. In vaccinated toddlers and children, vaccination with heptavalent PS-protein conjugate followed by a boost with plain PS vaccine containing PS from 23 serotypes did not prevent acute otitis media in children older than age 1 yr who had recurrent episodes before vaccination *(1218)*.

The pneumococcal vaccine induces the production of low-avidity IgM antibodies and in 50–60% of subjects a twofold increase of IgG antibodies. The protection is related to an enhanced opsoin-mediated killing of bacteria.

4.3. Neisseria Meningitidis Vaccines

The meningococci are strict microbes in humans that can be found in the nasopharynx of carriers. In a small percentage of cases, meningococci may enter into the bloodstream and cause acute otitis, meningitis, and in rare cases meningococcemia resulting in explosive Waterhouse–Frederichsen syndrome or disseminated intravascular coagulation syndrome. Based on the structure of capsular PS, the meningococci were classified into seven serotypes. Among them, serotypes A and C are the more frequent bacteria that cause disease in children.

The development of menigococcal PS-conjugate vaccines provided a new opportunity for prevention of meningococcal diseases in children, because, unlike the plain PS vaccines, they are immunogeneic in infants and memory primers.

In 1974, a quadrivalent vaccine consisting of purified PS from serotypes A, C, Y, and W-135 was successfully used to stop an epidemic in Brazil. The immunogenicity of meningococcal PS in assorted age groups varied. Whereas serotype A PS elicits bactericidal antibodies in 3-mo-old children, children younger than age 2 yr respond poorly to C, Y, and W-135 serotypes. Serotype B PS is not immunogeneic in humans.

New generations of the meningococcal vaccine consist of PS covalently linked to CRM_{197} protein absorbed onto aluminum hydroxide. The vaccine is safe and it does not cause serious side effects among groups of children with different vaccination schedules. There are important differences in the induction of the immune response in infants between plain PS and PS-protein conjugate vaccines.

Serotype C PS vaccine induces a largely T-independent response characterized by low, short-lived antibody response and short-lived protection. There are data that indicate that plain serogroup C PS vaccine may induce a hyperresonsiveness that is not observed after vaccination with serotype A vaccine *(1219)*. In contrast, the thymic-dependent PS-conjugate vaccines are more immunogeneic in toddlers and infants. These vaccines induce a mucosal immune response and immunological memory.

The induction of mucosal immunity is an important advantage because meningococcus is a mucosal pathogen colonizing nasopharynx and, therefore, may play a role in the defense reaction against infection and carriers. In a study of pre- and postvaccination concentrations of salivary IgG and IgA antibodies after primary vaccination with serotype C PS-protein conjugate vaccine, a significant increase of specific IgG antibodies was found, but there was no significant increase of IgA *(1220)*. An increase of salivary IgA antibodies was observed in a study in which a bivalent serotype A and C PS-conjugate vaccine was used *(1220)*. Salivary IgA is likely to be locally produced as a secretory form, because no increase of serum IgA concentration was observed after vaccination *(1221)*. Increased concentrations of salivary PS-specific IgG and IgA antibodies resulted in reduction of nasopharyngeal carriage after vaccination *(1222)*.

Vaccination of toddlers with menigococcal C conjugate vaccine induced high titers of anti-PS and bactericidal antibodies, which persisted for at least 12 mo *(1219)*. After the first boost, the bactericidal titer in 90% of vaccinees was low; however, the second dose given 2 mo after the primary immunization increased the titer more than eightfold.

Longlasting memory induced by vaccination with meningococcal A/C conjugate was demonstrated in a study in which the infants were revaccinated at age 5 yr *(1223)*. The induction of memory probably is related to recruitment of T-cell help by revaccination, providing the necessary signals to maintain the memory B cells. Therefore, these vaccines have the potential to provide long-term protection of infants *(1220)*.

5. RECOMBINANT PROTEIN VACCINES

The preparation of recombinant protein is based on cloning a microbial gene encoding a protein that bears protective epitopes linked to a promoter and inserted into a suitable plasmid replicon. The plasmid replicon is used to transform a bacterium such as *E. coli* or to stabilize transfected mammalian cells, insect cells, or yeast. The proteins are then purified from transfected cells or from the culture if the gene in the construct is linked to a secretory sequence.

Recombinant proteins are safe and induce strong protective antibody responses; however, they generally are unable to stimulate CTL responses because the recombinant protein is processed via the exogenous pathway, generating peptides recognized by CD4 T cells in the context of MHC class II antigens.

HBV causes acute hepatitis, a disease that can vary anywhere from a mild form to a destructive disease leading to cirrhosis or liver cancer. About 300 million people worldwide are thought to be carriers of HBV; of those carriers, 40% are expected to die of liver diseases. Vaccination provides a tool for the control of HBV. The vaccine consists of yeast-derived recombinant containing hepatitis B surface antigen (HbsAg). In the case of unresponsiveness to the current vaccine, an experimental vaccine containing both HbsAg recombinant protein and pre-S proteins are under evaluation *(1124)*.

The HbsAg vaccine is highly immunogeneic and given soon after birth. Successful vaccination induces high levels of protective antibodies, dramatically reducing the HBV infection rate and preventing chronic infection and the life-threatening sequelae (reviewed in ref. *1225*).

Immunoprophylaxis can be achieved by vaccination during pregnancy. Vaccination during pregnancy is safe and highly immunogeneic. The passive transfer of maternal antibodies to newborns confers protection for the first 4 mo of life. In offspring born to mothers vaccinated with three doses, the level of antibodies is 95 mIU/mL at birth, 57 mIU/mL at a 2-mo follow-up, and 37 mIU/mL at a 4-mo follow-up *(1226)*.

HBV can be transmitted vertically from infected mothers to newborns. In this case, it is recommended that immune Ig be administered within 12 h of birth, with three doses of vaccine administered at ages 1, 2, and 6 mo.

HBV vaccine is also very efficient in preterm babies. Good anti-HBV levels of antibody were detected in 60% of preterm babies after primary vaccination and in 100% of preterm babies after the third dose *(1227)*. Different studies clearly demonstrated that immunization at birth with HbsAg recombinant vaccine is beneficial in endemic area injection.

6. DNA VACCINES

The principle of the use of naked DNA as vaccines is based on observations that injection of plasmids containing a foreign gene may lead to in vivo transfection of cells. Wolff et al. *(640)* demonstrated that a foreign gene contained in a plasmid was transcribed and translated in muscle cells subsequent to intramuscular based on the use of plasmid that contained microbial genes bearing protective epitopes. Soon after this finding, Johnston et al. *(641)* showed that the intramuscular injection of a plasmid expressing the bovine growth hormone gene induced the production of antibodies specific for the hormone. This basic information galvanized a new research area, because it opened a new avenue for the development of vaccines that induce a longlasting antibody response.

Several advantages made genetic immunization very appealing for vaccinologists:

1. DNA is as stable as subunit vaccines and more stable than live-attenuated vaccines.
2. The immunogeneic dose is small, in terms of micrograms.
3. Manufacturing procedures are low-cost and, therefore, suitable for global vaccine programs—in particular, for developing countries that can not afford the high cost of some vaccines.
4. The DNA vaccines can be rapidly constructed. This is an important property for preparation of vaccines against microbes that exhibit natural genetic variation such as influenza virus, HIV, trypanosome, etc.
5. There is the possibility to express in the same plasmid genes encoding protective epitopes from different microbes.
6. Lack of proteins in plasmids precludes the induction of side effects such as allergic reaction, brain damage, and inflammatory reaction at the site of injection.
7. Genetic immunization does not require adjuvants because the plasmids are themselves endowed with immunostimulatory sequences rich in CpG motifs, which bind to Toll-R9.
8. Genetic immunization induces not only protective antibody response but also CTL response, which can not be elicited by inactivated, subunit, and recombinant protein vaccines.
9. Longlasting persistence of plasmids, as episome results in sustained synthesis of antigens at low levels, which precludes the induction of high-dose tolerance, and drives the immune response to memory.
10. Plasmid DNA does not integrate into host DNA by homologous recombination.

Numerous studies have addressed the ability of DNA vaccines to induce immune responses in neonates. These studies demonstrated that neonatal inoculation of DNA vectors expressing a wide range of microbial antigens into mice or non-human primates overcame the neonatal immune unresponsiveness and resulted in efficient priming of B cells, CD4, and cD8 T cells. Table 34 lists the animal models in which the genetic immunization of neonates induced humoral and CMI responses.

There are qualitative and quantitative differences between the immune responses induced by genetic immunization in neonates and adults. In neonates, the antibody response is generally low, however, the priming of B cells is very efficient. In spite of the fact that the magnitude of the antibody response elicited by DNA neonatal immunization is lower compared to adult DNA immuni-

Table 34
DNA Vaccines Inducing Immune Response in Neonates

Microbe	Gene-encoding protein	Species tested	Type of induced immune response
Clostridium tetanii	C fragment	Mouse	Humoral
Plasmodium yoelii	CSP	Mouse	Humoral, CTL
Influenza virus	Hemagglutinin, nucleoprotein	Mouse, babboon	Humoral ,CTl
		Mouse	CTL, humoral
Rabies virus	glycoprotein	Mouse	Humoral, Th1
Pseudorabies	gD glycoprotein	Pig	Humoral
Hepatitis B virus	HbsAg	Monkey	Humoral
Murine retrovirus	Cas-Br-M protein	Mouse	CTL, Th1
Measles virus	Hemaoglutinin	Mouse	Humoral, Th1
Herpes simplex virus	gB glycoprotein	Mouse	Humoral, Th1
Bovine hereps virus	gD glycoprtin	Sheep	Humoral, Th1
LCMV	Nucleoprotein	Mouse	CTL
Sendai virus	Nucleoprotein	Mouse	CTL, humoral
Respiratory syncitial virus F antigen	Mouse	Humoral, CTL	
HIV	Envelope gag-pol proteins	Monkey	Humoral

zation, the protection against a challenge with infectious agents carried out during adulthood was similar in mice immunized as newborns and as adults.

Whereas the neonatal response induced by various antigens is characterized by Th2 dominance, the profile elicited by neonatal immunization with naked DNA comprises an important Th1 component similar to that described after immunization at birth with BCG live-attenuated vaccine. Our studies carried out in mice demonstrated that immunization after birth with a plasmid containing the HA gene of influenza virus induced a mixed Th1/Th2 response *(951)*. The polarization toward a Th1 response can be induced by co-injection of plasmid containing a microbial gene with plasmids containing IL-12 or IFN-γ genes *(1228)*.

Although immunization of newborns with viruses induced a meager or no CTL response, the neonatal immunization with plasmids containing gene-encoding proteins that bear epitopes recognized by CD8 CTL efficiently primed the CTL. This was well illustrated in our study in which we measured the frequency of CTL precursors in mice immunized at birth with a plasmid containing influenza virus nucleoprotein (NP) gene. We found that memory CTL pool was expanded between 1 and 3 mo *(1076)*. This finding strongly suggests that exposure to antigens secreted by transfected cells continues after neonatal immunization with a plasmid and expanded the CTL precursors. Based on the long persistence of plasmids in transfected cells, it was assumed that DNA vaccines should generate memory cells. Using sensitive techniques such as measuring the frequency of precursors of antigen-specific lymphocytes or intracellular staining of cytokines producing T cells, various groups showed a remarkable lifelong persistence of memory T cells after neonatal immunization with naked DNA (reviewed in ref. *651*).

The studies on immunity induced by DNA vaccines clearly demonstrated that DNA vaccines administered after birth are immunogeneic rather than tolerogeneic. The neonatal immunity conferred by neonatal vaccination resembles that elicited in adults by DNA or live-attenuated vaccines. This is remarkable, taking into account the low response induced by vaccination of newborns with inactivated or subunit vaccines and the induction of tolerance by neonatal immunization with foreign antigens and alloantigens.

Efficient induction of immunity by DNA immunization of neonates may be related to several factors:

    a. Long persistence of plasmids as episomes in transfected cells allows the exposure and priming of newly emerging B cells from the bone marrow and T cells from the thymus to small amounts of antigens, circumventing the possibility to induce high-dose tolerance.

    b. The plasmid has intrinsic adjuvant properties, which contain CpG motifs able to bind to Toll-R9 and to activate immature neonatal APCs. Co-injection of CpG oligonucleotide with plasmid induced higher responses and crosspriming *(1068)*.

In addition, we have shown that CpG oligonucleotide can induce the expression of MHC class II and the increased production of chemokines in myocytes, which acquired the ability to present to CD4 T cell a peptide derived from a protein encoded by corresponding genes expressed in the plasmid *(965)*.

c. The plasmids rich in CpG motifs may accelerate the maturation of APCs, leading to upregulation of genes encoding MHC molecules; upregulation of costimulatory molecules such as CD40, B7.1, and B7.2; and production of IL-12, which is required for the activation of IFN-γ in Th1 cells. The coadministration of CpG motif-rich plasmids with plasmids containing GM-CSF accelerates the maturation of dendritic cells, which are the major target of in vivo transfection by plasmids *(88–91)*. Thus, the recruitment and the activation/maturation of APCs by immunostimulatory CpG motifs overcome the limiting number and immaturity of neonatal APCs.

d. There exists a lack of interference of genetic immunization with maternal antibodies *(697–702)*.

The efficacy of DNA vaccination of neonates in rodents and non-human primates was well established in various studies (reviewed in ref. *1230*). The findings generated from these preclinical trials represent a basis for the use of DNA vaccines for the immunization of newborns and infants.

We believe that ensuing years will see the use of DNA vaccines in infants.

7. THERACINES

Vaccines have been developed to prevent infectious diseases. The fervent development of immunobiology and molecular biology has led to an expansion of vaccines to prevent or alter the course of immunity-mediated diseases, including autoimmune, allergic, and some inflammatory diseases. These therapeutic vaccines are called theracines.

The basic principle of theracines is to use different platforms to deliver peptides that either suppress the T cells, which mediate such diseases, or expand regulatory T cells, exerting an inhibitory effect on pathogenic T cells.

Such vaccines can be used in autoimmune diseases mediated by T cells, such as multiple sclerosis, type I diabetes, uveitis, Crohn's disease, and allergic diseases.

Because the synthetic peptides corresponding to epitopes recognized by T cells have a short half-life, several new methods of delivery of peptides have been developed. The ideal delivery system of T-cell epitopes consists of the use of self-molecules as platforms. In our laboratory, we have developed three main approaches:

a. The expression of foreign or self-epitopes in CDRs of V_H genes that encode an antibody molecule *(1072)*.
b. Enzymatically engineered immunoglobulins expressing T-cell epitopes linked to oligosaccharide moiety of Ig molecules *(1231)*.
c. Soluble chimeric peptide-class II molecules *(855,1232)*.

The construction of such molecules and their properties was recently described *(1229–1231)*.

Peptides corresponding to epitopes of self-protein antigens inducing autoimmune diseases alone or presented on self-platforms were used in various experimental models of autoimmune diseases. Of particular interest is the use of theracines in neonates to prevent autoimmune or allergic diseases.

Experimental allergic encephalomyelitis (EAE) is an animal model of antigen-specific Th1-mediated disease. The characteristic clinical and histological features of chronic relapsing paralysis and demyelination with perivascular lymphocyte infiltration of the central nervous system resembles human multiple sclerosis. The pathogenic T cells initiating EAE are specific for myelin basic protein (MBP). The EAE can be induced by immunization with MBP as well as with synthetic peptides corresponding to different regions of MBP. The α-acetylated *N*-terminal peptide corresponding to nine amino acids is the dominant encephalitogenic T-cell epitope in certain strains of mice expressing H-2^u or H-2^s MHC haplotype. Neonatal administration of the peptide 1152de greatly reduced not only the response to MBP but also prevented the induction of EAE *(1151)*. These results demonstrated that the immunodominant peptide administered after birth can tolerize pathogenic T cells.

In our laboratory, we constructed a chimeric immunoglobulin molecule in which the CDR3 of a murine V$_H$ gene was replaced with an immunodominant epitope derived from influenza virus NP recognized by the CD8 T cell in the context of MHC class I molecules or from HA recognized by CD4 T cells in association with MHC class II molecules. These chimeric Ig molecules activate NP- or HA-specific T cells *(1072,1232)*.

Zagouhani's laboratory constructed a chimeric Ig molecule in which the CDR3 of the same V$_H$ gene was replaced with a peptide derived from encephalitogenic proteolipid protein (PPL). The Ig-PPL peptide is presented to T cells 100-fold better than the free PPL peptide *(1162)*. Neonatal exposure to chimeric Ig-PPL peptide confers resistance to EAE by polarizing the response toward Th2 and IFN-γ-mediated T cell anergy *(1162)*. T cells from neonatal tolerized mice failed to proliferate and produce IFN-γ upon incubation with peptide but secreted significant amounts of IL-2. The pathogenic PPL-specific T cells tolerized subsequent to neonatal exposure to Ig-PPL peptide chimeric molecules are defective in the expression of CD40 ligand; this leads to noneffective interaction with APCs and lack of production of IL-12, which is required for the production of IFN-γ by pathogenic Th1 cells.

These findings demonstrated that neonatal exposure to a PPL-derived peptide presented on an Ig platform can anergize pathogenic Th1 cells, thereby preventing the induction of EAE later in adult animals.

The role of T cells in pathogenesis of type I autoimmune diabetes has been overtly demonstrated by studies in animal models. Thus, it was shown that (a) neonatal thymectomy in genetically prone mice for diabetes prevents the occurrence of disease *(1233)*; (b) athymic nonobese diabetic (NOD) nu/nu mice do not develop diabetes *(1234)*; (c) T cells are the majority of early infiltrating lymphocytes in the pancreatic islets of NOD mice *(1235)*; (d) diabetes is transferred in neonates, adult F1 mice, and SCID mice either by bone marrow cells, splenic T cells, or pancreatic T cells from diabetic mice *(1236–1238)*; (e) transplantation of pancreatic islets in the thymus of genetically prone mice for diabetes, or administration of diabetogenic synthetic peptides, leads to negative selection of diabetogenic T-cell precursors with subsequent prevention of the disease onset *(1239,1240)*; (f) treatment of prediabetic NOD mice with anti-CD4 antibodies prevents the insulitis *(1241)*; and (g) treatment of diabetic NOD mice with anti-CD4 monoclonal antibodies followed by grafting homologous islets can restore the normoglycemia *(1242)*.

In humans and animal models for spontaneous autoimmune diabetes, the T-cell reactivity against β-cell antigens (i.e., glutamic acid decarboxylase 65 (GAD65) *(1243)*, insulin *(1244)*, tyrosine phosphatase IA-2 *(1245)*, heat shock protein 60 (hsp60) *(1246)*, and the islet-cell antigen 69 (ICA69) *(1247)*) were demonstrated. The high-risk susceptibility to type 1 diabetes in humans is genetically associated with the expression of HLA-DR*0301, HLA-DR*0401, and HLA-DQ8 haplotypes. Similarly, the expression of I-A^{g7} but not I-E allele leads to the development of type 1 diabetes in NOD mice *(1248–1250)*.

The pathogenicity of CD4 T cells in diabetes is much related to the Th1 cells, whereas protection is associated with the Th2 and CD4 T regulatory cells *(1251,1252)*. The pathogenic role of Th1 cells was demonstrated by induction of diabetes in adoptive transfer experiments using Th1 clones specific for islet antigens *(1253,1254)* or by polarization of T cells toward a Th1 response upon injection of rIL-12 *(1255)*..Alternatively, downregulation of Th1 cells by anti-IFN-γ monoclonal antibodies or the expansion of Th2 cells in the pancreas by expression of the IL-4 gene in pancreatic β-islets abrogated the insulitis and autoimmune diabetes in NOD mice *(1256,1257)*. The CD4 T regulatory cells (e.g., CD4$^+$CD25^{hi}), IL-10-secreting CD4 Tr1-cells, and/or TGF-β-secreting CD4 T cells can suppress the diabetogenic process *(1258–1262)*.

The diabetogenic role of Th1 cells is much related to the activation of CD8 T cells, which ultimately lyse the pancreatic β-islets. Wang et al. showed that knocking out the CD8 T cells in NOD mice during a discrete age window could inhibit the development of insulitis *(1256)*. Alternatively, Katz et al. and Skyler et al. showed that autoimmune diabetes does not occur in NOD β2m-deficient mice, which are unable to mount an efficient CD8 T-cell response *(1263,1264)*.

Although diabetic mice and humans manifest pleiotropic humoral responses to the islet antigens *(1265)*, the autoantibodies do not play a pathogenic role in type I diabetes, as demonstrated in passive immunity experiments in animal models.

Several approaches have been undertaken to develop reagents aimed at preventing the occurrence of autoimmune diabetes. These approaches have been performed in animal models of type I diabetes through induction of neonatal tolerance to antigens expressed on B cells.

The effect of theracines in the prevention of type I diabetes was studied in experimental models.

An NOD mouse is a model in which the disease is prevalent in females and overt diabetes occurs at age 8 wk. Like in human type CD4 T cells *(1258)* mediate 1 diabetes, the IDDM in NOD mice. It is believed that some diabetogenic T cells in NOD mice are specific for GAD65 antigen, because antibodies and GAD65-specific T cells were detected in the majority of patients with recent-onset of type 1 diabetes (1253,1265). The administration of 100 mg GAD65 into female NOD mice 24 h after birth delayed the onset of overt diabetes compared to NOD mice injected after birth with PBS or bovine serum albumin *(1266)*. NOD mice from the GAD65-injected group displayed nearly complete absence of insulitis, suggesting that neonatal tolerization with GAD65 prevented not only hyperglycemia but also islet cell autoimmunity during the first 18 wk of life. It is noteworthy that the prevention of type 1 diabetes was temporary, because 60% of mice developed diabetes during the 60-wk observation period.

The insulin B chain (InsB) also bears a major epitope recognized by diabetogenic human and NOD T cells. The injection of a plasmid containing the gene that encodes InsB protein in NOD neonates resulted in a substantial protection of female NOD mice against type 1 diabetes. This was associated with a polarization of the response toward Th2 cells, which are considered to have protective properties. In the same mice, the Th2-associated cytokine IL-4 production was critical for protection. This concept was strongly supported by demonstration of development of type 1 diabetes in IL-4-deficient NOD mice injected with the InsB plasmid *(1270)*.

In our laboratory, we characterized a transgenic mouse model of juvenile type 1 diabetes. This transgenic model consists of double-transgenic mice expressing the HA of A/PR8/8/34 influenza virus under the control of rat insulin promoter in β-cells (INS-HA) and the TCR recognizing the immunodominant HA110-120 peptide in association with I-E^d MHC molecule (TCR-HA). Double-transgenic mice exhibited perinsulitis beginning 3 d after birth, hyperglycemia at age 7 to 14 d, and hypoinsulinemia at age 28 d. The occurrence of diabetes was associated with a gradual accumulation of T cells specific for HA in the pancreas *(948)*.

We have generated a soluble dimeric class II peptide chimeric molecule consisting of the extracellular domains of I-E^d-α and -β chains dimerized trough a murine Fcγ2 region at the C-terminus of I-E -β chain. This molecule, called DEF, stimulates the proliferation of T cells, induces the differentiation of T cells toward Th2, and binds complement *(1269)*.

The administration of soluble DEF in 7-d-old prediabetic mice prevented the onset of hyperglycemia and normalized glycemia values as long as DEF was injected every 5 d. The prevention of type 1 diabetes after the administration of DEF is related to the expansion of Tr1 cells producing IL-10 *(1269)*.

In summary, the prevention of type 1 diabetes by administration of DEF in young mice depends on several factors, among which the TCR/CD4 occupancy and ligand valence plays a key role in determining the resultant effects.

The generation of theracines containing peptides recognized by pathogenic T cells that mediate will open new avenues for the prevention and/or alteration of the course of human immune-mediated diseases.

REFERENCES

1. Metchnikoff E. Sur la lutte des cellules de l'organisme contre l'invasion des microbes. Ann Inst Pasteur 1887;1:321–330.
2. Savill J, Fadock V, Henson P, et al. Phagocytosis of cells undergoing apoptosis. Immunol Today 1993;14:131–136.
3. Mesrobeanu I, Bona C, Ioanid L, et al. Pinocytosis of some exotoxines by leucocytes. Exp Cell Res 1966;43:490–499.
4. Mesrobeanu I, Bona C, Vranialici D, et al. Pinocytosis of *Salmonella typhimurium* "O" endotoxin by the leucocytes of immunized animals. Z Immunitatsforsch Allerg Klin Immunol 1967;133:108–125.
5. Mesrobeanu I, Mesrobeanu L, Bona C, et al. Immunogenicity of lysosomal fractions prepared from leucocytes which pinocytized endotoxin. Z Immunitatsforsch Allerg Klin Immunol 1970;113:301–311.
6. Cooper EL, Kaushke E, Cossarizza A. Digging for innate immunity since Darwin and Metchinikoff. BioEssays 2002;24:319–333.
7. Medzhitov R, Preston-Hurlburt P, Janeway C. A human homologue of the Drosophila Toll protein signal activation of innate immunity. Nature 1997;388:394–397.
8. LeMaitre B, Nicholas E, Michaut L, et al. The dorsoventral regulatory gene cassette spatsle/Toll/cactus controls the potent anti-fungal response in Drosophila adults. Cell 1996;86:973–983.
9. Bona C, Ghyka G, Vranialici D. Alteration of the ability to take up foreign matter in neutrophils submitted to the effect of chemical and enzymatic agents. Exp Cell Res 1968;53:519–524.
10. Skogh MS, Blomoff R, Esklid W, et al. Hepatic uptake of circulating IgG immune complexes. Immunology 1985;55:585–594.
11. Delaunay A, Lebrun J, Barber M. Factors involved in chemotactism of leucocytes in vitro. Nature 1967:216:774–779.
12. Seternes T, Sorensen K, Smedsrod B. Scavenger endothelial cells in vertebrates: a no peripheral leukocytes system for high capacity elimination of waste molecules. Proc Natl Acad Sci USA 2002;99:7594–7597.
13. Smedsrod B, Petroff H. Intracellular fate of endocytized collagen in rat liver cells. Exp Cell Res 1996;223:39–49.
14. Smedsrod B, Johanson S, Petroff H. Studies in vivo and in vitro on the uptake and degradation of soluble collagen alpha (I) chains in rat liver endothelial cells. Biochem J 1985;228:415–424.
15. Melkko J, Hellevik T, Risteli L, et al. Clearance of propeptides of typeI and II procollagen is a physiological function of the scavenger receptor of endothelial cells. J Exp Med 1994;179:405–412.
16. Van Berkel TJC, De Rijke L, Risteli J. Different fate of oxydatively modified low density lipoprotein and acetylated low density protein in rats. Recognition

From: *Contemporary Immunology: Neonatal Immunity*
By: Constantin Bona © Humana Press Inc., Totowa, NJ

by various scavanger receptors on Kupffer and endothelial cells. J Biol Chem 1991;266:2282–2289.

17. Medzhitov R, Janeway C. Innate immune recognition: mechanisms and pathways. Immunol Rev 2000;173:89–97.

18. Bona C, Sulica A Dumitrescu M Vranialici D. Recognition of altered autologous constituents as foreign by phagocytic cells. Nature 1967;213(78):824–825.

19. Hashimoto C, Hudson K, Anderson KV. The Toll gene of Drosophilla required for morphogenesis for dorsal-ventral embryonic polarity, appears to encode a transmembrane protein. Cell 1988;52:269–279.

20. Mitcham JL, Parnet P, Bonnert TP, et al. T1/ST2 signaling establishes it as member of an interleukin-1 receptor family. J Biol Chem 1966;271:5777–5783.

21. Kopp E, Medzhitov R, Carrothers J, et al. EXSIT is an evolutionary conserved intermediate in the Toll/IL-1 signal transduction pathway. Genes Dev 1999;13:2059–2071.

22. Stein D, Toth S, Vogelsung E, et al. The polarity of the dorsoventral axis in the Drosophila embryo is defined as an extracellular signal. Cell 1991;65:725–753.

23. Takeuki O, Kawai T, Sanjo H, et al. TLR6: a novel member of an expanding Toll-like family. Gene 1999;213:59–65.

24. Chadhary PM, Ferguson C, Nguyen O, et al. Cloning and characterization of two Toll/interleukin 1 receptor-like genes Toll 3 and Toll 4: evidence for a multi-gene receptor family in humans. Blood. 1998;91:4020–4027.

25. O'Neill LAJ, Dinarello CA. The IL-1 receptor/toll-like receptor superfamily:crucial receptor for inflammation and cell defense. Immunol Today 2000;21:206–209.

26. Akira S, Takeda K, Kaish T. Toll-like receptor: critical proteins linking innate immunity and acquired immunity. Nat Immunol 2001;8:675–680.

27. Underhill DM, Ozinsky A, Hajar AM, et al. The Toll-like receptor 2 is recruited to macrophage phagosomes and discriminates between pathogens. Nature 1999;401:811–815.

28. Alexopoulou L, Holt AC, Medzhitov R, et al. Recognition of double-stranded RNA and activation of NF-kB by Toll-like receptor 3. Nature 2001;413:732–738.

29. Poltorak A. Defective LPS signaling in C3H/HeJ and C57BL/10ScCrb mice mutation in TLR4 gene. Science 1998;282:2085–2088.

30. Hoshino K. Toll-like receptor 4-deficient mice are hyporesponsive to lipopolysaccharide evidence for TLR4 as *Lps* gene product. J Immunol 1999;162:3749–3752.

31. Means TK, Golembock DT, Fenton MJ. The biology of Toll-like receptors. Cytokine Growth Factor Rev 2000;11:219–232.

32. Hayashi F. The innate immunity to bacterial flagellin is mediated by Toll-like receptor 5. Nature 2001;410:1099–1103.

33. Hemmi H. Toll-like receptor recognizes bacterial DNA. Nature 2000;408:740–745.

34. Shelton CA. Wasermann SA. Pelle encodes a protein kinase required to establish dorsoventral polarity of Drosophila embryo. Cell 1993;72:515–525.

35. Groshans J. Activation of the kinase Pelle by tube in the dorsoventral signal pathway of Drosophila embryo. Nature 1994;372:563–566.

36. Belvin MP, Anderson KV. A conserved signaling pathway: the Drosophila toll-dorsal pathway. Annu Rev Cell Dev Biol 1996;12:393–416.

37. Suzuki N, Suzuki S, Yeh W-C. IRAK-4 as the central TIR signaling mediator of innate immunity. Trends Immunol 2002;23:503–506.

38. Camano J, Hunter CA. NF-kB family of transcription factors: central regulators of innate and adaptive immune functions. Clin Micr Rev 2002;15:414–429.

39. Brown GB, Scazlo AA, Matusomo K, et al. The natural killer gene complex: a genetic basis for understanding natural killer cell function and innate immunity. Immunol Rev 1997;155:53–65.

40. Karlhofer FM, Ribaudo RK, Yokohama WM. MHC class I alloantigen specificity of Ly-49 in IL-2 activated natural killer cells. Nature 1992;358:66–70

41. Campbel KS, Colonna M. Human natural killer cell receptors and signaling transduction. Intern Rev Immunol 2001;20:333–371.

42. Von Bering I, Kitasato S. Uber das Zustandekommen der Diphterie immunitat und dei tetanus immunitat bei Thieren. Dtsch.Med. Wochenschr. 1890;16:1113–1114.

43. Ehrlich P. On immunity with special reference to cell life. Proc Roy Soc Lond 1889;66:424–428.

44. Gowans JL. The life history of lymphocytes. Br Med Bull 1959;15:50–53.

45. Burnet FM. The Clonal Theory of Acquired Immunity. Cambridge University Press. London: 1959.

46. Nemazee DA, Burk K. Clonal deletion of B lymphocytes in a transgenic mouse bearing anti-MHC class I antibody genes. Nature 1989;33:562–566.

47. Goodnow CC, Crosby J, Jorgensen H, et al. Induction of self-tolerance in mature peripheral B lymphocytes. Nature 1989;342:385–391.

48. Jerne N. Towards a network theory of the immune response. Ann Immunol (Paris) 1974;125C:373–379.

49. Bona C. Regulatory Idiotypes. John Wiley & Sons, Inc. New York: 1987.

50. Gwinn MR. Single nucleotide polymorphism of the N-formyl-peptide receptor in localized juvenile peridontitis. J Peridentol 1999;70:1994–1201.

51. Robineaux R, Nelson RA. Etude par la microcinematographie en contrast de phase du phenomen d'immunoadherance de la phagocytose secondaire. Ann Inst Pasteur 1955;89:254–261.

52. Mollinedo F, Borregaard N, Boxer LA. New trends in neutrophil structure, function and development. Immnol Today 1999;20:535–537.

53. Cassatella MA. The production of cytokines by polymorphonuclear neutrophils. Immunol Today 1995;16:21–26.

54. Del Pozo V, De Andreas B, Martin E, et al. Eosinophils as antigen-presenting cell: activation of T cell clones and T hybridoma by eosinophils after antigen processing. Eur J Immunol 1992;22:1919–1925.

55. Weller PF, Rand TH, Barrett T, et al. Accessory cell function of human eosinophils. J Immunol 1991;150:1554–1562.

56. Arock M, Ross E, Lai-Kuen R, et al. Phagocytic and tumor necrosis factor alpha response of human mast cells following exposure to Gram-negative and Gram-positive bacteria. Infect Immun 1998;66:6030–6034.

57. Malaviya R, Ross EA, MacGregor JI, et al. Mast phagocytosis of FimH-expressing bacteria. J Immunol 1994;152:1907–1914.

58. Echtenacher B, Mannel DN, Hultner L. Critical protective role of mast cells in a model of acute septic peritonitis. Nature 1996;381:75–77.

59. Sher A, Hein A, Moser G, et al. Complement receptors promote the phagocytosis of bacteria by rat peritoneal mast cells. Lab Invest 1979;263:334–336.

60. Kitamura Y, Hirota S, Morii E, et al. Gain-of- function mutations of c-kit in human diseases. In: Mast cells and basophils (Marone G, Lichenstein LM, Galli SJ, eds.) Academic Press NewYork 2000 pp. 21–29.

61. Feger F, Varadaradjalou S, Gao Z, et al. The role of mast cells in host defense and their subversion by bacterial pathogens. Trends Immunol 2002;23:151–158.

62. Ehrenreich H, Burd PR, Rottem M, et al. Endothelines belong to the assortment of mast cells-derived and mast-cell-bound cytokoines. N Biol 1992;4:147–156.

63. Malaviya R, Abraham SN. Role of mast-cell leukotriens in neutrophil recruitment and bacterial clearance in infectious peritonitis. J Leuk Biol 2000;67:841–846.

64. Malaviya R, Ikeda T, Ross E, et al. Mast cell modulation of neutrophil influx and bacterial clearance at site of infection through TNF-alpha. Nature 1996;181:77–80.

65. Malavyia R, Twesten NJ, Ross AE, et al. Mast cells process bacterial antigens through a phagocytic route for class I MHC presentation to T cells. J Immunol 1996;156,1490–1496.

66. Fox CC, Jewell SD, Whitacre CC. Rat peritoneal mast cell present antigen to PPD specific T cell line. Cell Immunol 1994;158:253–264.

67. Bona CA, Bonilla FA. Textbook of Immunology. Harwood Academic Publishers. NewYork, London: 1990.

68. Steinman RM, Cohn ZA. Identification of a novel cell type in peripheral lymphoid organs of mice I morphology, quantition, tissue distribution. J Exp Med 1973;137:1142–1162.

69. Van Voorhis WJ, Valinsky J, Hoffman M, et al. Relative efficacy of human monocytes and dendritic cells as accessory cells for T cell replication. J Exp Med 1983;158:174–191.

70. Freudenthal PS, Steinman RM. The distinct surface of human blood dendritic cells, as observed after an improved isolation method. Proc Natl Acad Sci USA 1990;87:7698–7702.

71. Witmer MD, Steinman RM. The anatomy of peripheral lymphoid organs with emphasis on accessory cells: light microscopic, immunocytochemical studies of mouse spleen, lymph node and Peyer's patch. Am J Anat 1991;170:465–481.

72. Drexhage HA, Mullink H, de Groot J, et al. A study of cells present in peripheral lymph of pigs with special reference to a type of cell resembling the Langerhans cells. Cell Tiss Res 1979;20:407–430.

73. Pugh CW, MacPherson GG, Steer HV. Characterization of nonlymphoid cells derived from rat peripheral lymph. J Exp Med 1983;15:1758–1779.

74. Holt PG, Haining S, Nelson DJ, et al. Origin and steady-state turnover of class II MHC-bearing dendritic cells in the epithelium of conducting airways. J Immunol 1994;153:256–261.

75. Bujdoso R, Hopkins H, Dutia BM, et al. Characterization of afferent lymph dendritic cells and their role in antigen carriage. J Exp Med 1989;170:1285–1302.
76. Rakasz E, Lynch RG. Female sex hormones as regulatory factors in the vaginal immune compartment. Intern Rev Immunnol 2002;21:497–513.
77. Pulendran B, Maraskovsky E, Banchereau J, et al. Modulating the immune response with dendritic cells and growth factors. Trends Immunol 2001;22:41–47.
78. Jiang W, Swiggard WJ, Heufler C, et al. The receptor DEC-205 expressed by dendritic cells and thymic epithelial cells is involved in antigen processing. Nature 1995;375:151–155.
79. Sallusto F, Cella M, Danieli C, et al. Dendritic cells use macropinocytosis and the mannose receptor to concentrate antigen in the major histocompatibility class II compartment. Downregulation by cytokines and bacterial products. J Exp Med 1995;182:389–400.
80. Olweus J, Bit I, Masour A, et al. Dendritic cell ontogeny: a human dendritic lineage of myeloid origin. Proc Natl Acad Sci USA 1997;94:12,551–12,256.
81. Tsuneyasu T, Shizuo A. Dendritic-cell function in Toll-like receptor and MyD88 knockout mice. Trends Immunol 2001;22:78–82.
82. Shortman K, Liu YI. Mouse and human dendritic cell subtypes. Nat Rev Immunol 2002;2:151–160.
83. Cella M, Jarrossay D, Facchetti F, et al. Plasmoid monocytes migrate to inflamed lymph nodes and produce large amount of type I interferon. Nat Med 1999;5:919–924.
84. Bachereau J, Briere F, Caux C, et al. Immunobiology of dendritic cells. Annu Rev Immunol 2000;18:767–811.
85. Steiman RM, Bona C, Inaba K. Dendritic cells: important adjuvants during DNA vaccination. In: DNA Vaccines. (Ertl G, ed.), Landes Bioscience. Georgetown, Texas: in press.
86. Ito T, Inaba M, Inaba K, et al. A CD1a⁻-CD11c⁺ subset of human blood dendritic cells is a direct precursor of Langerhans cells. J Immunol 1999;163:1409–1419.
87. Larsen CP, Steinman RM, Witmer-Pack M, et al. Migration and maturation of Langerhans in skin transplants and explants J Exp Med 1990;172:1483–1493.
88. Casares S, Inaba K, Brumeanu T-D, et al. Antigen presentation by dendritic cells after immunization with DNA encoding a MHC class II-restricted viral epitope. J Exp Med 1998;186:1481–1486.
89. Bot A, Stan AC, Inaba K, et al. Dendritic cells at a DNA vaccination site express the encoded influenza nucleoprotein and prime MHC class I-restricted cytolytic lymphocytes upon adoptive transfer. Int Immunol 2000;12:825–832.
90. Akbari O, Panjwami N, Garcia S, et al. DNA vaccination:transfection and activation of dendritic cells as key events for immunity. J Exp Med 1999;189:169–178.
91. Porgador A, Irwine KR, Iwasaki A, et al. Predominant role for directly transfected dendritic cells in antigen presentation to CD8(+) T cells after gene gun immunization. J Exp Med 1998;188:1075–1082.
92. Geijtenbeek TBH, Torensma R, van Vliet SJ, et al. Identification of DC-SIGN, a novel dendritic cell-specific ICAM-3 receptor that supports primary immune responses. Cell 2000;100:575–585.

93. Inaba K, Witmer-Pack M, Inaba M, et al. The tissue distribution of the B7-2 costimulator in mice: abundant expression on dendritic cells in situ and during maturation in vitro. J Exp Med 1994;180:849–1860.

94. Pierre P, Mellman I. Developmental regulation of invariant chain proteolysis controls MHC class II trafficking in mouse dendritic cells. Cell 1998;93:1135–1145.

95. Hochrein H, O'Keeffe M, Luft T, et al. Interleukin (IL)-4 is a major regulatory cytokine governing bioactive IL-12 production by mouse and human dendritic cells. J Exp Med 2000;192:823–834.

96. Schulz O, Edwards AD, Schito M, et al. CD40 triggering of heterodimeric IL-12 p70 production by dendritic cells in vivo requires a microbial priming signal. Immunity 2000;13:453–462.

97. Ebner S, Ratzinger G, Krosbacher B, et al. Production of interleukin-12 by human monocyte-derived dendritic cells is optimal when the stimulus is given at the onset of maturation, and is further enhanced by interleukin-4. J Immunol 2001;166:633–641.

98. Cyster JG. Chemokines and homing dendritic cells to T cell areas of lymphoid organs. J Exp Med 1999;189:447–450

99. Penna G, Vulcano M, Roncari A, et al. Differential chemokine production by myeloid and plasmacytoid dendritic cells. J Immunol 2002;169:6673–6676

100. Trichineri G, Scott P. Interleukin-12: basic principle and clinical application. Curr Top Microbiol Immunol 1999;238:57–78.

101. Ferlazzo G. Human Dendritic cells activate resting natural killer cells and are recognized via the NKp30 receptor by activated NK cells. J Exp Med 2002;195:343–351.

102. Rescigno M. Dendritic cells and the complexity of microbial infection. Trends Microbiol 2002;100:425–431.

103. Kosko-Vilbois MH, Gray D, Scheidegger D, et al. Follicular dendritic cells help resting B cells to become effective antigen presenting cells. J Exp Med 1993;178:2055–2066.

104. Lindhout E, Lakeman A, Mevissen LCM, et al. Functionally active EBV-transformed follicular dendritc cell-like lines. J Exp Med 1994;17:1773–1180

105. Sulica A, Morel P, Metes D, et al. Ig-binding receptors on human NK cells as effector and regulatory surface molecules. Intern Rev Immunol 2001;20:371–415.

106. Fehniger TA, Caliguri MA. Ontogeny and expansion of human natural killer cells: clinical implications. Intern Rev Immunol 2001;20:503–534.

107. Hayakawa K, Hardy RR, Honda M, et al. Ly-1 B cells: functionally distinct lymphocytes that secrete IgM autoantibodies. Proc Natl Acad Sci USA 1984;81:2494–2498.

108. Lundkvist I, Couthino A, Varela F, et al. Evidence for a functional idiotypic network among natural antibodies in normal mice. Proc Natl Acad Sci USA.1989;86:5074–5078.

109. Bona C, Stevenson F. B cells producing pathogenic antibodies. In: Molecular Biology of B cells. (Alt F, Honjo T, Neuberger M, eds.), Elsevier and Academic Press. London: 2003, pp. 381–401.

110. Bendelac A, Rivera MN, Paek S-H, et al. Mouse CD1-specific NK1 T cells: development, specificity and function. Annu Rev Immunol 1997;15:535–562

111. Beckman EM, Porcelli SA, Morita CT. Recognition of a lipid antigen by CD1-restricted alpha beta+ T cells. Nature1994;372:691–694.

112. Sieling PA, Chapperjee D, Porcelli SA, et al. CD-1 restricted T cell recognition of microbial antigens. Science 1995;269:227–270.

113. Allisson JP, Havran WL. The immunology of T cells with invariant γδ antigen receptors. Annu Rev Immunol 1991;6:679–705.

114. Poccia F, Gougeon M-L, Bonneville M, et al. Innate T-cell immunity to non-peptidic peptides. Trends Immunol 1998;19:253–256.

115. Bona C, Revillard JP, eds. Cytokines and Cytokine Receptors in Physiology and Pathological Disorders. Harwood Academic PublIshers. New York: 2000.

116. Zaghouani H, Kuzu Y, Kuzu H, et al. Contrasting efficacy of presentation by major histocompatibility complex class I and class II products when peptides are administrated within a common protein carrier, self-immunoglobulin. Eur J Immunol 1993;23:2746–2750.

117. Davies DM. Assembly of immunological synapse for T cells and NK cells. Trends Immunol 2002;23:356–362.

118. Underitz E. Die Plasma zellen in Fierrich und iber anz unehmende Bedentung als Drussen Zellen fur Bildung der Blutei weisskorper. Helvet Med Acta 1938;5:548–559.

119. Mosier DE. Cell interactions in the primary immune response in vitro: a requirement for specific cell clusters. J Exp Med 1969;129:351–362.

120. Cline M, Sweet VC. The interaction of human monocytes and lymphocytes. J Exp Med 1968;128:1309–1320.

121. Lipski PE, Rosenthal AS. Macrophage-lymphocyte interaction. I. Characterization of the antigen-independent biding of guinea pig thymocytes to syngeneic macrophages. J Exp Med 1973;138:900–909.

122. Wulfing C, Sjaastad MD, Davis MM. Visualizing the dynamics of T cell activation: intracellular adhesion molecule 1 migrates rapidly to T cell/B cell interface and acts sustaining calcium levels. Proc Natl Acad Sci USA 1998;95:6302–6307.

123. Qi SY, Groves JT, Chakraborty AK. Synaptic pattern formation during cellular recognition. Proc Natl Acad Sci USA 2001;89:6548–6553.

124. Austyn JM, Weinstein DE, Steiman RM. Clustering with dendritic cells precedes and is essential for T-cell proliferation in a mitogenesis model. Immunology 1988;63:691–699.

125. Inaba K, Steinman RM. Accessory cell-T lymphocyte interaction:antigen–dependent and -independent clustering. J Exp Med 1986;163:247–255.

126. Revy P, Sospendra M, Barbour B, et al. Functional antigen-independent synapses formed between T cells and dendritic cells. Nat Immunol 2001;2:925–931.

127. Al-Alwan MM, Rowden G, Lee TDG, et al. The dendritic cell cytoskeleton is critical for the formation of the immunological synapse. J Immunol 2001;166:1452–1456.

128. Bromely SK, Dustin ML. Stimulation of naïve T-cell adhesion and immunological synapse formation by chemokine-dependent and -independent mechanisms. Immunology 2002;106:289–298.

129. Bona C, Robineaux R, Anteunis A, et al. Transfer of antigen from macrophages to lymphocytes II. Immunological significance of the transfer of lipopolysaccharide. Immunology 1973;24:831–840.

130. Batista FD, Iber D, Neuberger MS. B cells acquire antigen from target cell after synapse formation. Nature 2001;411:489–494.

131. Nossal GJV, Abbot A, Mitchell J, et al. Antigen immunity. XV. Ultrastructural feature of antigen captation in primary and secondary follicles. J Exp Med 1968;127:277–293.

132. Dustin MLm Dustin LD. The immunological relay race: B cells take antigen by synapse. Nature 2001;41:480–482.

133. Carlin LM, Eleme K, McCann FE, et al. Intracellular transfer and supra molecular organization of human leukocyte antigen C at inhibitory natural killer cell immune synapses. J Exp Med 2001;194:1507– 1517.

134. Ottavani E. The evolutionary paradox of invertebrate cytokines. Mol Asp Immunol 2002;2:215–217.

135. Dick JE, Magli MC, Huszar D, et al. Introduction of a selectable gene into primitive cells capable of long-term reconstitution of the hematopoietic system in W/Wv mice. Cell 1985;42:71–79.

136. Zapata AG, Tororoba M, Sacedon R, et al. Structure of lymphoid organs of elasmobranches. J Exp Zool 1996;275:125–143.

137. Al-Adhami MA, Kunz YW. Hematopoietic centers developing angelfish, *Perophillum scalare*. Roux Arch Dev Biol 1976;179:393–401.

138. El Deeb SO, Saad AH. Ontogenic maturation of the immune system in reptiles. Dev Comp Immunol 1990;14:151–159.

139. Leder A, Kuo A, Shen MM, et al. *In situ* hybridization reveals co-expression of embryonic and adult a globin gene in the earliest murine erythrocyte progenitors. Development 1992;116:1041–1049.

140. Cumano A, Dieterlen-Lievre F, Godin I. Lymphoid potential, probed before circulation in mouse, is restricted to caudal intraembryonic splanchnopleura. Cell 1996;86:907–916.

141. Palacio R, Imhof BA. A day 8-8.5 of mouse development the yolk sac, not the embryo proper, has lymphoid potential in vivo and in vitro. Proc Natl Acad Sci USA 1993;90:6581–6585.

142. Liu CP, Auerbach R. In vitro development of T cells from prethymic and preliver enbryonic yolk sac hematopoietic stem cells. Development 1991;113:1315–1323.

143. Moore MA, Metcalf D. Ontogeny of the hematopoietic system:yolk sac origin of in vivo and in vitro colony forming cells in the developing mouse embryo. Br J Haematol 1970;18:279–296.

144. Yoder MC, Hyatt K. Engraftment of embryonic hematopoietic cells in conditioned newborn recipients. Blood 1997;89:2176–2183.

145. Dieterlen-Lievre F, Martin C. Diffuse intraembryonic hematopoiesis in normal and chimeric avian development. Dev Biol 1981;88:180–191.

146. Dieterlen-Lievre F. Hematopoiesis during avian development. Poultry Sci Rev 1994;5:273–305.

147. Cormier F, Dieterlen-Lievre F. The wall of chick embryo aorta harbors M-CFC, G-CFC, GM-CFC and BFU-E. Development 1988;102:279–285.

148. Godin I, Garcia Porrero JA, Coutinho A, et al. Paraaortic splanochopleura from early mouse embryos contains B1a cell progenitors. Nature 1993;364:67–70.

149. O'Neill JG. Ontogeny of the lymphoid organs in an Antartic, teleost, Hapagiforer antarticua. Dev Comp Immunol 1989;13:25–33.

150. Kimmel CB, Ballard WW, Kimmel SR, et al. Stages of embryonic development of the zebrafish. Dev Dyn 1995;203:253–310.

151. Hansen JD, Zapata AG. Lymphocyte development in fish and amphibians Immunol Rev 1998;166:199–220.

152. Iuchi I, Yamamoto M. Erythropoiesis in the developing rainbow trout, Salmgairdneri irideus: histochemical and immunochemical detection of erythropoietic organs. J Exp Zool 1983;226:409–417.

153. Turpen JB, Knudsaon CM. Ontogeny of hematopoietic cells in Rana pipensis: precursor cell migration during embryogenesis. Dev Biol 1998;22:265–278.

154. Morrison SJ, Uchida N, Weissman I. Biology of hematopoietic stem cells. Ann Rev Cell Dev Biol 1995;11:35–71.

155. Medvinsky AL, Dzierzak EA. Development of definitive hematopoiesis hierachy in the mouse. Dev Comp Immunol 1988;22:289–301.

156. Mukouyama Y, Hara T, Xu M-J, et al .In vitro expansion of murine multipotential hematopoietic progenitors from embryonic aorta-gonad-mesonephros region. Immunity 1998;8:105–114.

157. Ogawa M, Fraser S, Fijimoto T, et al. Origin of hematopoietic progenitors during embryogenesis. Int Rev Immunol 2001;20:21–45.

158. Nishikawa SI, Nishikawa S, Hirashima M, et al. Progressive lineage analysis by cell sorting and culture identifies FLK-1+ cadherin + cells a diverging point of endothelial and hematopoietic cells. Development 1998;125:1747–1757.

159. Pardanaud L, Luon D, Prigent M, et al. Two distinct endothelial lineages in ontogeny, one of them related to hematopoiesis. Development 1996;122:1363–1371.

160. Palis J, McGarth KE, Kingsley M. Initiation of hematopoiesis and vasculogenesis in murine yolk sac explants. Blood 1995;86:156–163.

161. Shalaby F, Rossant J, Yamagichi TP. Failure of blood-island formation and vasculogenesis in Flk-1 deficient mice. Nature 1995;376:62–66.

162. Cho SK, Bourdeau A, Latarte M, et al. Expression and function of CD105 during the onset of hematopoiesis from Flk-1 precursors. Blood 2001;98:3635–3642.

163. Tavian M, Robin C, Coulombel L, et al. The human embryo, but not its yolk sac, generates lymphomyeloid stem cells: mapping multipotent hematopoietc cell fate in intraembryonic mesoderm. Immunity 2001;15:487–495.

164. Partanen J, Puri MC, Scwarttz L, et al. Cell autonomous functions of the receptor tyrosinase TIE in a late phase of angiogenetic capillary growth and endothelial cell survival during murine development. Development 1996;122:3013–3021.

165. Tsai FY, Keller G, Kuo FC, et al. An early hematopoietic defect in mice lacking the transcription factor GATA-2. Nature 1994;371;221–226.

166. Katsura Y, Kawamoto H. Stepwise lineage restriction of progenitors in lymphomyelpoiesis. Intern Rev Immunol 2001;20:1–20.

167. Morales-Alcelay S, Copin SG, Martinez JA, et al. Developmental hematopoiesis. Crit Rev Immunol 1998;18:485–501.

168. Akashi K, Traver D, Myamoto T, et al. A clonogenic common myeloid progenitor that give rise to all myeloid lineages. Nature 2000;404:193–197.

169. Traver D, Miyamoto T, Christensen J, et al. Fetal liver myelopoiesis occurs through distinct, prospectively isolatable progenitor subsets. Blood 2001;98:627–625.

170. Traver D, Miyamoto T, Christensen J, et al. Fetal liver myelopoisis occurs through distinct, prospectively isolable progenitors subsets. Blood 2001;88:627–636

171. Liesschke GJ. CSF-deficient mice—what have they taught us. In: The Molecular Basis of Cellular Defense Mechanisms. (Bock GB, Goode JA, eds.), John Wiley & Sons. West Sussex: 1997, pp. 60–77.

172. Dong F, van Buitenen C, Powels K, et al. Distinct cytoplasmic regions of the human granulocyte colony-stimulating factor receptor involved in induction of proliferation and maturation. Mol Cell Biol 1993;13:7774–7781.

173. Dong F, Dale DC, Bonilla MA, et al. Mutations in the granulocyte colony-stimulating factor receptor gene in patients with severe congenital neutropenia. Leukemia 1997;11:120–125.

174. Ward AC, Loeb DM, Soede-Bobok AA, et al. Regulation of granulopoiesis by transcription factors and cytokine signals. Leukemia 2000;14:973–990.

175. Friedman AD. Transcriptional regulation of granulocyte and monocyte development. Oncogene 2002;21:3377–3390.

176. Mucenski ML, McClain K, Kier AB, et al. A functional c-Myb gene is required for normal murine fetal hematopoiesis. Cell 1991;65:677–689.

177. Sasaki K, Yagi H, Bronson RT, et al. Absence of fetal liver hematopoiesis in mice deficient in transcriptional coactivator core binding factor. Proc Natl Acad Sci USA 1996;92:12,359–12,363.

178. Shivadsani RA, Orkin SH. The transcriptional control of hematopoiesis. Blood 1996;87:4025–4039.

179. Heyworth C, Gale K, Dexter M, et al. A GATA 2/estrogen receptor chimera functions as ligand-dependent negative regulator of self-renewal. Gene Dev 1999;13:1847–1860.

180. Bies J, Mukkopadhyaya R, Pierce J, et al. Only late, nonmitotic stages of differentiation in 32Dcl3 cells are blocked by ectopic expression of c-Myb and its truncated form. Cell Growth Differ 1995;6:59–68.

181. Nagamura-Inoue T, Tamura T, Ozato K. Transcription factors that regulate growth and differentiation of myeloid cells. Intern Rev Immunol 2001;20;83–106.

182. Zang P, Radomska HS, Iwasaki-Arai J, et al. Induction of granulocyte differentiation by 2 pathways. Blood 2002;99:4406–4412.

183. Bavisotto L, Kaushansky L, Lin N, et al. Antisense oligonucleotides from the stage-specific myeloid zinc finger gene MZF-1 inhibit granulopoiesis in vitro. J Exp Med 1991;174:1097–1101.

184. Morris JF, Hromans R, Rauscher FJ. Characterization of DNA-binding properties of the myeloid zinc finger protein MZF-1: two independent DNA-binding domains recognize two DNA consensus sequences with a common G-rich core. Mol Cell Biol 1994;14:1786–1795.

185. Schroeder T, Just U. Notch signaling via RBP-J promotes myeloid differentiation. EMBO J 2000;19:2558–2568.

186. Capron M, Morita M, Woerly G, et al. Differentation of eosinophils from cord blood cell precursors: kinetics of Fc epsilon and Fc epsilon RII expression. Int Arch Allergy Immunol 1997;113:48–50.

187. Rosenberg HF, Dyer KD, Li F. Characterization of eosinophils generated in vitro from CD34⁺ peripheral blood progenitor cells. Exp Hematol 1996;24:888–893.

188. Lundhal J, Sehmi R, Moshfengh A, et al. Distinct phenotype adhesion molecule expresssion on human cord blood progenitor during eosinophilic commitment: upregulation of β7 integrin. Scand J Immunol 2002;56161–167.

189. McNagny KM, Sieweke MH, Doderlein G, et al. Regulation of eosinophil-specific expression by a C/EBT-Ets complex and GATA-1. EMBO J 1998;17:3669–3380.

190. Hirasawa R, Shimizu R, Tkahashi S, et al. Essential and instructive roles of GATA factors in eosinophil development. J Exp Med 2002;195:1379–1386.

191. Braccioni F, Dorman SC, O'Byrne PM, et al. The effect of cystenyl leukotrienes on growth of eosinophil progenitor from peripheral blood and bone marrow of atopic subjects. J Allergy Clin Immunol 2002;110:96–101.

192. Rais M, Wild JS, Chouhury K, ct al. Interleukin-12 inhibits eosinophil differentiation from bone marrow stem cells in an interferon-γ-dependent manner in a mouse model of asthma. Clin Exp Allerg 2002;32:627–632.

193. Arock M, Schneider E, Boissan M, et al. Differentiation of human basophils: an overview of recent advances and pending questions. J Leuk Biol 2002;71:557–564.

194. Buhring HJ, Simmons PJ, Pudney M, et al. The monoclonal antobody 97A6 defines a novel surface antigen expressed on human basophils and their multipotent and unipotent progenitors. Blood 1999;94:2343–2256.

195. Sillader C, Geissler K, Scherrer R, et al. Type beta transforming growth factors promote IL-3 dependent of human basophils but inhibits IL-3 dependent differentiation of human eosinophils. Blood 1992;80:634–641.

196. Valente P. Cytokines involved in growth and differentiation of human basophils and mast cells. Exp Dermatol 1995;4:255-259.

197. Quackenbush EJ, Wershil BK, Aguirrfe V, et al. Eotoxin modulates myelopoiesis and mast cell development from embryonic hematopoietic progenitors. Blood 1998;92:1887–1897.

198. Hoffman JA, Zachary D, Hoffman D, et al. Post-embryonic development and differentiation: hematopoietic function in some insects. In: Insect Hemocytes. (Gupta AP, ed.), Cambridge University Press. Cambridge, UK: 1979.

199. Tepass U, Fessler LI, Aziz A, et al. Embryonic origin of hemocytes and their relationship with cell death in Drosophila. Development 1994;120:1829–1837.

200. Luciani M, Chimini G. The ATP binding cassette transporter ABC1 is required for the engulfment of corpses generated by apoptosis. EMBO J 1996;15:226–235.

201. Amatruda JF, Zon LI. Dissecting hematopiesis and disease using zebrafish. Dev Biol 1999;216:1–20.

202. Ohinata H, Tochinai S, Katagiri C. Occurrence of nonlymphoid leukocytes that are not derived from blood islands in Xenopus laevis larvae. Dev Biol 1990;141:123–129.

203. Takahashi K, Yamamura F, Nato M. Differentiation, maturation, and proliferation of macrophages in the rat yolk sac. Tissue Cell 1989;45:87–96.

204. Shepard JL, Zon LI. Development derivation of embryonic and adult macrophages. Curr Opin Hematol 2000;7:3–8.

205. Kim J, Feldman RA. Activated Fes protein tyrosine kinase induces terminal macrophage differentiation of myeloid progenitors (U937 cells) and activation of transcription factor PU.I. Mol Cell Biol 2002;22:1903–1918.

206. Miranda MB, Mc Guire TF, Johnson DE. Importance of MEK1/2 signaling in monocytic and granulocytic differentiation myeloid cell lines. Leukemia 2002;16:683–692.

207. Krishnaraju K, Hoffman B, Lieberman DA. Early growth respose gene stimulates development of hematopoietic progenitor cells along the macrophage lineage at the expense of the granulocye and erythroid lineages. Blood 2001;97:1298–1305.

208. Smith LT, Hohaus S, Gonzalez DA, et al. PU.1 (Spi-1) and C/EBP alpha regulate the granulocyte colony-stimulating factor promoter in myeloid cells. Blood 1996;88:1234–1247.

209. Faust N, Bonifer C, Sippel AE. Differential activity of the –2.7kb chicken lysozyme enhancer in macrophages with different ontogenic origins is regulated by C/EBP and PU.1 transcription factors. DNA Cell Biol 1999;18:631–642.

210. Servet-Delpart C, Arnaud S, Judic P, et al. Flt3$^+$ macrophage precursors commit sequentially to osteoclast dendritic cells and microglia. BMC Immunol 2002;3:15–26.

211. Randolph GJ, Beaulieu S, Lebecque S, et al. Differentiation of monocytes into dendritic cells in a model of transendothelial trafficking. Science 1998;282;480–483.

212. Sordet O, Rebe C, Pienchette S, et al. Specific involvement of capsases in the differentiation of monocytes into macrophages. Blood 2002;100:4446–4453.

213. Senju S, Hirata S, Matsuyoshi H, et al. Generation and genetic modification of dendritic cells derived frm mouse embryonic cells. Blood 2003;101:3501–3508.

214. Jackson SH, Candido A, Owens A, et al. Characterization of an early dendritic cell precursor derived from murine lineage-negative hematopoietic progenitor cells. Exp Hematol 2002;30:430–439.

215. Inaba K, Inaba M, Deguchi M, et al. Granulocytes, macrophages and dendritic cells arise from a common major class II-negative progenitor in mouse bone marrow. Proc Natl Acad Sci USA 1993;3038–3042.

216. Reid CD, Stackpole A, Meager A, et al. Interactions of tumor necrosis factor with granulocyte-macrophage colony-stimulating factor and other cytokines in the regulation of dendritic cell growth in vitro from early bipotent CD34$^+$ progenitors in human bone marrow. J Immunol 1992;149:2681–2688.

217. Caux C, Vanbervliet B, Massacrier C, et al. Dendritic cells. J Hematol Cell Ther1996;38:463–471.

218. Wu L, Vandenabelle S, Georgopoulos K. Derivation of dendritic cells from myeloid and lymphoid precursors. Intern Rev Immunol 2001;20:117–135.

219. Strunk D, Egger C, Leitner G, et al. A skin molecules defines the Langerhans cell progenitor in human peripheral blood. J Exp Med 1997;185:1131–1136.

220. Wu L, Vremev D, Ardavin C, et al. Mouse thymus dendritic cells: kinetics of development and changes in surface markers. Eur J Immunol 1995;25:418–425.
221. Vremec D, Zorbas M, Scollay R, et al. The surface phenotype of dendritic cells purified from mouse thymus and spleen: investigation of CD8 expression by a population of dendritic cells. J Exp Med 1992;176:47–58.
222. Ardavin C, Wu L, Li C-L, et al. Thymus dendritic cells and T cells develop simultaneously in the thymus from a common precursor. Nature 1993;362:761–763.
223. Wu L, Antica M, Johnson GR, et al. Developmental potential of eraliest precursor cells from adult mouse thymus. J Exp Med 1991;178:1617–1627.
224. Brawand P, Fitzpatrick DR, Greenfield BW, et al. Murine plasmoacytoid pre-dendritic cells generated from Flt3 ligand-supplememted bone marrow cultures are immature APCs. J Immunol 2002;169:6711–6719.
225. Hochrein H, O'Keeffe M, Wagner H. Human and mouse plasamacytoid dendritic cells. Human Immunol 2002;63:1103–1110.
226. Strobl H, Scheinecker C, Riedl E, et al. Identification of a CD68⁺ lin⁻ peripheral blood cells with dendritic precursors characteristics. J Immunol 1998;161:740–748.
227. Briere F, Bendriss-Vermare N, Deale T, et al. Origin and filation of human plasmacytoid dendritic cells. Human Immunol 2002;63:1081–1093.
228. Liu Y-J. Uncover the mystery of plamacytoid dendritic cell precursors or type I interferon producing cells by serendipity. Human Immunol 2002;63:1067–1071.
229. Kadowaki N, Liu Y-J. Natural type I interferon-producing cells as a link between innate and adaptive immunity. Human Immunol 2002;63:1126–1132.
230. Del Hojo GM, Martin P, Vargas HH, et al. Characterization of a common precursor population for dendritic cells. Nature 2002;415:1043–1047.
231. Sivakumar PV, Gunturi A, Salcedo M, et al. Expression of functional CD94/NKG2A inhibitory receptors on fetal NK.1.1⁺ Ly-49⁻ cells: a possible mechanism of tolerance during NK cell development. J Immunol 1999;162:6976–6980.
232. Van Beneden K, Stevenaert F, De Creus A, et al. Expression of Ly49E and CD94/NKG2 on fetal and adult NK cells. J Immunol 2001;166:4302–4311.
233. Leclercq G, Debacker V, de Smed M, et al. Differential effects of IL-15 and IL-2 on differentation of bipotential T/natural killer progenitor cells. J Exp Med 1996;184:325–336.
234. Fraser KP, Gays F, Robinson JH, et al. NK cells developing in vitro from fetal mouse progenitors express at least one member of the Ly49 family that is acquired in a time-dependent and stochastic manner independently of CD94 and NKG2. Eur J Immunol 2002;32:868–878.
235. Moore T, Bennett M, Kumar V. Transplantable NK cell progenitors in murine bone marrow. J Immunol 1995;154:1653–1663.
236. Roth C, Carlyle JR, Takizawa H, et al. Clonal acquisition of inhibitory Ly49 receptors on developing NK cells is succesively restricted and regulated by stromal cells. Immunity 2000:13:143–152
237. Williams NS, Moore TA, Schaltze JD, et al. Generation of lytic natural killer 1.1⁺ Ly-49⁻ cells from multipotential murine bone marrow progenitors in a stroma-free culture: definition of cytokine requirments and developmental intermediates. J Exp Med 1997;186:1609–1614.

238. Vance RE, Jamieson AM, Raulet DH. Recognition of the class Ib molecule Qa-1a by putative activating receptors CD94/NKG2C and CD94/NKG2E on mouse natural killer cells. J Exp Med 1999;190:1801–1812.

239. Lian RH, Maeda M, Lohwasser S, et al. Orderly and nonstochastic acquisition of CD94/NKG2 receptors by developing NK cells derived from embryonic stem cells in vitro. J Immunol 2002;168:4980–4987.

240. Raulet DH. Development and tolerance of natural killer cells. Curr Opin Immunol 1999;11:129–141.

241. Raff MC, Megason M, Owen JJT, et al. B cell differentation. Nature 1976;259:224–226.

242. Osmond DG, Rolink A, Melchers F. Murine B lymphopoiesis; toward a unified model. Immunol Today 1998;19:65–68.

243. Lloyd-Evans C. Development of the lymphomyeloid system in the dog fish. Dev Comp Immunol 1993;17:501–514.

244. Kobayashi K, Tomonaga S, Teshima K, et al. Ontogenetic studies on the appearance of two classes of immunoglobulin-forming cells in the spleen of the Aleutian skate, Bathyraja aleutica, a cartilaginous fish. Eur J Immunol 1985;15:952–956.

245. Miracle AL, Anderson MK, Litman RT, et al. Complex expression patterns of lymphocyte-specific genes during the development of cartilaginous fish implicate unique lymphoid tissues in generating an immune repertoire. Intern Immunol 2001;13:567–580.

246. Dagfeldt A, Bengten E, Pilstrom LA. Cluster type organization of the loci of the immunoglobulin light chain in Atlantic cod (*Gadus morhua L*) and rainbow trout (*Oncorhynchus mykiss Walbaum*) indicated by nucleotide sequence of cDNA and hybridization analysis. Immunogenetics 1993;38:199–209.

247. Hansen JD, Strassburger P, Du Pasquier L. Conservation of master hematopoietic switch gene during vertebrate evolution: isolation and characterization of Ikaros from teleost and amphibian species. Eur J Immunol 1997;27:3049–3058.

248. Hansen JD, Kaattari SL. The recombination activation gene 1 of rainbow trout: cloning, expression and phylogenetic analysis. Immunogenetics 1995;42:188–195.

249. Ellis AE. Ontogeny of the immune system in Samo solar. Histogenesis of lymphoid organs and appearance of immunoglobulin and mixed lymphocyte reactivity. In: Developmental Immunology. (Solomon JB, Horton JD, eds.), Amsterdam Elsevier, North Holland Biomedical Press: 1977, pp. 225–232.

250. Secombes CJ, van Groningen JJ, van Muiswinkel WB, et al. Ontogeny of the immune system in carp (*Cyprinus carpio*). Dev Comp Immunol 1983;7:455–464.

251. Thompson MA. The cloche and spadtail genes differentially affect hematopoiesis and vasculogenesis. Dev Biol 1998;197;248–269.

252. Schroder MB, Villena AJ, Jorgesen TO. Ontogeny of lymphoid organs and immunoglobulin producing cells in Atlantic cod (*Gadus morhua L*). Dev Comp Immunol 1998;22:707–517.

253. Petrie-Hanson L, Answorth AJ. Ontogeny of channel catfish lymphoid organs. Vet Immunol Immunopathol 2001;81:113–127.

254. Du Pasquier L, Robert J, Courtet M, et al. B-cell development in the amphibians. Immunol Rev 2000;175:201–213.

255. Hadji-Azimi I, Schwagner J, Thiebaud C. B-lymphocyte differentiation in Xenopus *laevis larvae*. Dev Biol 1982;90:253–258.

256. Natarajan K, Muthukkaruppan VR. Distribution and ontogeny of B cells in garden lizard, Calotes versicolor. Dev Comp Immunol 1985;9:301–310.

257. El Deeb S, el Ridi R, Zada S. The development of lymphocytes with T or B membrane determinants in the lizard embryo. Dev Comp Immunol 1986;10:353–364.

258. Cooper MD, Cain WA, Van Alten PJ, et al. Development and function of the immunoglobulin producing system I. Effect of buresectomy at different stages of development on germinal centers, plasma cells and immunoglobulin production. Int Arch Allergy 1969;35:242–261.

259. Moore MAS, Owen JJT. Experimental studies on the development of bursa of Fabricius. Dev Biol 1966;14:40–52.

260. Olah I, Nagy N, David C, et al. Ontogeny of the dendritic and follicle-associated epithelial cells in the bursa of Fabricius of guinea fowl. Ital J Anat Embryol 2001;106:271–277.

261. Lassilla O, Eskola J, Tovanien P. Prebursal stem cells in the intraembryonic mesenchyme of chick embryo at 7 day of incubation. J Immunol 1979;123:179–188.

262. Reynaud CA, Imhof BA, Anques V, et al. Chicken D locus and its contribution to the immunoglobulin heavy chain repertoire. EMBO J 1992;11:4349–4360.

263. Pickel JM, McCormack WT, Chen CL-H, et al. Differential regulation of V(D)J recombination during development of avian B and T cells. Intern Immunol 1993;5:919–927.

264. Houssaint E, Lassila O, Vaino O. Bu-1 antigen as a marker for B cell percursors in chicken embryo. Eur J Immunol 1989;19:239–247.

265. Bando Y, Higgins DA. Duck lymphoid organs: their contribution to the ontogeny of IgM and IgY. Immunology 1996;89:8–12.

266. Masteller EL, Pharr GT, Funk PE, et al. Avian cell development. Int Rev Immunol 1997;15:185–206.

267. Meibius RE, Miyamoto T, Christensen J, et al. The fetal liver counterpart of adult common lymphoid progenitors give rise to all lymphoid lineages CD45$^+$ CD4$^+$ CD3$^-$ as well as macrophages. J Immunol 2001;166:6593–6601.

268. Shimitzu T, Mundt C, Licence S, et al. VpreB1/VpreB2/λ5 triple-deficient mice show impaired B cell development but functional alleleic exclusion of the IgH locus. J Immunol 2002;168:6286–6293.

269. Kearny JF, Woon W-J, Benedict C, et al. B cells development in mice. Int Rev Immunol 1997;15:207–243.

270. Clarke SH, Arnold LW. B-1 cell development: evidence for an uncommitted immunoglobulin IgM$^+$ B cell precursor on B-1 cell differentiation. J Exp Med 1998;187:1325–1334.

271. Haykawa K, Hardy RR. Development and function of B-1 cells. Curr Opin Immunol 2000;12:346–353.

272. Knight KL, Winstead CR. B Lymphocyte development in rabbit. Int Rev Immunol 1997;15:129–164.

273. Bona C, Chedid L, Damais C, et al. Blast transformation of rabbit B-derived lymphocytes by a mitogen extracted from Nocardia. J Immunol 1975;114:348–353.

274. Cazenave PA Juy D Bona C. Ontogeny of lymphocyte function during embryonic life of the rabbit. J Immunol 1978;120:444–448.

275. Solvason N, Kearney JF. The human fetal omentum: a site of B c ell differantiation. J Exp Med 1992;175:397–404.

276. Dixon FJ, Weigle WO. The nature of the immunologic inadequacy of neonatal rabbits. J Exp Med 1959:110:139–146.

277. Sinkora M, Smirnova J, Buttler JE. B cell development and VDJ rearrangement in the fetal pig. Vet Immunol Immunopathol 2002;87:341–346.

278. Press CM, Hein WR, Landsverk T. Ontogeny of leucocyte populations in the spleen of fetal lambs with emphasis of the early prominence of B cells. Immunology 1993;80:598–604.

279. Reynolds J. The genesis, tutelage and exodus of B c ells in the ileal Peyer's patches of sheep. Int Rev Immunol 1997;15:265–299.

280. Makori N, Tarantal AF, Lu FX, et al. Functional and morphological development of lymphoid tissues and immune regulatory and effector functions in Rhesus monkey. Clin Diagn Lab Immunol 2003;10:140–153.

281. Youinou P, Janin C, Lydyard PM. CD5 expression in human B cell population. Immunol Today 1999;20:312–316.

282. Thoma SL, Lamping CP, Zigler BL. Phenotype analysis of hematopoietic CD34+ cell population derived from umbilical cord blood using flow cytometry and cDNA-polymerase chain reaction. Blood 1994;83:2103–2114.

283. Bender JG, Unverzagt KL, Walker DE, et al Identification and comparison of CD34+ cells and their subpopulation from normal peripheral blood and bone marrow using multicolor cytometry. Blood 1991;77:25,961–25,966.

284. Ghia P, Boekel E, Sanz E, et al. Ordering of human bone marrow lymphocyte precursors by a single-cell polymerase chain reaction analyses of the rearrangement status of the immunoglobulin H and L chain gene loci. J Exp Med 1996;184:2217–2229.

285. Fluckiger A-C, Sanz E, Garcia-Loret M, et al. In vitro reconstitution of human B-cell ontogeny: from CD34+ multipotent progenitors to Ig-secreting cells. Blood 1998;92:4509–4520.

286. Wang YH, Stephan RP, Schenfold A, et al. Differential surrogate light chain expression governs B cell differentiation. Blood 1992;99:2458–2467.

287. Schultz C, Reiss I, Bucsky P, et al. Maturational changes of lymphocyte surface antigens in human blood: comparison between fetuses, neonates and adults. Biol Neonate 2000;78:77–82.

288. Georogopoulos K, Bigby M, Wang JH, et al. The Ikaros gene is required for the development of all lymphoid lineages. Cell 1994;79:143–156.

289. Wang J-H, Nichogiannopoulou A, Wu L, et al. Selective defects in the development of the fetal and adult lymphoid system in mice with an Ikaros null mutation. Immunity 1996;5:537–549.

290. Molnar A, Georogopoulos K. The Ikaros gene encodes a family of functionally diverse zinc finger DNA binding proteins. Mol Cell Biol 1994;83:785–7994.

291. Kristetter P, Thomas M, Dietrich A, et al. Ikaros is critical for B cell differentiation and function. Eur J Immunol 2002;32:720–730.

292. Hansen JD, Strassburger PB, Du Pasquier L. Generation of master hematopoietic switch gene during vertebrate evolution: isolation and characterization of Ikaros from teleost and amphibian species. Eur J Immunol 1997;27:3049–3058.

293. Durand C, Kerfourn F, Charlemagne J, et al. Identification and expression of Helios, a member of the Ikaros family, in the Mexican axolotl: implications for the embryonic origin of lymphocyte progenitors. Eur J Immunol 2002 32;1748–1752.

294. Hahm K, Ernst P, Lo K, et al. The transcription of LyF-1 is encoded by specific, alternatively spliced mRNAs derived from Ikaros gene. Mol Cell Biol 1994;14:7111–7123.

295. Okabe T, Bauer SR, Kudo A. Pre-B lymphocyte-specific transcriptional control of the mouse VpreB gene. Eur J Immunol 1992;12:31 36.

296. Staal FJT, Clevers HC. Regulation of lineage commitment during lymphocyte development. Int Rev Immunol 2001;20:45–64

297. Lin H, Grosschedel R. Failure of B cell differentiation in mice lacking the transcription factor EBF. Nature 1995;376:263–269.

298. Liberg D, Sigvardsson M. Transcriptional regulation in B cell differentiation. Crit Rev Immunol 1999;19:127–153.

299. Hagaman J, Gutch MJ, Lin H, et al. EBF contains a zinc coordination motif and multiple dimerization and transcriptional activation domains. EMBO J 1995;14:2907–2916.

300. Gisler R, Sigvardsson M. The human V-pre B promoter is a target for coordinated activation by early B cell factor and E47. J Immunol 2002;168:5130–5138.

301 Kozmick Z, Wang S, Dorfler P, et al. The promoter of CD19 gene is a target for the B cell specific transcription factor BSAP. Mol Cell Biol 1992;12:2662–2672.

302. Yang H, Chang JF, Parnes JR. PU.1 is essential for the B cell-specific activity of the mouse CD72 promoter. J Immunol 1998;160:2287–2296.

303. Himmelmann A, Riva A, Wilson GL, et al. PU.1/Pip and basic helix loop helix zipper transcription factor interact with binding sites in CD20 promoter to help confer lineage- and stage-specific expression of CD20 in B lymphocytes. Blood 1997;90:3984–3995.

304. Threvenin C, Lucas BP, Kozlow EJ, et al. Cell type- and stage-specific expression of the CD20/B1 antigen correlates with the activity of a diverged octamer DNA motif present in its promoter. J Biol Chem 1993;268:5949–5956.

305. Wilson GL, Najfeld V, Kozlow E, et al. Genomic structure and chromosomal localization of the human CD22 gene. J Immunol 1993;150:5013–5024.

306. Nutt SL, Eberhard D, Horcher M, et al. Pax5 determines the identity of B cells from the beginning to the end of B-lymphopoiesis. Intern Rev Immunol 2001;20:65–82.

307. Nutt SL, Heavy B, Rolink AG, et al. Committment to the B-lymphoid lineage depends on transcription factor Pax5. Nature 1999;401:556–562.

308. Rolink AG, Nutt SL, Melchers F, et al. Long-term in vivo reconstitution of T-cell development by Pax5-deficient B cell progenitors. Nature 1999;401:603–606.

309. Liao F, Birshtein BK, Busslinger M, et al. The transcription factor BSAP(NF-kB) is essential for immunoglobulin germ-line epsilon. J Immunol 1994;152:2904–2911.

310. Nieman P, Liippo J, Lassila O. Pax-5 and EBF are expressed in committed B-cell progenitors prior to colonization of embryonic Bursa of Fabricius. Scand J Immunol 2000;52:465–469.

311. Cordier AC, Hammond SM. Development of thymus, parathyroid and multibrachial bodies in NMR1 and nude mice. Am J Anat 1980;157:157:227–254.

312. Kirby ML, Waldo KL. Role of neural crest in congenital heart diseases. Circulation 1990;82:332–340.

313. Manley NR. Thymus oragnogenesis and molecular mechanisms of thymic epithelial cell differentiation. Semin Immunol 2000;12:421–428.

314. Gill J, Malin M, Hollander GA, et al. Generation of a complete thymic microenvironment by MTS24+ thymic epithelial cells. Nat Immunol 2002:3:635–642.

315. Klug DB, Carter C, Gimenez-Conti IB, et al. Thymocyte-independent and thymocyte-dependent phases of epithelial patterning in the fetal thymus. J Immunol 2002;169:2842–2845.

316. Snodgrass HR, Dembic Z, Steinmetz M, et al. Expression of T cell antigen receptor genes during fetal development of thymus. Nature 1985;315:232–233.

317. Sain-Ruf C, Ungewiss K, Groettrup M, et al. Analysis and expression of a cloned pre-T cell receptor gene. Science 1994;266:1208–1212.

318. Castillo A, Lopez-Fierro P, Zapata A, et al. Post-hatching development of the thymic epithelial cells in the rainbow trout *Salmo garidineri*: an ultrastructural study. Am J Anat 1991;190:299–307.

319. Grace MF, Manning MJ. Histogenesis of the lymphoid organs in rainbow trout. Dev Comp Immunol 1980;4:255–264.

320. Hansen JD, Zapata AG. Lymphocyte development in fish and amphibians. Immunol Rev 1998;166:199–220.

321. Trede NS, Zon LI. Development of T cells during fish embryogenesis. Dev Comp Immunol 1998;22:253–263.

322. Clothier EM, Balls M. Structural changes in the thymus gland of Xenopus laevis during development. In: Metamorphosis. (Ball M, Bownes M, eds.), Oxford University Press. Oxford: 1985, pp. 332–359.

323. Turpen J, Smith PB. Precursor immigration and thymocyte succession during larval development and metamorphosis in Xenopus. J Immunol 1989;142:42–47.

324. Jurgen JB Gartland LA Du Paquier L Horton JD Gobel TW Cooper MD. Identification of candidate CD5 homologue in the amphibian Xenopus laevis. J Immunol 1995;155:4218–4223.

325. Le Douarin NM, Joterau FV. Origin and renewal of lymphocytes in avian thymuses studied in interspecies combinations. Nature 1973;208:956–960.

326. Le Douarin NM, Joterau FV. Tracing of cells of the avian thymus through embryonic interspecific chimeras. J Exp Med 1975;142:17–28.

327. Coltey M, Joterau FV, Le Douarin NM. Evidence for a cyclic renewal of lymphocyte precursor cell in the embryo chick thymus. Cell Differ 1987;22:71–83.

328. Pickel JM, McCormack WT, Chen C-IH, et al. Differential regulation of V(D)J recombination during development of avian B and T cells. Int Immunol 1993;5:919–927.

329. Sinkora M, Sinkora J, Rehakova Z, et al. Early ontogeny of thymocytes in pigs: sequential colonization of thymus by T cell progenitor. J Immunol 2000;165:1832–1839.

330. Stites DP, Pavia CS. Ontogeny of human T cells. Pediatrics 1979 64:795–802.

331. Barcena A, Galy AH, Punnonen J, et al. Lymphoid and myeloid differentiation of fetal liver CD45+ lineage cells in human thymic organ culture. J Exp Med 1994;180:123–132.

332. Res P, Martinez Caceres E, Jaleco AC, et al. CD34$^+$ CD38^{dim} cells in human thymus can differentiate into T, Natural killer and dendritic cells but are distinct from stem cells. Blood 1996;87:5196–5211.

333. Plum J, De Smedt M, Verhasselt B, et al. Human T lymphopoiesis. In vitro and in vivo study models. Ann New York Acad Sci 2000;917:724–731.

334. Vanheecke DB, Leclercq G, Plum J, et al. Characterization of different stages during diferentiation of human CD69$^+$ CD3$^+$ thymocytes and identification of thymic immigrants. J Immunol 1993;150:8–19.

335. Ramiro AR, Trigueros C, Marquez C, et al. Regulation of pre-T cell receptor gene expression during human thymic development. J Exp Med 1996:185;519–528.

336. Blom B, Verschuren MCM, Heemskerk MHM, et al. TCR gene rearrangement and expression of the pre-T cell receptor complex during human differentiation. Blood 1999;93:3033–3043.

337. Gardner LP, Rosenzweig M, Marks DF, et al. Lymphopoietic capacity of cord blood derived CD34$^+$ progenitor cells. Exp Hematol 1998;26:991–999.

338. Salemo A, Dieli F. Role of γδ T lymphocytes in immune response in humans and mice. Crit Rev Immunol 1998;18:327–358.

339. Six A, Rast JP, McCormack WT, et al. Characterization of avian T-cell receptor genes. Proc Natl Acad Sci USA 1996;93:15,329–15,334.

340. Itohara S, Nakanishi N, Kanagawa O, et al. Monoclonal antibodies specific to native T-cellreceptor γ/δ:Analysis of γ/δ T cells during thymic ontogeny and peripheral lymphoid organs. Proc Natl Acad Sci USA 1989;86:5094–5098.

341. Heiling JS, Tonegawa S. Diversity of murine γ genes and expression in fetal and adult T lymphocytes. Nature 1986;322:834–840.

342. Houlden BA, Cron RQ, Colligan JE, et al. Systematic development of distinct T cell receptor-γδ T cell subsets during fetal ontogeny. J Immunol 1988;141:37753–3759.

343. Leclercq G, Plum J, Nandi D, et al. Intrathymic differentiation of Vγ3 T cells. J Exp Med 1993;178:309–318.

344. Van Beneden K, De Creus A, Stevenaert F, et al. Expression of inhibitory receptor Ly49E and CD94/NKG2 on fetal and thymic and adult epidermal TCR Vγ3 lymphocytes. J Immunol 2002;168:3295–3302.

345. Correa I, Bix M, Liao NS, et al. Most of γδ T cells develop normally in β2-microglobulin-deficient mice. Proc Natl Acad Sci USA. 1992;89:653–658.

346. Rocha B, Vassali P, Guy-Grand D. The extrathymic T-cell development pathway. Immunol Today 1992;13:449–458.

347. McVay LD, Jaswal SS, Kennedy C, et al. The generation of human γδT cell repertoires during fetal development J Immunol 1998;160:5851–5860.

348. Carding SR, McNamara JG, Pan M, et al. Characterization γδ T cell clones isolated from human fetal liver and thymus. Eur J Immunol 1990;20:1327–1341.

349. Makino Y, Kanno R, Koseki H, et al. Development of Vα14 NK T cells in the early stages of embryogenesis. Proc Natl Acad Sci USA 1996;93:6516–6520.

350. Wienand S, Engels N. Multitasking of Ig-α and Ig-β to regulate B cell antigen receptor function. Int Rev Immunol 2001;20:679–696.

351. Wienand S, Schweikert J, Wollscheid B, et al. SLp-65: a new signaling component in B lymphocytes which requires expression of antigen receptor and phosphorylation. J Exp Med 1998;188:791–795.

352. Fu C, Turck CW, Kurosaki T, et al. BLNK: a central linker protein in B cell activation. Immunity 1998;9:93–103.
353. Kraus M, Saijio K, Torres RM, et al. Ig-alpha cytoplasmic truncation renders immature B cells more sensitive to antigen contact. Immunity 1999;11:537–545.
354. Hashimoto A, Okada H, Jiang A, et al. Involvement of guanosine triphosphate and phospholipase C-γ2 in extracellular signal-related kinase, c-Jun NH2-terminal kinase and p38 mitogen activated kinase J Exp Med 1998;188:1287–1295.
355. Jiang A, Craxton A, Kurosaki T, et al. Different protein tyrosine signal-related kinase, c-Jun NH2-terminal kinase, and p38 mitogen activated kinase. J Exp Med 1998;188:1297–1306.
356. Tan JE, Wong SC, Gan SK, et al. The adaptor protein BLNK is required for B cell antigen receptor-induced activation of nuclear factor-kappa β and cell cycle entry and survival of B lymphocytes. J Biol Chem 2001;276:20,055–20,063.
357. Langlet C, Bernard A-M, Drevot P, et al. Membrane rafts and signaling by the multichain immune recognition receptors. Curr Opin Immunol 2000;12:250–261.
358. Justement LB. The role of protein thyrosine phosphatase CD45 in regulation of B lymphocyte activation. Int Rev Immunol 2001;20:731–738.
359. Benatar T, Carsetti R, Furlonger C, et al. Immunoglobulin-mediated signal transduction in B cells from CD45-deficient mice. J Exp Med 1996;183:329–334.
360. Byth KF, Conroy LA, Howlett S, et al. CD45-null transgenic mice reveal a positive regulatory role for CD45 in early thymocyte development, in selection of CD4$^+$ CD8$^+$ thymocytes and B cell maturation. J Exp Med 1996;183:1701–1718.
361. Penninger VA, Wallace TM, Kishihara K, et al. The role of p56lck and p59 fyn tyrosine kinases and CD45 proteintyrosine phosphataeses in T cell development and clonal selection. Immunol Rev 1993;135:183–214.
362. Poe JC, Hasegawa M, Tedder TS. CD19, CD21 and CD22: multifaced response regulators of B lymphocyte signal transduction. Intern Rev Immunol 2001;20:739–742.
363. El-Hillal O, Kurosaki T, Yamamura H, et al. Syk kinase activation by asrc-kinase activation loopphosphorylated chain reaction. Proc Natl Acad Sci USA 1997;94:1919–1924.
364. Hasegawa M, Fujimoto M, Poe JC, et al. CD19-dependent signaling pathway regulates autoimmunity in Lyn-deficient mice. J Immunol 2001;167:2469–2478.
365. Lankester GMV, van Schijndel PML, Rood AJ, et al. B cell antigen receptor cross-linking induces phosphorylation and membrane translocation of a multimeric Shc complex that is augmented by CD19 co-ligation. Eur J Immunol 1994;24:2818–2825.
366. Beckwith M, Jorgesen G, Longo DL. The protein product of the protooncogen c-cbl forms a complex with phosphatidy inositol 3-kinase p85 and CD19 in anti-IgM-stimulated human lymphoma cells. Blood 1996;88:3502–3507.
367. Fujimoto M, Fujimoto Y, Poe JC, et al. CD19 regulates Src family protein tyrosinase kinase in B lymphocytes through processive amplification. Immunity 2000;13:47–57.
368. Brooks SR, Li X, Volanskis EJ, et al. Systemic analysis of the role of CD19 cytoplasmic tyrosinases in enhancement of activation in human Daudi cells: clustering of phospholipase C and Vav and of Grb2 and Sos with different CD19 tyrosines. J Immunol 2000;164:3123–313.

369. Peaker CJ, Neuberger MS. Association of CD22 with the B cell antigen receptor. Eur J Immunol 1993;23:1358–1365.
370. Yohannnan J, Wienands J, Coggeshall KM, et al. Analysis of tyrosine phosphorylation-dependent interaction between stimulatory effector proteins and B cell co-receptor CD22. J Biol Chem 1999;274:18,768–18,776.
371. Tuscano JM, Engel P, Tedder TF, et al. CD22 cross-linking generates B-cell antigen receptor-independent signals that activates JNK/SAPK signaling cascade. Blood 1996;87:4723–4730.
372. Tuscano JM, Engel P, Tedder TF, et al. Involvement of p72syk kinase, p53/56lyn kinase and phosphatidylinositol kinase-3 signal transduction via the human B lymphocyte antigen CD22. Eur J Immunol 1996;26:1246–1252.
373. Lajaunias F, Nitschke L, Moll T, et al. Differentially regulated expression and function of CD22 in activated B-1 and B-2 lymphocytes. J Immunol 2002;168:6078–6083.
374. Pillai S. The chosen few? Positive selection and generation of naïve B lymphocytes. Immunity 1999;10:493–502.
375. Juma H, Wollscheid B, Mitterer M, et al. Abnormal development and function of B lymphocytes in mice deficient for signaling adaptor protein SLP-65. Immunity 1999;11:547–554.
376. Lam KP, Rajewsky K. B cell antigen receptor specificity and surface density together determine B-1 versus B-2 cell development. J Exp Med 1999;190:471–477.
377. Uliveri C, Valensin S, Majolini MB, et al. Normal B-1 cell development but defective BCR signaling in LCK–/– mice. Eur J Immunol 2003;33:441–445.
378. Freeman GJ, Gribben JG, Boussiotis VA, et al. Cloning of B7-2: a CTLA-4 counter-receptor that costimulates human T cell proliferation. Science 1993;203:909–911.
379. Suvas S, Singh V, Sahdev S, et al. Distinct role of CD80 and CD86 in the regulation of the activity of B cell and B cell lymphoma. J Biol Chem 2002;277:7766–7775.
380. Doty RT, Clark EA. Two regions in the CD80 cytoplasmic tail regulate CD80 redistribution and T cell costimulation. J Immunol 1998;161:2700–2707.
381. Ikemizu S, Gilbert RJ, Fennelly JA, et al. Structure and dimerization of a soluble form of B7-1. Immunity 2002;12:51–60.
382. Clark EA, Shu G, Ledbetter JA. Role of Bp35 cell surface peptide in human B cell activation. Proc Natl Acad Sci USA 1985;82:1766–1770.
383. Ledbetter JA, Shu G, Gallanger M, et al. Augmentation of normal and malignant B cell proliferation by monoclonal antibody to the B cell specific antigen BP50 (Cdw40). J Immunol 1987;138:788–796.
384. Pauli S, Rosen A, Eblin-Henriksson B, et al. The human B-lymphocyte and carcinoma antigen CD40 is a phosphoprotein involved in growth signal transduction. J Immunol 1989;142:590–595
385. Fessus E. Biochemical events in naturally occurring forms of cell death. FEBS Lett 1993;328:1–12.
386. Bishop GA, Hostager BS. Molecular mechanisms of CD40 signaling. Arch Immunol Ther Exp 2001;24:97–108.

387. Sutherland CL, Heath AW, Pelch SL, et al. Differential activation of the ERK, JNK and p38 mitogen-activated protein kinase by CD40 and B cell antigen receptor. J Immunol 1996;157:3381–3385.

388. Francis DA, Karras JG, Ke XY, et al. Induction of transcription of NF-kB, AP-1 and NF-AT during B cell stimulation through CD40 receptor. Int Immunol 1995;7:151–159.

389. Dadgostar H, Zarnegar B, Hoffman A, et al. Cooperation of multiple signaling pathways in CD40-regulated gene expression in B lymphocytes. Proc Natl Acad Sci USA 2002;99:1487–1502.

390. Goldstein MD, Watts TH. Identification of distinct domains in CD40 involved in B7-1 induction and growth inhibition. J Immunol1996;157:2837–2843.

391. Haxhinasto SA, Hostager BS, Bishop GA. Molecular mechanisms of synergy between CD40 and B cell antigen receptor: role for TNF receptor-associated factor 2 in receptor interaction. J Immunol 2002;169:1145–1149.

392. Leo E, Zapata JM, Reed JC. CD40-mediated activation of IgCγ1 and IgCε germline promoters involves multiple TRAF family proteins. Eur J Immunol 1999;29:3908–3913.

393. Muta T, Kurosaki T, Misulovin Z, et al. A 13-amino acid motif in cytoplasmic domain of Fc gamma RIIB modulates B cell receptor signaling. Nature 1994;369:350–346.

394. Brooks DG, Qiu WQ, Luster AD, et al. Structure and expression of human IgG FcRII (CD32). J Exp Med 1989;170:1368–1385.

395. Ravetch JV, Bolland S. IgG Fc receptors. Ann Rev Immunol 2001;19:275–290.

396. Tonegawa S. Somatic generation of antibody diversity. Nature 1983;302:571–581.

397. Sakano H, Huppi K, Heinrich G, et al. Sequencees at the somatic receecombination sites of immunoglobulin light chain genes. Nature 1979;280:288–293.

398. Max EE, Seidman JG, Leder P. Sequences of five recombination sites encoded close to an immunoglobulin k constant region gene. Proc Nat Acad Sci USA 1979;76:3450–3455.

399. Kurosawa Y, Tonegawa S. Organization, structure and assembly of immuno-globulin heavy chain diversity segments. J Exp Med 1982;155:201–208.

400. Bassing CH, Swat W, Alt FA. The mechanisms and regulation of chromo-somal V(D)J recombination. Cell 2002;109:S45–S55.

401. Khanna KK, Jackson SP. DNA double strand breaks: signaling, repair and can-cer connection. Nat Gen 2001;27:247–254.

402. Blackwell TK, Alt FA. Site specific recombination between immunoglobulin D and JH segments that were introduced into the genome of a murine pre-B cell line. Cell 1984;37:105–112.

403. Nagoka H, Yo W, Nussenzweig MC. Regulation of RAG expression in devel-oping lymphocytes. Curr Opin Immunol 2000;12:187–190.

404. Papavasillou F, Misulovin Z, Suh H, et al. The role of Igβ in precursor B cell transition and allelic exclusion. Science 1995;268:408–411.

405. The YM, Neuberger MS. The immunoglobulin Igα and Igβ cytoplasmic do-mains are independently sufficient to signal B cell maturation and activation in transgenic mice. J Exp Med 1977;185:1753–1758.

406. Torres RM, Haften KA. Negative regulatory role for Ig-α during B cell development. Immunity 1999;11:527–563.
407. Macardle PJ, Weedon H, Fusco M, et al. The antigen receptor complex on cord B lymphocytes. Immunology 1997;90:376–382.
408. Golding B, Muchmore AV, Blaese RM. Newborn and Wiskott–Aldrich patients B cells can be activated by TNP-*Brucella abortus*: evidence that TNP-*Brucella abortus* behaves as T-independent type I antigen in humans. J Immunol 1984:2966–2305.
409. Viemann D, Schlenke P, Hammers H-J, et al. Differential expression of the B-cell restricted molecule CD22 on neonatal B lymphocytes depending upon antigen stimulation. Eur J Immunol 2000;30:550–559.
410. Sproul TW, Malapati S, Kim J, et al. B cell antigen receptor signaling occurs outside lipid rafts in immature B cells. J Immunol 2000;165:6020–6023.
411. Birkeland ML, Monroe JG. Biochemestry of antigen receptor signaling in mature and developing B lymphocytes. Crit Rev Immunol 1997;17:353–385.
412. Papavasilou F, Jankovic M, Suh H, et al. The cytoplasmic domains of imunnoglobulin Igα and Igβ can independently induce precursor B cell transition and allelic exclusion. J Exp Med 1995;182:1389–1394.
413. Wechsler RJ, Monroe JG. Immature B lymphocytes are deficient in expression of the src-family kinase p59^tyn and p55^fgr1 J Immunol 1995;154:1919–1929.
414. Yellen-Shaw AJ, Monroe JG. Developmentally regulated association of 56kD member of the surface immunoglobulin M complex. J Exp Med 1992;176;129.
415. Hashimoto A, Takeda K, Inaba M, et al. Essential role of phospholipase C-γ2 in B cell development and function. J Immunol 2000;165:1738–1742.
416. Ling V, Munroe RC, Murphy EA, et al. Embryonic stem cells and embryoid bodies express lymphocyte costimulatory molecules. Exp Cell Res 1998;241:55–65.
417. Elliot SR, Macardle PJ, Roberton DM, et al. Expression of the costimulatory molecules, CD80, CD86, CD28 and CD152 on lymphocytes of neonates and young children. Human Immunol 1999;60:1039–1048.
418. Durandy A, De Saint Basile G, Lisowska-Grospierre B, et al. Undetectable CD40 ligand on T cells and low B cell response to CD40 binding agonists in human newborn. J Immunol 1995;154:1560–1571.
419. Elliot SR, Roberton DM, Zolla H, et al. Expression of the costimulatory molecules CD40 and CD154 on lymphocytes from neonates and young children. Human Immunol 2000;61:378–388.
420. Philips NE, Parker DC. Fc-dependent inhibition of mouse B celll activation by whole anti-mu antibodies. J Immunol 1983;130:602–609.
421. Ashman RF, Peckman D, Stunz LL. Fc receptor off-signal in the B cell involved apoptosis. J Immunol 1996;157:5–11.
422. Jessup CF, Ridings J, Ho A, et al. The Fc receptor for IgG (CD23) on human neonatal lymphocytes. Human Immunol 2001;62:678–685.
423. Lima JO, Zang L, Atkinson TP, et al. Early expression of epsilon CD23, IL-4R alpha and IgE in human fetus. J Allergy Clin Immunol 2000;106:911–917.
424. King CL, Malhorta I, Mungai P, et al. B cell sensitization to helmitic infection develops *in utero* in humans. J Immunol 1998;160:3578–3584.

425. Furuhashi M, Suguira K, Katsumata Y, et al. Cord blood against milk and egg proteins. Biol Neonate 1977;72:210–215.

426. Bonnefoy JY, Gauchat JF, Life P, et al. Pairs of surface molecules involved in human IgE regulation: CD23-CD21 and CD40-CD40L. Eur Respir 1996;9:63s–66s.

427. Texido G, Eibel H, Le Gros G, et al. Transgene CD23 expression on lymphoid cells modulates IgE and IgG1 responses. J Immunol 1994;153:3028–3043.

428. Thornton CA, Halloway JA, Warner JO. Expression of CD21 and CD23 during human fetal development. Ped Res 2002;52:245–250.

429. Howard LM, Reen DJ. CD72 ligation regulates defective naïve newborn B cell responses. Cell Immunol 1997;175:179–188.

430. Lee HC, Graeff RM, Walseth TF. ADP-ribosyl cyclase and CD38. Multi-functional enzymes in Ca^{+2} signaling. Adv Exp Med Biol 1999;419:411–419.

431. Lee HC, Munshi C, Graeff RM. Structure and activities of cyclic ADP-ribose NAADP and their metabolic enzymes. Cell Biochem 1999;193:89–98.

432. Santos-Argumedo L, Texeira C, Preece G, et al. A B lymphocyte surface molecule mediating activation and protection from apoptosis via calcium channels. J Immunol 1993;193 89–98.

433. Donis- Heranadez FR, Mike R, Parkhouse RME, et al. Ontogeny distribution and function of CD38-expressing B lymphocytes in mice. Eur J Immunol 2001;31:1261–1267.

434. Muramatsu M, Sankaranand VS, Anant S, et al. Specific expression of activation-induced cytidine deaminase (AID), a novel member of the RNA-editing deaminase family in germinal center B cells. J Biol Chem 1999;274:18,470–18,476.

435. Cyster JG, Healy JI, Kishihara KM, et al. Regulation of B lymphocyte positive and negative selection by tyrosine phosphatase CD45. Nature 1996;381:325–328.

436. O'Keefe TL, Williams GT, Neuberger MS. Hyperresponsive B cells in CD22 deficient mice. Science 1996;274:798–801.

437. Weissman IL. Development switches in the immune system. Cell 1994;76:207–218.

438. Osmond DG. Population dynamics of bone morrow B lymphocytes. Immunol Rev 1986;93:103–124.

439. Schittek B, Rakewsky K. Maintenanace of B cell memory by long-lived cells generated from proliferating precursors. Nature 1990;346:749–751.

440. Gu H, Tartilon D, Muller W, et al. Most peripheral B cells are ligand selected. J Exp Med 1991;173:1357–1371.

441. Heltemes LM, Manser T. Level of B cell antigen receptor surface expression influence both positive and negative selection of B cells during development. J Immunol 2002;169:1283–1292.

442. Goodnoww CC. Balancing immunity, autoimmunity and self-tolerance. Ann. NY Acad Sci 1997;815:55–66.

443. Mercolin TJ, Arnold LW, Hawkins LA, et al. Normal mouse peritoneum contains a large population of Ly-1+(CD5) B cells that recognize phosphatidyl choline. J Exp Med 1988;168:687–698.

444. Pennel CA. Selection for S107-V11 expression by peritoneal B cells in adult mice. J Immunol 1995;155:1264–1275.

445. Mayer R, Zaghouani H, Usuba O, et al. The Ly-1 expression in murine hybrydomas producing autoantibodies. Autoimmunity 1990;6:293–305.

446. Painter CJ, Monestier M, Chew A, et al. Specificities and V genes encoding monoclonal antibodies from viable motheaten mice. J Exp Med 1988;167:1137–1153.

447. Kasturi KN, Mayer R, Bona CA, et al. Germline V genes encode viable moth eaten mouse autoantibodies against thymocytes and red blood cells. J Immunol 1990;154:2304–2311.

448. Pennell CA, Arnold LW, Haughton G, et al. Restricted Ig variable region gene expression among Ly1+ B cell lymphomas. J Immunol 1988;141:2788–2796.

449. Reininger I, Ollierr P, Kaushik A, et al. Novel V genes encode virtually identical and variable regions of six murine monoclonal anti-bromalain-treated red blood cells autoantibodies. J Immunol 1987;138:316–323.

450. Karas JG, Wang Z, Huo L, et al. STAT 3 is constitutively activated in normal self-renewing B-1 cells, but only inducible expressed in conventional B1 cells. J Exp Med 1997;185:1035–1042.

451. Brombacher F, Kohler G, Eibel H. B cell tolerance in mice transgenic for anti-CD8 immunoglobulin μ chain. J Exp Med 119;174:1335–1346.

452. Tiegs SL, Ussel DM, Nemazee D. Receptor editing in self-reactive bone mar row B cells. J Exp Med 1993;177:1009–1020.

453. Lortan JE, Roobottom-Oldfields CA, McLeanan IC. Newly produced virgin B cells migrate to secondary lymph nodes but their capacity to enter foliclles is restricted. Eur J Immunol 1987;17:1311–1316.

454. Makela O, Karajalienen K. Inherited immunoglobulin idiotype of mouse. Immunol Rev 1977;34:119–138

455. Eichmann K. Genetic control of antibody specificity in mouse. Immunogenetics 1975;2:491–506.

456. Gerhart P, Cebra JJ. Idiotype sharing by murine strains differing in immunoglobulin allotype. Nature 1978;272:264–268.

457. Cancro M, Klinman NR. B cell repertoire ontogeny: heritable but dissimilar development of parental and F1 repertoires. J Immunol 1981;126:1160–1164.

458. Tiffany LJ, Riblet R, Stein KE. The Sr1 gene that controls diversity of the anti-inulin antibody response maps to chromosome 14. Immunogenetics 2003;55:80–86.

459. Keller MA, Calandra G, Song C, et al. Neonatal A/J response to HEL. In: The Immune Response to Structurally Defined Proteins: The Lysozyme Model. (Smith-Gill S, Sercaz EE, eds.), Academic Press. New York: 1989, pp. 381–387.

460. Cancro MP, Thompson MA, Raychaudhuri S, et al. Ontogeny of the HA-responsive B-cell repertoire: interaction of heritable and inducible mechanisms in the establishment of phenotype. In: Idiotype in Biology and Medicine. (Kohler H, Urabain J, Cazenave P-A, eds.), Academic Press. New York, London: 1984; pp. 143 170.

461. Mussmann R, Wilson M, Marcuz A, et al. Membrane exons sequences of three Xenopous Ig classes explain the evolutionary origin of mammalian isotypes. Eur J Immunol 1996;26:409–419.

462. Raff MC, Owen JJ, Cooper MD, et al. Differences in susceptibility of mature and immature mouse B lymphocytes to anti-immunoglobulin suppression in vitro. Possible implications for B-cell tolerance to self. J Exp Med 1975;142:1052–1064.

463. Gu H, Kitamura D, Rajewsky K. B-cell development regulated by gene rearrangement: arrest of maturation by membrane bound D(protein and selection of D_H element reading frame. Cell 1991;65:47–54.

464. Schwager J, Burckert N, Courtet M, et al. The ontogeny and diversification at the heavy chain locus in Xenopous. EMBO J 1991;10:2461–2470.

465. Du Pasquier L. Phylogeny of B-cell development. Curr Opin Immunol 1993;5:185–193.

466. DuPasquier L, Wilson M, Greenberg A, et al. Somatic mutation in ectodermic vertebrates: using on selection and origins. Curr Top Microbiol Immunol 1998;229:199–216.

467. Reynaud C-A, Anquez V, Weill J-C. The chicken D locus and its contribution to the immunoglobulin heavy chain repertoire. Eur J Immunol 1991;21:2661–2670.

468. Benatar T, Tkalek L, Ratcliffe JH. Stochastic rearrangement of immunoglobulin varable region genes in chicken B-cell development. Proc Natl Acad Sci USA 1992;89:7615–7619.

469. Thompson CD. Creation of immunoglobulin diversity by intrachromosomal gene conversion. Trends Genet 1992;8:416–423.

470. Reynaud C-A, Anquez V, Grimal H, et al. A hyperconversion mechanism generated in the chicken light chain preimmune repertoire. Cell1987;48:379–388.

471. McCormack WT, Thompson CB. Chicken IgL varaible region gene conversion display pseudogene donor prefernce and 5_ to 3_ polarity. Genes Dev 1990;4:548–558.

472. Arakawa K, Hauschild J, Buerstedde J-M. Requirement of activation-induced deminase (AID) gene for immunoglobulin gene conversion. Science 2002;295:1301–1306.

473. Ekino S, Suginohara K, Urano T, et al. The Bursa of Fabricius: a trapping site for environmental antigens. Immunology 1985;55:405–410.

474. Arkawa H, Kuma K, Yasuda M, et al. Effect of environmental antigens on the Ig diversification and selection of productive V-J joints in the Bursa. J Immunol 2002;169:818–828.

475. D'Hoostelaere LA, Huppi K, Mock B, et al. The Ig kappa L chain allelic groups among the Ig kappa haplotypes and Ig kappa crossover populations suggest a gene order. J Immunol 1988;141:652–661.

476. Brodeur P, Riblett R. The immunoglobulin heavy chain variable region (IgH-V) in the mouse I. 100 IgH-V genes comprise 7 families of homologous genes. Eur J Immunol 1984;14:922–930.

477. Kofler R, Strohal R, Balderas S, et al. Ig kappa-light chain varable gene complex organization and immunoglobulin gene encoding anti-DNA autoantibodies in lupus mice. J Clin Invest 1988;82:852–866.

478. Shefener R, Mayer R, Kaushik AD, et al. Identification of a new Vk gene family that is highly expressed in hybridomas from an autoimmune strain. J Immunol 1991;145:1609–1614.

479. Dildrop R, Krawinkel U, Winter E, et al. V_H gene expression in murine li-popolysaccharide blasts distributes over the nine known V_H-gene groups may be random. Eur J Immunol 1985;15:1154–1161.

480. Schultze DH, Kelsoe G. Genotypic analysis of B cell colonies by *in situ* hybridization. Stoichiometric expression of three VH families in adult C56Bl/6 and Balb/c mice. J Exp Med 1987;166:162–172.

481. Jeong HD, Komisar JL, Kraig E, et al. Strain dependent expression of V_H families. J Immunol 1988;140:2436–2441.

482. Kaushik AK, Bona CA. Genetic Origin of murine autoantibodies. In: Molecular Pathology of Autoimmune Disease. (Theophilopoulos AN, Bona CA, eds.), Taylor and Francis. New York, London: 2002 pp. 53–67.

483. Wu G, Paige C. V_H gene family utilization in colonies derived from B and pre-B cells detected by RNA colony blot assay. EMBO J 1986;5:3475–1481.

484. Yancopoulos GC, Desiderio SV, Paskind M, et al. Preferential utilization of the most J_H-proximal segments in pre-B cell line. Nature 1984:311:724–733.

485. Perlmutter RM, Kearney JF, Chang SP, et al. Developmentally controlled expression of V_H genes. Science 1985;227:1597–1601.

486. Reth MG, Jackson S, Alt FW. $V_H DJ_H$ formation and DJ_H replacement during pre-B differentiation: non-random usage of gene segments. EMBO J 1986;5:2131–2138.

487. Decker D, Boyle N, Klinman N. Predominance of non-productive rearrangements of $V_H 81X$ gene segments evidences a dependence of B cell clonal maturation on the structure of nascent H chains. J Immunol 1991;147:1406–1411.

488. Huetz F, Carlsson L, Tomberg U, et al. V-region directed selection in differentiating B lymphocytes. EMBO J 1993;12:1819–1826.

489. Martin F, Chen X, Kearney JF. Development of $V_H 81X$ transgene-bearing B cells in fetus and adult:sites for expansion and deletion in conventional CD5/B1 cells. Int Immunol 1997;9:493–505.

490. Kenya U, Beck-Engeseer GB, Jongstra J, et al. Surrogate light chain-dependent selection of Ig heavy chain V regions J Immunol 1995;155:5536–5542.

491. Marshall AJ, Wu GE, Paige CJ. Frequency of $V_H 81X$ usage during B cell development: initial decline in usage is independent of Ig heavy chain cell surface expression. J Immunol 1996;156:2077–2084.

492. Huetz F, Tornberg U-C, Malanchere E, et al. Targed disruption of the $V_H 81X$ gene: influence on the B cell repertoire. Eur J Immunol 1997;27:307–314.

493. Alt FW, Blackwell K, Yancopoulos GD. Development of the primary antibody repertoire. Science 1987;238:1079–1087.

494. Jeong HD, Teale JM. Comparison of fetal and adult functional B cell repertoire by analysis of V_H gene expression. J Exp Med 1988;168;589–603.

495. Malynn BA, Yancopoulos GD, Barth JE, et al. Biased expression of J_H-proximal V_H genes occurs in the newly generated repertoire of neonatal and adult mice. J Exp Med 1990;171:843–859.

496. Carlsson L, Overmo C, Holmberg D. Developmentally controlled selsection of antibody genes: characterization of individual V_H 7183 genes and evidence for stage-specific somatic diversification. Eur J Immunol 1992;22:71–78.

497. Dighiero G, Lymberi P, Holmberg D, et al. High frequency of natural autoantibodies in normal newborn mice. J Immunol 1985;134:765–771.

498. Bellon B, Manheimer-Lory A, Monestier M, et al. High frequency of autoantibodies bearing cross-reactive idiotype among hybrydomas using $V_H 7183$ gene from normal and autoimmune murine strains. J Clin. Invest 1987;79:1044–1053.

499. Kienker LJ, Korostoff JM, Cancro MP. Patterns of Ig V region expression among neonatal hemagglutinin-responsive B cells. J Immunol 1988;141:3634–3641.

500. Gu H, Forster I, Rajewsky K. Sequence homology, N sequence insertion and JH gene utilization in VHDJH joining: implication for the joining mechanism and ontogentic timing of Ly1 B-CLL progenitor generation. EMBO J 1990;9:2133–2140.

501. Hartman AB, Rudikoff S. V_H genes encoding the immune response to β-(1,6) galactan:somatic mutation in IgM molecules. EMBO J I984;3:3023–3030.

502. Klonowski KD, Primiano LL, Monestier M. Atypical V_H–D–J_H rearrangements in newborn autoimmune MRL mice. J Immunol 1999;162:1566–1572.

503. Connor A, Fanning LJ, Celler JW, et al. Mouse $V_H 7183$ recombination signal sequences mediate recombination more frequently than those of $V_H J558$. J Immunol 1955;155:5268–5272.

504. Tsukuda S, Sugyama H, Oka Y, et al. Estimation of D segment usage in initial D to J joinings in an immature B cell line:preferential usage of $D_{FL16.1}$, the most 5_D segment and Q52 the most J_H–proximal segment. J Immunol 1990;144:4053–4059.

505. Teale JM, Medina CA. Comparative expression of adult and fetal Vgene repertoire. Intern Rev Immunol 1992;8:95–112.

506. Desiderio SV, Yancopoulos GD, Paskind M, et al. Insertion of N-regions into heavy-chain genes is correlated with the expression of terminal deoxytransferase in B cells. Nature 1984;311:752–755.

507. Alt FW, Baltimore D. Joining of immunoglobulin heavy chain genes segments: implications for a chromosome with evidence of three D-J_H fusions. Proc Natl Acad Sci USA 1982;79:4118–4122.

508. Komori T, Pricop ,L Hatakeyama A, et al. Repertoire of antigen receptors in TdT congenitally defected mice. Intern Rev Immunol 1996;13:317–326.

509. Fenny AJ. Lack of N regions in fetal and neonatal mouse immunoglobulin V-D-J junctional sequences. J Exp Med 1990;172:1377–1390.

510. Bangs LA, Sanz IE, Teale JM. Comparison of DJH and junctional diversity in the fetal, adult and aged B cell repertoire. J Immunol 1991;141:1996–2004.

511. Malynn BA, Berman JE, Yamcopoulos GD, et al. Expression of the immunoglobulin heavy-chain variable gene repertoire. Curr Top Microbiol Immunol 1987;135:75–94.

512. Boss NA, Meeuwsen CG. B cell repertoire in adult antigen-free and conventional neonatal Balb/c mice I. Preferential utilization of C_H-proximal V_H gene family PC7183. Eur J Immunol 1989;19:1811–1815.

513. Komori T, Minami Y, Sakato N, et al. Biased usage of two restricted V_H gene segments in VH development. Eur J Immunol 1993;23:517–522.

514. Arnold LW, Pennell CA, McCray SK, et al. Development of B-1 cells: segregation of phosphatidyl choline-specific B cells to the B-1 population occurs after immunoglobulin-gene expression. J Exp Med 1994;179:1585–1595.

515. Teale J, Morris E. Comparison of V_K gene family in adult and fetal B cells. J Immunol 1989;143:2768–2772.

516. Kaushik A, Schulze DH, Bona C, et al. Murine V_K gene expression does not follow the V_H paradigm. J Exp Med 1989;169:1859–1864.

517. Kaushik A, Schulze DH, Bonilla FA, et al. Stochastic pairing of heavy-chain and κ-light-chain variable gene families occurs in polyclonally activated B cells. Proc Natl Acad Sci USA 1990;87:4932–4936.

518. Kim S, Davis M, Sin E, et al. Antibody diversity: somatic mutation of rearranged Vh genes. Cell 1981;27:573–581.

519. Wilson PC, de Bouteiller O, Liu Y-J, et al. Somatic hypermutation introduces insertation and deletion into immunoglobulin V genes. J Exp Med 1998;187:59–70.

520. Gerhart P, Bogenhagen DF. Clusters of point mutation are found exclusively around rearranged antibody variable genes. Proc Natl Acad Sci USA 1983;80:3439–3443.

521. Chien NC, Pollock RR, Desaymard C, et al. Point mutations cause the somatic diversification of IgM and IgG2a antiphosphorylcholine antibodies. J Exp Med 1998;167:954–973.

522. Clarke SH, Huppi K, Bell M, et al. Inter- and intraclonal diversity in the response to influenza hemagglutinin. J Exp Med 1985;161:187–194.

523. Press J. Neonatal Immunity and somatic mutation. Intern Rev Immunol 2000;19:265–287.

524. Erikson J, Radic MZ, Camper SΛ, et al. Expression of anti-DNA immunoglobulin transgenes in non-autoimmune mice. Nature 1991;349:331–334.

525. Radic MZ, Erikson J, Litwin S, et al. B lymphocytes may escape tolerance by revising their antigen receptors. J Exp Med 1993;177:1165–1173.

526. Casellas R, Yang Shih T-A, Kleinewietfeld M, et al. Contribution of receptor editing to the antibody repertoire. Science 2001;291:1541–1544.

527. Magari M, Sawatari T, Kawano Y, et al. Contribution of light chain rearrangement in peripheral B cells to the generation of high affinity of antibodies. Eur J Immunol 2002;32:957–966.

528. Hikida M, Mori M, Takai T, et al. Re-expression of RAG-1 and RAG-2 genes in activated mature mouse B cells. Science 1996;274:2092–2094.

529. Hikida M, Mori M, Kawabata T, et al. Characterization of B cells expressing recombination activating genes in germinal centers of immunized mouse lymph nodes. J Immunol 1997;158:2509–2512.

530. Han S, Zheng B, Schatz DG, et al. Neoteny in lymphocytes: Rag1 and Rag2 expression in germinal center B cells. Science 1996;274:2094–2097.

531. Han S, Dillon SR, Zheng B, et al. V(D)J recombinase activity in a subset of germinal center B cell lymphocytes. Science 1997;278:301–305.

532. Knight KL, Becker RS. Molecular basis of allelic inheritance of rabbit immunoglobulin V_H allotypes. Implication for the generation of antibody diversity. Cell 1990;60:963–970.

533. Stepankova R, Kovaru F. Immunoglobulin-producing cells in lymphatic tissue of germfree and conventional rabbits detected by immunofluorescence method. Folia Microbiol 1985;30:291–294.

534. Tunyaplin C, Knight KL. Fetal VDJ gene repertoire in rabbits: evidence for preferential rearrangement of V_H1. Eur J Immunol 1995;25:2582–2587.

535. Friedman ML, Tunyaplin C, Zahai SK, et al. Neonatal V_H D and JH gene usage in rabbit B-lineage cells. J Immunol 1994;152:632–641.

536. Staerzl J, Trnka Z. Effect of very large doses of bacterial antigen on antibody production in newborn rabbits. Nature 1957;179:918–919.

537. Bridges RA, Condie RM, Zak SJ, et al. Clinical and experimental: the morphologic basis of antibody formation development during the neonatal period. J Lab Clin Med 1959;53:331–357.

538. Knight KL, Crane MA. Generation of antibody repertoire in rabbits. Adv Immunol 1994;56:179–218.

539. Chien HT, Alexander CB, Chen FF, et al. Rabbit DQ52 and DH gene expression in early B-cell development. Mol Immunol 1996;33:1313–1321.

540. Short JA, Sethupathi P, Zhai SK, et al. VDJ genes in Vha2 allotype-suppressed rabbits. J Immunol 1991;147:4014–4018.

541. Wienstein PD, Anderson AO, Mage RG. Rabbit IgH sequences in appendix germinal centers: V_H diversification by gene conversion-like and hypermutation mechanisms. Immunity 1994;1:647–659.

542. Dufour V, Malinge S, Nau F. The sheep Ig variable region repertoire consists of a single V_H family. J Immunol 1996;156:2163–2170.

543. Jeong Y, Osborne BA, Goldsby RA. Early Vλ diversification in sheep. Immunology 2001;103:26–34

544. Fahey KJ, Morris B. Humoral response in foetal sheep. Immunology 1978;38:651–661.

545. Motyka B, Reynolds JG. Apoptosis is associated with extensive B cell death in sheep ileal Peyer's patches and in the chicken bursa of Fabricius. Eur J Immunol 1991;21:1951–1959.

546. Hein WR, Dudler L. Diversity of Ig light chain variable region gene expression in fetal lambs. Int Immunol 1998;10:1251–1259.

547. Jenne CN, Kennedy LJ, McChllagh P, et al. A new model of sheep Ig diversification: shifting the emphasis toward combinatorial mechanisms and away from hypermutation. J Immunol 2003;170:3739–3750.

548. Reynaud CA, Garcia C, Hein R, et al. Hypermutation generating sheep immunoglobulin repertoire is antigen-independent. Cell 1995;80:1115–1125.

549. Hansal SA. B cell development and immunoglobulin gene. In: Cattle PhD Thesis. University of Massachusetts: 1994.

550. Meyer A, Parng C-L, Hansal SA, et al. Immunoglobulin gene diversification in cattle. Int Rev Immunol 1997;15:165–183.

551. Berens SJ, Wylie DE, Lopez OJ. Use of a single V_H family and long CDR3 in the varaible region of cattle Ig heavy chain. Int Immunol 1997;9:189–199.

552. Sinclaire MC, Gilchrist J, Aitken R. Bovine IgG repertoire is dominated by a single diversified V_H family. J Immunol 1997;159:3883–3889.

553. Parng C-L, Hansal S, Goldsby RA, et al. Gene conversion contributes to Ig light chain diversity in catttle. J Immunol 1996,157:5478–5486.

554. Matsuda F, Ishii K, Bourvagnet P, et al. The complete nucleotide sequence of the human immunoglobulin heavy chain locus. J Exp Med 1998;188:2151–2262.

555. Zachau HG. The immunoglobulin κ locus. Gene 1993;135:167–173.
556. Tomilson IM, Cox PL, Gherardi E, et al. The structural repertoire of the human V$_k$ doamain. EMBO J 1995;14:4628–4638.
557. Frippiat HJP, Williams SC, Tomilson IM, et al. Organization of the human lambda-chain locus on chromosome 22q11.2. Hum Mol Genet 1995;4:983–991.
558. Kawasaki K, Minoshima S, Nakato E, et al. One-megabasc of the human immunoglobulin λ gene locus. Genome Res 1995;7:250–261.
559. Schiff C, Milli M, Bossy D, et al. Organization and expression of the pseudo-light chain gene in human B cell ontogeny. Int Rev Immunol 1992;8:135–146.
560. Raaphorst FM, Timmers E, Kenter MJH, et al. Restricted utilization of germ-line V$_H$3 genes and short diverse third complementary-determining region (CDR3) in human fetal B lymphocytes immunoglobulin heavy chain rearrangements. Eur J Immunol 1992;22:247–251.
561. Cuisiner AM, Guigou V, Boubli L, et al. Preferential expression of VH5 and VH6 immunoglobulin genes in early human B-cell ontogeny. Scand J Immunol 1989;30:493–487.
562. Berman JE, Nickerson KG, Pollock RR, et al. VH gene usage in humans: biased usage of the V$_H$6 gene in immature B lymphoid cells. Eur J Immunol 1991;21:1311–1314.
563. Schroder HW, Wang JY. Preferential utilization of conserved immunoglobulin heavy chain variable gene segments during human fetal life. Proc Natl Acad Sci USA 1990;87:6146–6150.
564. Schroder HW, Perlmutter RM. Development of the human antibody repertoire. In New Concepts. In: Immunodeficiency Diseases. (Gupta S, Griscelli C, eds.), John Wiley & Sons. New York: 1993, pp. 3–22.
565. Mortari F, Wang JY, Schroder HW. The human cord blood antibody repertoire. Frequent usage of VH7 gene family. Eur J Immunol 1992;22:241–246.
566. Mageed RA, MacKenzie LE, Stevenson FK, et al. Selective expression of a V$_H$IV subfamily of immunoglobulin genes in human CD5$^+$ B lymphocytes from cord blood J Exp Med 1991;174:109–113.
567. Bauer K, Zemlin M, Hammel M, et al. Diversification of Ig heavy chain genes in human preterm neonates prematurely exposed to environmental antigens. J Immunol 2002:168:1349–1356.
568. Ridings J, Nicholson IC, Coldsworthy W, et al. Somatic hypermutation of immunoglobulin genes in human neonates. Clin Exp Immunol 1997;108:336–374.
569. Ridings J, Dinan L, Roberson DM, et al. Somatic mutations of immunoglobulin V$_H$6 gene in human infants. Clin. Exp Immunol 1998;114:33–39.
570. Weber JC, Blaison G, Martin T, et al. Evidence that the V kappa III gene usage is non-stochastic in both adult and newborn peripheral B cells and that periperal CD5$^+$ adult B cells are oligoclonal. J Clin Invest 1994;93:2093–2015.
571. Feeney AJ, Lugo G, Escuro G. Human cord blood kappa repertoire. J Immunol 1997;158:3761–3768.
572. Girschick HJ, Lipsky PE. The kappa repertoire of human neonatal B cells. Mol Immunol 2001;38:1113–1127.
573. Lee J, Monson NL, Lipsky PE. The VλJλ repertoire in human fetal spleen: evidence for positive selection and extensive receptor editing. J Immunol 2000;165:6322–6333.

574. Silverstein AM, Uhr JW, Kraner KL. Fetal response to antigen stimulus. II. Antibody production by fetal lamb. J Exp Med 1963;117:799–812.

575. Rowlands DT, Blakeslee D, Angala E. Acquired immunity in opossum embryos. J Immunol 1974;112:2148–2153.

576. Yung LL, Wyn-Evans TC, Diener E. Ontogeny of the murine immune system: development of antigen recognition and immune responsiveness. Eur J Immunol 1973;3:224–228.

577. Sherwin WK, Rowlands DT. Development of humoral immunity in lethally irradiated mice reconstituted with fetal liver cells. J Immunol 1974;113:1353–1360.

578. Sherwin WK, Rowlands DT. Determinants of the hierarchy of humoral immune responsiveness during ontogeny. J Immunol 1975;115:1549–1554.

579. Teale JM. B cell immune repertoire diversifies in a predictable temporal order in vitrol. J Immunol 1985;135:954–958.

580 Press JL, Klinman NR. Enumeration and analysis of antibody-forming cell precursors in the neonatal mouse. J Immunol 1973;111:829–835.

581. Press JL, Klinman NR. Frequency of hapten-specific B cells in neonatal an adult murine spleens. Eur J Immunol 1974;4:155–159.

582. Klinman NR, Press JL. The characterization of the B cell repertoire specific for the 2,4 dinitrophenyl and 2,4,6-trinitrophenyl determinants in neonatal Balb/c mice. J Exp Med 1975;141:1133–1146.

583. Sigal N. The frequency of p-azophenylarsonate and dimethylaminonaphtalene-sulfonyl-speceific B cells in neonatal and adult Balb/c mice. J Immunol 1977;119:1129–1133.

584. Cancro MP, Gerhard W, Klinman NR. The diversity of the influenza-specific primary B cell repertoire in Balb/c mice. J Exp Med 1978;147:776–787.

585. Mushinski EB, Potter M. Idiotypes on galactan binding myeloma proteins and anti-galactan antibodies in mice. J Immunol 1997;119:1888–1893.

586. Bona C. Idiotypes and Lymphocytes. Academic Press. New York: 1981, pp. 45–58.

587. Bona C, Liberman R, Chien CC, et al. Immune response to levan. I. Kinetics and ontogeny of anti-levan and anti-inulin antibody response and of expression of cross-reactive idiotype. J Immunol 1978;120:1436–1442.

588. Bona CA, Victor C. Ontogeny of anti-levan and inulin antibody responses. In: Idiotypy in Biology and Medicine. (Kohler H, Urbain J, Cazenave PA, eds.), Academic Press. New York: 1984, pp. 173–185.

589. Bona CA. Sequential activation of V genes during postnatal life. Am J Reprod. Immunol 1980;1;35–39.

590. Lieberman R, Potter M, Mushinski EB, et al. Genetics of a new IgVH (T15 idiotype) marker in the mouse regulating natural antibody to phosphorylcholine. J Exp Med 1974;139:983–997.

591. Segal N, Gearhart PJ, Press JL, et al. Late acquisition of a germ line antibody specfcity. Nature 1976;159:51–52.

592. Fung J, Kohler H. Late clonal selectoion and expansiom of the TEPC-15 germline specificity. J Exp Med 1980;153:1262–1273.

593. Mond JJ, Liberman R, Inman JK, et al. Inability of mice with a defect in B-lymphocyte maturation to respond to phosphorylcholine on immunogenic carriers. J Exp Med 1977;146:1138–1142.

594. Nisonoff A, Bangasser SA. Immunological suppression of idiotypic specificities. Transplant Rev 1975;27:100–134.

595. Nutt NB, Wiesel AN, Nisonoff A. Neonatal expression of cross-raective idiotype associated with anti-phenyl arsonate antobodies in strain A mice. Eur J Immunol 1979:864–868.

596. Zeldis JB, Konigsberg WH, Richards FF, et al. Location and expression of idiotypic determinants in the immunoglobulin variable region. Mol Immunol 1979;16:371–378.

597. Bona C, Paul WE. Cellular basis of idiotype expression. T suppressor cells specific for MOPC460 idiotype regulte the expression of cells secreting anti-TNP antibodies bearing 460 idiotype. J Exp Med 1979;149:592–600.

598. Stein KE, Bona C, Lieberman R, et al. Regulation of the anti-inulin antibody response by nonallotype linked gene. J Exp Med 1980;151:1088–1102.

599. Lieberman R, Potter M, Humphrey W, et al. Idiotyes of inulin-binding antibodies and myeloma proteins controlled by genes linked to the alloype locus of the mouse. J Immunol 1976;117;2105–2111.

600. Bona C, Mond JJ, Stein KE, et al. Immune response to levan III. The capacity to produce anti-inulin antibodies and cross-reactive idiotypes appears late in ontogeny. J Immunol 1979;123:1484–1490.

601. Bona C. Modulation of immune responses by Nocardia immunostimulants . Prog Allergy 1979;26:97–136.

602. Shahin RD, Cebra JJ. Rise in inulin-sensitive B cells during ontogeny can be prematurely stimulated by thymus-dependent and thymus-independent antigens. Inf Immun 1981;32:211–215.

603. D'Hoostelaere L, Potter M. Genetics of the (1-6 dextran response:expression of the QUPC52 idiotype in different inbred and congenic strains of mice. J Immunol 1982;128:492–500.

604. Howard JG, Hale C. Lack of neonatal susceptibility to induction of tolerance by polysacchride antigens. Eur J Immunol 1976;6:486–492.

605. Stein KE, Zopf DA, Miller CB, et al. Immune response to a thymus-dependent form of B512 dextran requires the presence of Lyb-5+ lymphocytes. J Exp Med 1983;157:7657–7666.

606. Bona C. Molecular characteristics of anti-polysaccharide antibodies. Springer Semin Immunopathol 1993;15:103–118.

607. Billingham RE, Brent L, Medawar PB. Actively acquired tolerance of foreign cells. Nature 1953;172:603–606.

608. Press CM, Hein WR, Landsverk T. Ontogeny of leukocyte populations in the spleen of fetal lambs with emphasis on early prominence of B cells. Immunology 1993;80:598–604.

609. Gerds V, Snider M, Brownlie R, et al. Oral vaccination in utero induces mucosal immunity and immune memory in the neonate. J Immunol 2002;168:1877–1885.

610. Gerds V, Babiuk LA, van Drunen Littel-van den Harke S, et al. Immunization by a DNA vaccine deliverd into oral cavity. Nature Med 2000 6:929–932.

611. Fennestad KL, Borg-Petersen C. Antibody and plasma cells in bovine fetuses infected with Leptospira saxkoebing. J Infect Dis 1962;110:63–69.

612. Sinkora M, Sun J, Sinkorova J, et al. Antibody repertoire development in fetal and neonatal piglets. VI. B cell lymphogenesis occurs at multiple sites with differences in the frequency of in-frame rearrangements. J Immunol 2003;170:1781–1788.

613. Fazio VM, Ria F, Franco E, et al. *In utero* naked gene transfer and anti-HBV DNA vaccination: protective response at birth, safety and long term responsiveness. 2002 DNA vaccine. (abstract).

614. Watts AM, Stanley JR, Shearer MH, et al. Fetal immunization of baboons induces a fetal-specific antibody response. Nat Med 1999;5:427–430.

615. Silverstein AM, Lukes RJ. Fetal response to antigenic stimulus. I. Plasmacellular and lymphoid reactions in the human fetus to intrauterine infection. Laboratory Invest 1962;11:918–932.

616. Wicher V, Baughan RE, Wicher K. Congenital and neonatal syphilis in guinea pigs show a different pattern of immune response. Immunology 1994;82:404–409.

617. Fitzgerald TJ, Froberg MK. Congenital syphilis in newborn rabbits: immune functions and susceptibility to challenge infections at 2 and 5 weeks of age. Infect Immun 1991;59:1869–1876.

618. Gamboa D, Miller JN, Lukhart SA, et al. Experimental neonatal syphilis. II. Immunologic response of neonatal rabbits following intradermal injection with Treponema palidum (Nicholas strain). Pediatr Res 1984;18:972–986.

619. Aasa JM, Noren GR, Reddy MV, et al. Mumps-virus infection in pregnant women and the immunlogic response of their offspring. N Engl J Med 1972;286:1379–1382.

620. King CL, Malhotra I, Wamachi A, et al. Acquired immune response to Plasmodium falciparum merozoite surface preotein-1 in the human fetus. J Immunol 2002;168:356–364.

621. Beeson JG, Reeder JC, Rogerson SJ, et al. Parasite adhesion and immune evasion in placental malaria. Trends Parasitol 2001;17:331–356.

622. King CL, Malhotra IJ, Mungai P, et al. B cell sensitization to helminthic infection develops *in utero*. J Immunol 1998;160:3578–3584.

623. Gill TJ, Reppetti CF, Metlay LA, et al. Transplacental immunization of the human fetus to tetanus by immunization of the mother. J Clin Invest 1983;72:987–996.

624. McCormick J, Gusmao HH, Nakamura S, et al. Antibody response to serogroup A and C meningococcal polysaccharide in infants born of mothers vaccinated during pregnancy. J Clin Invest 1908;65:1141–1144.

625. Blackall DP, Liles LH, Talati AI. *In utero* development of a warm-reactive autoantibody in a severely jaundiced neonate. Transfusion 2002;42:44–47.

626. Snapper CF, Roasa FR, Moorman MA, et al. Restoration of T cell-dependent type 2 induction of Ig secretion by neonatal B cells in vitro. J Immunol 1997;158:2731–2735.

627. Chelvarajan RL, Gilbert NL, Bondada S. Neonatal murine B lymphocyte response to polysaccharide antigens in the presence of IL-1 and IL-6. J Immunol 1998;161:3315–3324.

628. Morse HC III, Prescott B, Cross SS, et al. Regulation of the antibody response to typeII pneumococcal polysaccharide. V. Ontogeny of factors influencing the magnitude of the plaque-forming cell response. J Immunol 1976;116:279–287.

629. Mosier DE. Induction of B cell priming by neonatal injection of mice with thymic-independent (type 2) antigens. J Immunol 1978;121:1452–1463.

630. Baker PJ, Hiernaux JR, Fauntleroy MB, et al. Ability of monophosphoryl lipid A to augment antibody response in young mice. Infect Immun 1988;56:3064–3077.

631. Arulanandam BP, Mittler JN, Lee WT, et al. Neonatal administration of IL-12 enhances the protective efficacy of antiviral vaccines. J Immunol 2000;164:3698–3704.

632. Antohi S, Bot A, Manfield L, et al. The reactivity pattern of hemagglutinin-specific clonotypes from mice immunized as neonates or adults with naked DNA. Intern Immunol 1998;10:663–668.

633. Montesano MA, Colley DG, Freeman GL, et al. Neonatal exposure to idiotype induces *Schistosoma mansoni* egg-specific cellular and humoral immune response. J Immunol 1999;163:898–905.

634. Hiernaux J, Bona C, Baker PJ. Neonatal treatment with low doses of anti-idiotypic antibody leads to the expression of a silent clone. J Exp Med 1981;131:1004–1008.

635. Gorczynski R, Baumal R, Boulanger M, et al. Protection of adult Balb/c mice against MOPC315 myeloma by neonatal administration of monoclonal anti-idiotypic antibody to MOPC315 IgA. J Natl Cancer Inst 1986;77:801–807.

636. Montgomery PC, Williamson R. Molecular restriction of anti-hapten antibody elicited in neonatal rabbits: antibody production in littermates. J Immunol 1972;109:1036–1045.

637. Butler JE, Weber P, Sinkora M, et al. Antibody repertoire development in fetal and neonatal piglets. VIII. Colonization is required for newborn piglets to make serum antibodies to T-dependent and type 2 T-independent antigens. J Immunol 2002;169:6822–6830.

638. Rijkers GT, Sanders EAM, Breukeles MA, et al. Infant B cell response to polysaccharide determinants. Vaccine 1998;16:1396–1400.

639. Rijkers GT, Dollekamp EG, Zegers BJM. The in vitro response to pneumococcal polysaccharides in adults and neonates. Scand J Immunol 1987;25:447–452.

640. Wolff JA, Kudtke JJ, Acsadi G, et al. Long-term persistence of plasmid DNA and foreign gene expression in mouse muscle. Hum Mol Genet 1992;1:363–369.

641. Tang DC, Dewit C, Johnston SA. Genetic immunization is a simple method for eliciting an immune response. Nature 1992;356:152–154.

642. Bot A, Bot S, Garcia-Sastre A, et al. DNA immunization of newborn mice with a plasmid-expressing nucleoprotein of influenza virus. Viral Immunol 1996;9:207–210.

643. Wang Y, Xiang Z, Pasquini S, et al. Immune response to genetic immunization. Virology 1997;228:278–284.

644. Bot A, Antohi S, Bot S, et al. Immune response of neonates elicited by somatic transgene vaccination with naked DNA. Front Biosci 1997;2:173–188.

645. Martinez X, Brandt C, Saddalah F, et al. DNA immunization circumvents deficient induction of T helper type I and cytotoxic T lymphocytes during responses in neonates and during early life. Proc Natl Acad Sci USA 1997;94:8726–8731.

646. Monteil M, Le Poitier MF, Guillotin J, et al. Genetic immunization of seronegative one-day-old piglets against pseudorabies induces neutarlizing antibodies but not protection and is ineffective in piglets from immune dams. Vet Res 1996;27:443–452.

647. Prince AM, Whalen R, Brotman B. Successful nucleic acid based immunization of newborn chimpazees against hepatitis B virus. Vaccine 1997;15:916–919.

648. Bagarazzi ML, Boyer JD, Javadian MA, et al. Safety and immunogenicity of intramuscular and intravaginal delivery of HIV-1 DNA constructs to infant chimpazees. J Med Primat 1997;26:27–33.

649. Bot A, Shearer M, Bot S, et al. Induction of antibody response by DNA immunization of newborn baboons against influenza virus. Viral Immunol 1999;12:91–96.

650. Bot A, Shearer M, Bot S, et al. Induction of immunological memory in baboons primed with DNA vaccines as neonates. Vaccine 2001;19:1960–1967.

651. Bot A, Bona C. Genetic immunization of neonates. Micr Inf 2002;4:511–520.

652. Albrecht P, Ennis FA, Saltzman EJ, et al. Persistence of maternal antibodies in infants beyond 12 months: mechanism of measles vaccine failure. J Pediatr 1977;91:715–718.

653. Perkins FT, Yetts R, Gaisford WA. A comparison of the responses of 100 infants to primary poliomyelitis immunization with two and with three doses of vaccine. Br Med J 1959;1:1083–1086.

654. Burstyn DG, Baraff LJ, Peppler MS, et al. Serological response to filamentous hemagglutinin and lymphocytosis-promoting toxin of *Bordetella pertussis*. Infec Immun 1983;41:1150–1156.

655. Barr M, Glenny AT, Randall KJ. Diphtheria immunization in young babies. Lancet 1950;6593:6–10.

656. Sarvas H, Kurikka S, Seppala IJ, et al. Maternal antibodies partly inhibit an active immune response to routine tetanus toxoid immunization in infants. J Infect Dis 1992;165:977–979.

657. Bjorkholm B, Granstrom M, Taranger J, et al. Influence of high titers of maternal antibody on serologic response of infants to diphtheria vaccination. Pediatr Inf Dis J 1995;14:846–850.

658. Ghetie V, Ward ES. FcRn, the MCH class I-related receptor that is more than an IgG transporter. Immunol Today 1997;18:592–598.

659. Kim JK, Firan M, Radu CG, et al. Mapping the site on human IgG for binding to the MHC class I-related receptor, FcRn. Eur J Immunol 1999;29:2819–2825.

660. Kohler PF, Farr RS. Elevation of cord over maternal IgG immunoglobulin: evidence for an active placental IgG transport. Nature 1966;210:1070–1071.

661. Arvola M. Immunoglobulin-secreting cells of maternal origin can be detected in B cell-deficient mice. Biol Reprod 2000;63:1817–1824.

662. Mayer B, Zolnai A, Frenyo LV, et al. Redistribution of the sheep Fc receptor in the mammary gland around the time of parturition in ewes and its localization in the small intestine of neonatal lambs. Immunology 2002;107:288–296.

663. Martin MG, Wu SV, Walsh JH. Ontogenic development and distribution of antibody transport and Fc receptor expression in rat intestine. Dig Dis Sci 1997;42:1062–1069.

664. Beryman M, Rodewald R. Beta 2-microglobulin codistributes with the heavy chain of the intestinal IgG-Fc receptor throughout the transepithelial transport pathway of the neonatal rat. J Cell Sci 1995;108:2347–2360.

665. Ghetie V, Hubbard JG, Kim JK, et al. Abnormally short serum half-lives of IgG in beta 2-microglobulin-deficient mice Eur J Immunol 1996;26:690–699.

666. Malanchere E, Huetz F, Couthino A. Maternal IgG stimulates B lineage cell development in the progeny. Eur Immunol J 1997;27:788–793.

667. Delassus S, Darche S, Kourilsky P, et al. Maternal immunoglobulins have no effect on the rate of maturation of the B cell compartment of the offspring. Eur J Immunol 1997;27:1737–1742.

668. Martin D, Rioux S, Gagnon E, et al. Protection from Group B Streptoccocal infection in neonatal mice by maternal immunization with recombinant Sip protein. Infect Immun 2002;70:4897–4901.

669. Offit PA, Clark HF. Maternal antibody-mediated protection against gastroenteritis duc to rotavirus in newborn mice is dependent on both serotype and titer of antibody. J Inf Dis 1985;152:1152–1158.

670. Reuman PD, Paganini MA, Ayoub EM, et al. Maternal-infant transfer of influenza-specific immunity in the mouse. J Immunol 1983;130:932–936.

671. Sweet C, Bird RA, Jakeman K, et al. Production of passive immunity in neonatal ferrets following maternal vaccination with killed influenza A virus vaccine. Immunology 1987;60:83–89.

672. Husseini RH, Sweet C, Overton H, et al. Role of maternal immunity in the protection of newborn ferrets against infection with a virulent influenza virus. Immunology 1984;5:389–394.

673. Sweet C, Jakeman KJ, Smith H. Role of milk-derived IgG in passive maternal protection of neonatal ferrets against influenza. J Gen Virol 1987;68:2681–2686.

674. Jakeman KJ, Smith H, Sweet C. Mechanism of immunity to influenza:maternal and passive neonatal protection following immunization of adult ferrets with a live Vaccinia-influenza virus hemagglutinin recombinant but not with recombinants containing other influenza virus proteins. J Gen Virol 1989;70:1523–1531.

675. Perryman LE, Kapil SJ, Jones ML, et al. Protection of calves against Cryptosporidium with bovine colostrum induced with a Criptosporidium parvum recombinant protein. Vaccine 1999;17:2142–2149.

676. Barman NN, Sarma DK. Passive immunization of piglets against entertoxinogenic colibacilosis by vaccinating dams with K88a pili bearing bacterins. Indian J Exp Biol 1999;37:1132–1135.

677. Barrandeguy M, Parreno V, Lagos Marmol M, et al. Prevention of rotavirus diarrhoea in foals by parenteral vaccination of marres: field trial. Dev Biol Stand 1998;92:253–257.

678. Englund JA, Mbawiuike IN, Hammil H, et al. Maternal immunization with influenza or tetanus toxoid vaccine for passive antibody protection in young infants. J Infect Disease 1993;168:647–656.

679. Glezen WP, Alper M. Maternal immunization. Clin Inf Dis 1999;28:219–224.

680. Cunningaham AS. Morbidity in breast-fed and artificially fed infants. J Ped 1977;90:7226–7229.

681. Englund JA, Glezezn WP, Turner C, et al. Transplacental antibody transfer following maternal immunization with polysaccharide and conjugate Hemophilus influenzae type b vaccine. J Inf Dis 1995;171:99–105.

682. Amstey MS, Insel R, Munoz J, et al. Fetal-neonatal passive immunization against Hemophilus influenzae type b. Am J Obstet Gynecol 1985;153:607–611.

683. Riley ID, Douglas RM. An epidemiological approach to pneumococcal disease. Rev Inf Dis 1981;3:233–245.

684. Englund JA. Passive protection against respiratory syncitial virus disease in infants: the role of maternal antibody. Pediatr Infect Dis J 1994;13:449–453.

685. Rossi P, Moschese V, Broliden PA, et al. Presence of maternal antibodies to human immunodeficiency virus 1 envelope glycopreoton gp120 epitopes correlates with uninfected ststus of children born to seropositive mothers. Proc Natl Acad Sci USA 1989;86:8055–8058.

686. Ugen KE, Srikantan V, Goedert JJ, et al. Vertical transmission human immunodeficiency virus 1 envelope glycopreotein gp120 epitopes: seroreactivity by maternal antibody to carboxy region of gp41 envelope glycoprotein. J Inf Dis 1997;175:63–69.

687. Palasanthiran P, Robertson P, Ziegler JB, et al. Decay of transplacental human immunodeficiency virus 1 antibodies in neonates and infants. J Inf Dis 1994;170:1593–1596.

688. Boppana SB, Miller J, Britt WJ. Transplacental acquired antiviral antibodies and outcome in congenital human cytomegalovirus infection. Viral Immunol 1996;9:211–218.

689. Chatterjee A, Harrison CJ, Britt WJ, et al. Modification of maternal and congenital cytomegalovirus infection by anti-glycoprotein B antibody transfer in guines pigs. J Inf Dis 2001;183:1546–1553.

690. Osborn JJ, Dancis J, Julia JF. Studies of the immunology of the newborn infant. II. Interference with active immunization by passive transplacental circulating antibody. Pediatrics 1952;10:328–334.

691. Uhr JW, Moller G. Regulatory effect of antibody on the immune response. Adv Immunol 1968;8:81–127.

692. Cerottini J-C, McCoanet PJ, Dixon FJ. Specificity of the immunosuppression caused by passive administration of antibody. J Immunol 1969;103:268–275.

693. Song CH, Calandra GB, Palmer CJ, et al. Inhibition of offspring response to HEL-CFA administation of anti-HEL MAB to the mother is not related to the predominant idiotype IdXE or specificity of the mAB. Cell Immunol 1990;131:311–324.

694. Siegrist CA, Cordiva M, Brandt C, et al. Determinants of infant response to vaccines in persenece of maternal antibodies. Vaccine 1998;16:1409–1414.

695. Xiang ZQ, Ertl HCJ. Transfer of maternal antibody results in inhibition of specific immune responses in the offspring. Virus Res 1992;24:297–314.

696. Englund JA, Anderson EL, Reed G. The effect of maternal antibody on the serologic response and the incidence of adverse reactions after primary immunization with accelular and whole-cell pertussis vaccine combine with diphtheria and tetanus toxoids. Pediatrics 1995;96:580–584.

697. Manickan E, Yu Z, Rouse BT. DNA immunization of neonates induces immunity despite the presence of maternal antibody. J Clin Invest 1997;100:2371–2375.

698. Van Druen Little-van Den Hurtk S, Braun RP, Lewis PJ, et al. Immunization of neonates with DNA encoding a bovine Herpes glycoprotein is effective in the presence of maternal antibodies. Viral Immunol 1999;12:67–77.

699. Premenko-Lanier M, Rota PA, Rhodes G, et al. DNA vaccination of infants in the presence of maternal antibody: a measles model in the primate. Virology 2003;307:67–75.

700. Siegrist C-A, Barrios C, Martinez X, et al. Influence of maternal antibodies on vaccine responses: inhibition of antibody but not T cell responses allows successful early prime-boost strategies in mice. Eur J Immunol 1998;28:4138–4148.

701. Pertmer TM, Oran AE, Moser JM, et al. DNA vaccines for influenza virus: differential effects of maternal antibody on immune response to hemagglutinin and nucleoprotein. J Virol 2000;54:7787–7793.

702. Radu DL, Antohi S, Bot A, et al. Effect of maternal antibodies on influenza virus-specific immune response elicited by inactivated virus and naked DNA. Scand J Immunol 2001;53:475–482.

703. Hassett DE, Zhang J, Whitton JL. Neonatal DNA immunization with plasmid encoding an internal viral protein is effective in the presence of maternal antibodies and protects against subsequent viral challenge. J Virol 1997;71:7881–7888.

704. Cazenave P-A. Immunoglobulin allotype. In: Lymphocytic Regulation by Antibodies. (Bona C Cazenave P-A, eds.), John Wiley & Sons. New York: 1981, pp. 109–138.

705. Dray S. Effect of amternal isoantibodies on the quantitative expression of two allelic genes controlling γ-globulin specificities. Nature 1962;195:677–679.

706. Lowe JA, Cross LM, Catty D. Humoral and cellular aspects of immunoglobulin suppression in rabbit. III Production of anti-allotypic antibodies by suppressed animals. Immunology 1975;28:469–476.

707. Sell S. Studies on rabbit lymphocyes in vitro. IX. The suppression of anti-allotype-induced blast transformation in lymphocyte cultures from allotypically suppressed donors. J Exp Med 1968;128:341–352.

708. Harrison MR, Mage RG, Davie JN. Deletion of b5 immunoglobulin bearing lymphocytes in allotype suppressed rabbits. J Exp Med 1973;137:254–266.

709. Harrison MR, Mage RG. Allotype suppression. I. The ontogeny of cells bearing paternal immunoglobulin allotype in neonatal rabbits and the fate of these cells during induction of allotype suppression by anti-allotype antisera. J Exp Med 1973;138:764–772.

710. Bona C, Cazenave P-A. Release from maternal-induced allotypic suppression in rabbit by Nocardia water-soluble mitogen. J Exp Med 1977;146:881–886.

711. Majelessi L, Marcos M-A, Benaroch P, et al. T cell-induced Ig allotypic suppression in mice. J Immunol 1994;152:3342–3352.

712. Cosenza H, Kohler H. Specific suppression of the antibody response by antibodies to receptors. Proc Natl Acad Sci 1972;69:2701–2705.

713. Bona C, Stein KE, Liberman R, et al. Direct and indirect suppression induced by anti-idiotype antibody in inulin-bacterial levan antigenic system. Mol Immunol 1979;16:1093–1101.

714. Weiler IJ, Weler E, Sprenger R, et al. Idiotype suppression by maternal influence. Eur J Immunol 1977;7:591–597.

715. Victor-Kobrin C, Bona C, Pernis B. Expansion of idiotype positive B cells in maternally suppressed mice. J Mol Cell Immunol 1984;1:331–343.
716. WiklerM, Demeur C, Dewasme G, et al. Immunoregulatory role of maternal idiotypes. Ontogeny of immune networks. J Exp Med 1980;152:1024–1035.
717. Rubinstein LJ, Victor-Kobrin CB, Bona CA. The function of idiotypes on the development of the immune repertoire. Dev Comp Immunol 1984;suppl 2:109–116.
718. Rubinstein LJ, Ming Y, Bona CA. Idiotype-anti-idiotype network. II Activation of silent clones by treatment at birth with idiotypes is associated with the expansion of idiotype-specific helper T cells. J Exp Med 1982;156:506–521.
719. Lemke H, Lange H, Berek C. Maternal immunization modulates the primary immune response to 2-phenyl-oxazolone in Balb/c mice. Eur J Immunol 1994;24:3025–3030.
720. Dighiero G, Lymberi P, Mazie J, et al. Murine hybridomas secreting natural antibodies reacting with self-epitopes. J Immunol 1983;131:2267–2272.
721. Casali P, Prabhakar S, Notkins AL. Characterization of multireactive autoantibodies and identificatiom of LEU-1 B lymphocytes as cells making antibodies binding multiple self and exogenous molecules. Int Rev Immunol 1998;3;17–47.
722. Hayakawa K, Hardy RR, Honda M, et al. Ly-1 B cells: functionally distinct lymphocytes that secrete IgM autoantibodies. Proc Natl Acad Sci USA 1984;81:2494–2498.
723. Schwartz RS. Polyvalent anti-DNA antibodies: immunochemical and biological significance. Int Rev Immunol 1998;3:97–117.
724. Davies T, Kendler DL, Martin A. Immunological mechanisms in Graves' disease. In: The Molecular Pathology of Autoimmune Diseases. (Theophilopoulos A, and Bona C, eds.), Taylor and Francis. New York, London: 2002, pp. 649–684.
725. Mariotti S, Caturegli P, Piccolo P, et al. Antithyroglobulin antibodies in thyroid diseases. J Clin Endocrinol Metab 1990;71:661–669.
726. Witebsky E, Rose NR, Terplan K, et al. Chronic thyroiditis and autoimmunization. J Amer Med Assoc 1957;164:1439–1447.
727. Bona CA. Postulates defining pathogenic autoantibodies and T cells. Autoimmunity 1991;10:162–172.
728. Rose NR, Bona C. Defining criteria for autoimmune diseases (Witebsky's postulates revisited). Immunol Today 1993;14:426–410.
729. Wang HB, Li HE, Bakhei M, et al. The role of B cells in experimental myasthenia gravis in mice. Biomed Pharmacother 1999;53:227–233.
730. Papazian O. Transient neonatal myasthenia gravis. J Clin Neurol 1992;7:135–141.
731. Gardenerova M, Eymard B, Morel E, et al. The fetal/adult acetylcholine antibodies ratio into mothers with myasthenia gravis as marker for transfer of disease to the newborn. Neurology 1997;48:50–54.
732. Brenner T, Shahin R, Steiner I, et al. Presence of anti-acetylcholine receptor antibodies in human milk: possible correlation with neonatal myasthenia gravis. Autoimmunity 1992;12:315–316.
733. Bartoccioni E, Evoli A, Casali C, et al. Neonatal myasthenia gravis: clinical and immunological study of seven mothers and their newborn infants. J Neuroimmunol 1986;12:155–161.

734. Arizono N, Yonezawa T, Yamaguchi K, et al. Transplacental transmission of experimental autoimmune myasthenia gravis. A morphological study. Acta Pathol Jpn 1983;33:507–513.
735. Vincent A, Newland C, Brueton L, et al. Arthrogryposis multiplex congenita with maternal autoantibodies specific for fetal antigen. Lancet 1995;346:24–25.
736. Baum H, Berg, PA. The complex nature of mitochondrial antibodies and their relation to primary biliary cirrhosis. Semin Liver Dis1981;1:309–320.
737. Coppel RL, Gershwin ME. Primary biliary cirrhosis: the molecule and the mimic. Immunol Rev 1995;144:17–49.
738. Hannam S, Bogdanos D-P, Davies E, et al. Neonatal liver disease associated with placental transfer of anti-mitochondrial antibodies. Autoimmunity 2002;35:545–550.
739. Zakarija M, McKenzie JM, Eidson MS. Transient neonatal hypothyroidism: characterization of maternal antibodies to the thyrotropin receptor. J Clin Endocrinol Metab 1990;70:1239–1246.
740. Smith C, Thomsett M, Choong C, et al. Congenital thyrotoxicosis in premature infants. Clin Endocrinol 2001;54:371–376.
741. Seetharamaiah GS, Wagle NM, Morris JC, et al. Generation and characterization of monoclonal antibodies to block thyrotropin receptor. Endocrinology 1995;136:2817–2824.
742. Adams DD, Fastier FN, Howie JB, et al. Stimulation of the human thyroid by infusions of plasma containing LATS protector J Clin Endocr Metab 1974;39:826–832.
743. Hojo M, Momotani N, Ikeda N, et al.T Prolonged suppresed thyroid-stimulating hormone levels in hyperthyroidism in a newborn to a mother with Graves' disease. Acta Pediatr Jpn 1998;40:483–485.
744. Fors P, Lifshitz F, Pugliese M, et al. Neonatal thyroiod disease: differential expression in three succesive offspring J Clin Endocrin Metab 1988;66:647–647.
745. Borras Perez MV, Moreno-Perez D, Zusanabar-Cotro A, et al. Neonatal hyperthyroidism in infants of mothers previously thyroidectomized due to Graves' disease. J Pediatr Endocrinol Metab 2001;14:1169–1172.
746. Nicase C, Gire C, Bremond V, et al. Neonatal hyperthyroidism in a premature infant born to a mother with Graves's disease. Arch Pediatr 2000;7:505–508.
747. Zimmerman D. Fetal and neonatal hyperthyiroidism. Thyroid 1999;9:727–723.
748. Peleg D, Cada S, Peleg A, et al. The relationship between maternal serum thyroid-stimulating immunoglobulin and fetal and neonatal thyrotoxicosis. Obstet Gynecol 2002;99:1040–1043.
749. Kohn LD, Suzuki K, Hoffman WH, et al. Characterization of monoclonal thyroid-stimulating and thyrotropin binding-inhibiting autoantibodies from a Hashimoto's patient whose children had intra uterine and neonatal thyroid. J Clin Endocrinol Metab 1977;8:3998–4001.
750. Harington WJ, Sprague CC, Minich V, et al. Immnologic mechanisms in neonatal thrombocytopenic purpura. Ann Intern Med 1953;38;433–469.
751. Kunicki TJ, Plow EF, Kekomaki F. Human monoclonal antibody 2E7 is specific for a peptide sequence of platelet glycoprotein IIb. Localization of the epitope to IIb231-238 with an immunodominant Trp235. J Autoimmun 1991;4:415–431.

752. Nugent DJ, Kijiniki TJ, Berglund C, et al. A human monoclonal antibody recognizes a neoantigen on glycoprotein IIIa expressed on stored and activated platelets. Blood 1987;70:16–22.
753. Van Leeuwen EF, van der Ven JTM, Engelfriet CP, et al. Specificity of autoantibodies in autoimmune thrombocytopenia. Blood 1982;59:23–26.
754. Uhrynowska M, Niznikowska-Marks M, Zupanska B. Neonatal and maternal trombocytopenia; incidence and immune background. Eur J Haematol 2000;64:42–46.
755. Williamson LM, Hackett G, Rennie J. The natural history of feto-maternal alloimmunization to platelet-specific antigen HPA1a as determined by antenatal screening. Blood 1998;68;2280–2287.
756. Schiltz JR, Michel B. Production of achantolysis in normal skin in vitro by the IgG fraction from pemphigus vulgaris serum. J Invest Dermatol 1976;67:254–260.
757. Fitzpatrick RE, Newcomer VD. The correlation of disease activity and antibody titer in pemphigus. Arch Dermatol 1980;116:282–290.
758. Lin MS, Artega LA, Warren SJP, et al. Pemphigus. In: Molecular Pathology of Autoimmune Disease. (Theophilopoulos AN, Bona CA, eds.), Taylor and Francis. New York, London: 2002, pp. 799–816.
759. Merlob P, Metzker A, Hazaz B, et al. Neonatal pemphigus vulgaris. Pediatrics 1986;78:1102–1105.
760. Avalos-Diaz E, Olague-Marchan L, Lopez Swiderski A, et al. Transplacental passage of maternal pemphigus foliaceus antibodies induces neonatal pemphigus. J Am Acad Dermatol 2000;43:1130–1134.
761. McCuistion CH, Schoch EP. Possible discoid lupus erythematosus in newborn infant. Arch Dermatol 1954;70:782–785.
762. Lee LA. Neonatal lupus erythematosus J Invest Dermatol 1993;100:9S–13S.
763. Miyagawa S, Fukamoto T, Hashimoto K, et al. Maternal autoimmune response to recombinant Ro/SSA and LA/SSB proteins in Japanese neonatal lupus erythematosus. Autoimmunity 1995;21:277–282.
764. Campos S, Campos-Carvalho AC. Neonatal lupus syndrome: the heart as a target of immune system. An Acad Bras Cienc 2000;72:83–89.
765. Eronen M, Siren MK, Ekblad H, et al. Short- and long-term outcome of children with congenital heart diagnosed as newborn. Pediatrics 2000;106:86–91.
766. Buyon JP, Slade SG, Reveille JD, et al. Autoantibody response to native 52kD SSA/Ro protein in neonatal lupus syndrome, systemic lupus erythematosus and Sjogren's syndrome. J Immunol 1994,152:3675–3684.
767. Miyagawa S, Yanagi K, Yoshioka A, et al. Neonatal lupus erythematosus: maternal antibodies bind to a recombinant NH2-terminal fusion protein encoded by human alpha-fodrin cDNA. J Invest Dermatol 1998;111:1189–1192.
768. Provost TT, Watson R, Gammon WR, et al. The neonatal lupus syndrome associated with UIRNP (nRNP) antibodies. N Engl J Med 1987;316:1135–1138.
769. Miyagawa S, Shinohara K, Kidoguchi K-I, et al. Neonatal lupus erythematosous: studies on HLA class II genes and autoantibody profiles in Japanese mothers. Autoimunity 1997;29:95–101.
770. Niedl LE, Silverman ED, Glenn PT, et al. Maternal anti-Ro and anti-La antibody-associated endocardial fibroelastosis. Circulation 2002;105:843–848.

771. Bouutjdir M, Chen L, Zang ZH, et al. Serum and IgG from the mother of a child with congenital heart block induce abnormalities and inhibit L-type calcium channels in a rat heart model. Pediatr Res 1998;80:354–362.
772. Buyon JP, Clancy RM. Neonatal lupus: review of proposed pathogensis and clinical data from the US-based research registery for neonatal lupus. Autoimmunity 2003;36:41–50.
773. Clancy RM, Askanaase AD, Kapur RP, et al. Transdifferantiation of cardiac fibroblsts, a fetal factor in anti-SSA/RO-SSB/LA antibody-mediated congenital heart block. J Immunol 2002;169:2156–2163.
774. Miranda-Carus ME, Askanaase AD, Clancy RM, et al. Anti-SSA/Ro and anti-SSB/La autoantibodies bind the surface of apoptotic fetal cardiocytes and promote secretion of TNF-α by macrophages. J Immunol 2000;165:5345–5351.
775. Mexkler KA, Kapur RP. Congenital heart block and associated cardiac pathology in neonatal lupus syndrome. Pediatr Dev Pathol 1998;58:291–303.
776. Maheshwari A, Christensen RD, Calhoun DA. Immune-mediated neutropenia in the neonate. Acta Paediatr 2002;suppl 438:98–103.
777. Nakamura K, Kobayashi M, Konishi N, et al. Defect of granulopoiesis in patients with severe congenital neutrpoenia. Hiroshima J Med Sci2002;51:63–74.
778. Hartman KR, LaRussa VF, Rothwell SW, et al. Antibodies to myeloid precursor cells in autoimmune neutropenia. Blood 1994;84:625–631.
779. LaBarbera AR, Miller MM, Ober C, et al. Autoimmune etiology in premature ovarian failure. Amer J Reprod Immunol Microbiol 1988;16:115–126.
780. Setiady YY, Samy ET, Tung KSK. Maternal autoantibodies triggers de novo T-cell mediated neonatal autoimmune disease. J Immunol 2003;170:4656–4664.
781. Atma S, Greely W, Katsumata M, et al. Elimination of maternally transmitted autoantibodies prevents diabetes in nonobese diabetic mice. Nat Med 2002;8:399–402.
782. McKeever U, Khandekar S, Jesson M, et al. Maternal immunization with soluble TCR-Ig chimeric protein: long-term, V-8 family-specific suppression of T cells by maternally transferred antibodies. J Immunol 1997;159:5936–5945.
783. Turka LA, Schatz DG, Oettinger MA, et al. Thymocytes expression of RAG1 and RAG2: termination by T cell receptor crosslinking. Science 1991;257:778–781.
784. Weiss A. T cell antigen receptor signal transduction: a tail of tails and cytoplasmatic protein-tyrosine kinases. Cell 1993;73:209–212.
785. Weiss A, Littman DR. Signal transduction by lympocyte antigen receptors. Cell 1994;76:263–274.
786. Samelson LE, Patel MD, Weissman AM, et al. Antigen activation of murine T cells induces tyrosine phosphorylation of a polypeptide associated with the antigen receptor. Cell 1986;46:1083–1090.
787. Reth M. Antigen receptor tail clue. Nature 1989;338:383.
788. Qian D, Griswold-Prenner I, Rosner MR, et al. Multiple components of the T cell antigen receptor complex become phosphorylated upon activation. J Biol.Chem. 1993;268:4488–4493.
789. Weiss A. The CD3 chains of the T cell antigen receptor associate with the ZAP-70 tyrosine kinase and are tyrosine phosphorylated after receptor stimulation. J Exp Med 1993;178:1523–1530.

790. Ardouin L, Boyer C, Gillet A, et al. Crippling of CD3-zeta ITAMs does not impair T cell receptor signaling. Immunity 1999;4:409–420.
791. Burkhardt AL, Stealey B, Rowley RB, et al.Temporal regulation of non-transmembrane protein tyrosine kinase enzyme activity following T cell antigen receptor engagement. J Biol Chem 1994;269:23,642–23,,647.
792. Iwashima M, Irving BA, van Oers NSC, et al. Sequential interactions of the TCR with two distinct cytoplasmatic tyrosine kinases. Science 1994;263:1136–1139.
793. Kersh EN, Shaw AS, Allen PM. Fidelity of T cell activation trough multistep T cell receptor phosphorylation. Science 1996;287:572–575.
794. Romeo C, Amiot T, Seed B. Sequence requirements for induction of cytolysis by the T cell antigen/Fc receptor ζ-chain. Cell 1992;68:889–897.
795. Zenner G, Vorherr T, Mustelin T, et al. Differential and multiple binding of signal transducing molecules to the ITAMs of the TCR-zeta chain. J Cell Biochem 1996;63:94–103.
796. Veillette A, Bookman MA, Horak EM, et al. The CD4 and CD8 T cell surface antigens are associated with the internal membrane tyrosine-proteine kinase p56lck. Cell 1998;55:301–308.
797. Barber EK, DasGupta JD, Schlossman SF, et al. The CD4 and CD8 antigens are couple to a protein-tyrosine kinase (p56lck) that phosphorylates the CD3 complex. Proc Natl Acad Sci USA. 1989;86:3277–3281.
798. Veillette A, Bookman MA, Horak EM, et al. Signal transduction through the CD4 receptor involves the activation of the internal membrane tyrosine-protein kinase p56lck. Nature 1989;338:257–259.
799. Luo K, Sefton BM. Cross-linking of the T-cell surface molecules CD4 and CD8 stimulates phosphorylation of the lck tyrosine protein kinase at the autophosphorylation site. Mol Cell Biol 1990;10:5305–5313.
800. Watts JDM, Sanghera JS, Pelech SL, et al. Phosphorylation of serine 59 of p56lck in activated T cells. J Biol Chem 1993;258:23275–2328.
801. Marth JD, Peet R, Krebs EG, et al. A lymphocyte-specific protein tyrosine kinase gene is rearranged and overexpressed in the murine T cell lymphoma LSTRA. Cell 1985;43:393–404.
802. Veillette A, Foss FM, Sausville EA, et al. Expression of the lck tyrosine kinase gene in human colon carcinoma and other non-lymphoid human tumor cell lines. Oncogene Res 1987;1:357–374.
803. Strauss DB, Weiss A. Genetic evidence for the involvement of the lck tyrosine kinase in signal transduction through the T cell antigen receptor. Cell 1992;70;585–593.
804. Karnitz L, Sutor SL, Torigoe T, et al. Effects of p56lck defficiency on the growth and cytolytic effector function of an interleukin-2-dependent cytotoxic T-cell line. Mol Cell Biol 1992;10:4521–4530.
805. Molina TJ, Kishihara K, Siderovski DP, et al. Profound block in thymocyte development in mice lacking p56lck. Nature 1992;357:161–165.
806. Weil E, Veillette A. Signal transduction by the lymphocyte-specific tyrosine protein kinase p56lck. Curr Topics Microbiol Immunol 1996;205:63–87.
807. Margolis B, Hu P, Katzav S, et al. Tyrosine phosphorylation of vav proto-oncogene product containing SH2 domain and transcription factor motifs. Nature 1992;356:71–74.

808. Donovan JA, Wange RL, Langton WA, et al. The protein product of the c-Cbl oncogene is the 120 kDa tyrosine phosphorylated protein in Jurkat cells activated via the T cell receptor. J Biol Chem 1994;269:22,921–22,924.

809. Ravichandran K, Lee KK, Songyang Z, et al. Interaction of Shc with zeta chain of the T cell receptor upon T cell activation. Science 1993;262:902–905.

810. Bruyns E, Marie-Cardine A, Kirchgessner H, et al. T cell receptor (TCR) interactim molecule (TRIM), a novel disulfide-linked dimer associated with the TCR-CD3-ζ complex, recruits intracellular signaling proteins to the plasma membrane. J Exp Med 1998;188:561–575.

811. Jackman JK, Motto DG, Sun Q, et al. Molecular cloning of SLP-76, a 76-kDa tyrosine phosphoprotein associated with Grb-2 in T cells. J Biol Chem 1995;270:7079–7032.

812. Wu J, Motto DG, Koretzky GA, et al. Vav and Slp-76 interact and functionally cooperate in IL-2 gene activation. Immunity 1996;4:593–602.

813. Raab M, da Silava AJ, Findell PR, et al. Regulation of Vav-SLP-76 binding by ZAP-70 and its relevance to TCR. Immunity 1997;6:155–164.

814. Prasad KVS, Kapeller R, Janssen O, et al. Phosphatidylinositol (PI) 3-kinase and PI 4-kinase binding to the CD4-p56(lck) complex:the p56(lck) SH3 domain binds to PI 3-kinase but not PI 4-kinase. Mol Cell Biol 1993;13:7708–7717.

815. Kapeller R, Prasad KVS, Janssen O, et al. Identification of two SH3-binding motifs in the regulatory subunit of phosphatidylinositol 3-kinase. J Biol Chem 1994;269:1927–1933.

816. Osman N, Lucas S, Turner SH, et al. A comparison of the interaction of Shc and tyrosine kinase ZAP-70 with the T cell antigen receptor z chain tyrosine-based activation motif. J Biol Chem 1995;270:13981–13986.

817. Zenner G, Vorherr T, Mustelin T, et al. Differential and multiple binding of signal transducing molecules to the ITAMs of TCR-ζ chain. J Cell Biochem 1996;63:94–103.

818. Zhang W, Sloan-Lancester J, Kitchen J, et al. LAT: the ZAP–70 tyrosine kinase substrate that links T cell receptor to cellular activation. Cell 1998;92:83–92.

819. Ward SG, Ley SC, Macphee C, et al. Regulation of D-3 phosphoinositides during T cell activation via the T cell antigen receptor/CD3 complex and CD2 antigen Eur J Immunol 1992;22:45–49.

820. Reif K, Gout I, Waterfield MD, et al. Divergent regulation of phoaphatidylinositol 3-kinase p85-alpha and p85-beta isoforms upon T cell activation. J Biol Chem 1993;268:10,780–10,788.

821. Osman N, Levy SC, Crumpton MJ. Evidence for an association between the T cell receptor/CD3 complex and the CD5 antigen in human T lymphocytes. Eur J Immunol 1992 22:2995–3000.

822. Egerton M, Burgess WH, Chen D, et al. Identification of ezrin as an 81-kDa tyrosine-phosphorylated protein in T cells. J Immunol 1992;149:1847–1852.

823. Egerton M, Ashe OR, Chen D, et al. VCP, the mammalian homolog of cdc48, is tyrosine phosphorylated in response to T cell antigen receptor activation. EMBO J 1992;11:3533–3540.

824. Finco TS, Kadlecek T, Zhang W, et al. LAT is required for TCR-mediated activation of PLCgamma1 and the Ras pathway. Immunity 1998;5:617–626.

825. Cantrell D. T cell antigen receptor signal transduction pathways. Annu Rev Immunol 1996;14:259–274.

826. McCormick F. Signal transduction-how receptors turns ras on. Nature 1993;363:15–16.

827. Osman N, Lucas S, Turner SH, et al. A comparison of the interaction of Shc and tyrosine kinase ZAP-70 with the T cell antigen receptor z chain tyrosine-based activation motif. J Biol Chem 1995, 270:13,981–13,986.

828. Sawasdikosol S, Ravichandran K, Lee K, et al. Crk interacts with tyrosine-phosphorylated p116 upon T cell activation. J Biol Chem. 1995;270:2893–2896.

829. Gulbins E, Coggeshall KM, Gottfried B, et al. Tyrosine kinase stimulated guanidine nucleotide exchange activity of Vav in T cell activation. Science 1993;260:822–825.

830. Bustelo XR, Suen KL, Leftheris K, et al. Vav cooperates with Ras to transform rodent fibroblasts but is not a Ras GDP/GTP exchange factor. Oncogene 1994;9:2405–2413.

831. Tarakhovski A, Turner M, Schaal S, et al. Defective antigen receptor mediated proliferation of B- and T-cells in the absence of Vav. Nature 1995;374:467–470.

832. Cooper JA. Straight and narrow or tortuous and intersecting? Curr Biol 1994;4:1118–1121.

833. Zhang X-F, Settleman J, Kyriakis JM, et al. Normal and oncogenic p21ras proteins bind to the amino-terminal regulatory domain of Raf-1. Nature 1993;364:308–313.

834. Izquierdo M, Leevers SJ, Williams DH, et al. A p21ras couples the T cell antigen receptor to extracellular signal regulated kinase in T cells. J Exp Med 1993;178:1199–1207.

835. Marshall CJ. MAP kinase kinase kinase, MAP kinase kinase and MAP kinase. Curr Opin Genet Dev 1994;4:82–89.

836. Boussiotis VA, Freeman GJ, Berezovskaya A, et al. Maintenance of human T cell anergy:blocking of IL-2 gene transcription by activated Rap1. Science 1997;278:124–128.

837. Marais R, Wynne J, Treisman R. The SRF accessory protein Elk-1 contains a growth factor-regulated transcriptional activation domain. Cell 1993;173:381–393.

838. Nunes J, Collette Y, Truneh A, et al. The role of p21ras in CD28 signal transduction: triggering of CD28 with antibodies but not the ligand B7-1 activates p21ras. J Exp Med. 1994;180:1067–1076.

839. Weiss A, Imboden JB. Cell surface molecules and early events involved in human T lymphocyte activation. Adv Immunol 1987;41:1–38.

840. Lewis RS, Cahalan MD. Potasium and calcium channels in lymphocytes. Annu Rev Immunol 1995;13:623–653.

841. Loh C, Shaw KT, Carew J, et al. Calcineurin binds the transcription factor NFAT1 and reversibly regulates its activity. J Biol Chem 1996;271:10,884–10,891.

842. Shaw KT, Ho AM, Raghavan A, et al. Immunosuppressive drugs prevent a rapid dephosphorylation of transcription factor NFAT1 in stimulated immune cells. Proc Natl Acad Sci USA 92:1995;11,205–11,209.

843. Rao A, Luo C, Hogan PG. Transcription factors of the NFAT family: regulation an function. Annu Rev Immunol 1997;15:707–747.

844. Jain J, Loh C, Rao A. Transcriptional regulation of the IL-2 gene. Curr Opin Immunol 1995;7:333–342.

845. Karin M, Liu Z, Zandi E. AP-1 function and regulation. Curr Opin Cell Biol 1997;9:240–246.

846. Weiss A, Imboden J, Shoback D, et al. Role of T3 surface molecules in human T cell activation: T3-dependent activation results in an increase in cytoplasmatic free calcium. Proc Natl Acad Sci USA 1984;81:4169–4173.

847. Gajewski TF, Lancki DW, Stack R, et al. Anergy of Th0 helper T lymphocytes induces downregulation of Th1 characteristics and a transition to a Th2-like phenotype. J Exp Med 1994;179:481–491.

848. Gajewski TF, Pinnas M, Wong T, et al. Murine Th1 and Th2 clones proliferate optimally in response to distinct antigen presenting cell populations. J Immunol 1991;146:1750–1758.

849. Genot MEP, Parker J, Cantrell DA. Analysis of the role of protein kinase C-α, ε, and ζ in T cell activation J Biol Chem 1995;270:9833 9839.

850. Izquierdo M, Reif K, Cantrell DA. The regulation and function of p21ras during T-cell activation and growth. Immunol Today 1995;16:159–64.

851. Kang SM, Beverly B, Tran AC, et al. Transactivation by AP-1 is a molecular target of T cell clonal anergy. Science 1992;257:1134–1138.

852. Carmella W, Mondino A, Mueller DL. Blocked signal transduction to the ERK and JNK protein kynases in anergic CD4+ T cells. Science 1996;271:1272–1275.

853. Kubo M, Kincaid RL, Webb DR, et al. Ca2+/calmodulin-activated, phosphoprotein phosphatase calcineurin is sufficient for positive reulation of the mouse IL-4 gene. Int Immunol 1994;6:179–188.

854. Sloan-Lancester J, Steinberg TH, Allen PM. Selective loss of the calcium ion signaling pathway in T cells maturing toward a T helper type 2 phenotype. J Immunol 1997;159:1160–1168.

855. Casares S, Bona CA, Brumeanu T-D. Engineering and characterization of a murine MHC class II-Immunoglobulin chimera expressing an immunodominant CD4+ T viral epitope. Protein Eng 1997;10:1295–1301.

856. Casares S, Zong CS, Radu DL, et al. Antigen-specfic signaling by a soluble, dimeric peptide/major histocompatibility complex class II/Fc chimera leading to T helper cel type 2 differentiation. J Exp Med 1999;190:543–553

857. Rivas A, Takada S, Koide J, et al. CD4 molecules are associated with antigen receptor complex on activated but not resting T cells. J Immunol 1988;140:2912–2918.

858. Mittler RS, Goldman SJ, Spitalny GL, et al. T-cell receptor-CD4 physical association in a murine T-cell hybridoma:induction by antigen receptor ligation. Proc Natl Acad Sci USA 1989;86:8531–8535.

859. Rojo JM, Saizawa K, Janeway CA, Jr. Physical association of CD4 and the T-cell receptor can be induced by anti-T-cell receptor antibodies. Proc Natl Acad Sci USA 1989;86:3311–3315.

860. Sleckman BP, Peterson A, Jones WK, et al. Expression and function of CD4 in a murine T-cell hybridoma. Nature 1987;328:351–353.
861. Boussiotis VA, Barber DL, Lee BJ, et al. Differential association of protein tyrosine kinases with the T cell receptor is linked to the induction of anergy and its prevention by B7 family-mediated costimulation. J Exp Med 1996;184:365–376.
862. Carrel S, Moretta A, Pantaleo G, et al. Stimulation and proliferation of CD4+ peripheral blood T lymphocytes induced by anti-CD4 monoclonal antibody. Eur J Immunol 1988;18:333–339.
863. Oyaizy N, McCloskey TW, Than S, et al. Cross-linking of CD4 molecules upregulates Fas antigen expression in lymphocytes by inducing interferon-gamma and tumor necrosis factor-alpha secretion. Blood 1994;84:2622–2631.
864. Baldari CT, Milia E, Di SM, et al. Distinct signaling properties indentify functionally different CD4 epitopes. Eur J Immunol 1995;25:1843–1850.
865. Milia E, Di Somma MM, Majolini MB, et al. Gene activating and proapoptotic potential are independent properties of different CD4 epitopes. Mol Immunol 1997 34:287–296.
866. Thuillier L, Hivroz C, Fagard R, et al. Ligation of CD4 surface antigen induces rapid tyrosine phosphorylation of the cytoskeletal protein erzin. Cell Immunol 1994;156:322–331.
867. Baldari CT, Pelicci G, Di Somma MM, et al. Inhibition of CD4/p56lck signaling by a dominant negative mutant of the Shc adaptor protein. Oncogene 1995;10:1141–1147.
868. Anderson P, Blue M-L, Morimoto C, et al. Cross-linking of T3(CD3) with T4(CD4) enhances the proliferation of resting T lymphocytes. J Immunol 1987;139:678–682.
869. Walker C, Bettens F, Pickler WJ. Activation of T cells by cross-linking an anti-CD3 antibody with a second anti-T cell antibody: mechanism and subset-specific activation. Eur J Immunol 1987;17:873–880.
870. Emmrich F, Kanz L, Eichmann K. Crosslinking of the T cell receptor complex with the subset-specific differentiation antigen stimulates interleukin-2 receptor expression in human CD4 and CD8 T cells. Eur J Immunol 1987;17:529–534.
871. Shen X, Hu B, McPhie P, et al. Pepetides corresponding to CD4-interacting regions of murine MHC class II molecules modulate immune responses of CD4+ T lymphocytes in vitro and in vivo. J Immunol 1996;157:87–100.
872. Leitenberg D, Boutin Y, Constant S, et al. CD4 regulation of TCR signaling and T cell differentiation following stimulation with peptides of different affinities for the TCR. J Immunol 1998;161:1194–1203.
873. Fowell DJ, Magram J, Turck CW, et al. Impaired Th2 subset development in the absence of CD4. Immunity 1997;6:559–569.
874. Brown DR, Moskowitz NH, Killen N, et al. A role for CD4 in peripheral T cell differentiation. J Exp Med 1997;186:101–107.
875. Fowell DJ, Magram J, Turck CW, et al. Impaired Th2 subset development in the absence of CD4. Immunity 1997;6:559–569.
876. Briant L, Signoret N, Gaubin M, et al. Transduction of activation signal that follows HIV-1 binding to CD4 and CD4 dimerization involves the immunoglobulin CDR3-like region of domain 1 of CD4. J Biol Chem 1997;272:19,441–19,450.

877. Eichmann K, Jonsson JI, Falk I, et al. Effective activation of mouse T lymphocytes by cross-linking submitogenic concentrations of the T cell antigen receptor with either Lyt-2 or L3T4. Eur J Immunol 1987;17:643–650.

878. Emmrich F, Strittmatter U, Eichmann K. Synergism in the activation of human CD8 T cells by cross-linking the T-cell receptor complex with the CD8 differentiation antigen. Proc Natl Acad Sci USA 1986;83;8298–8302.

879. Lin RS, Rodriguez C, Veillette A, et al. Zinc is essential for binding p56(lck) to CD4 and CD8 alpha. J Biol Chem 1998;273:32,878–32,882.

880. Huse M, Eck MJ, Harrison SC. A Zn^{+2} ion links the cytoplasmatic tail of CD4 and the N-terminal region of Lck. J Biol Chem 1988;273:18,729–18,733.

881. Gross J, Callass E, Alison J. Identification and distribution of the costimulatory receptor CD28 in the mouse. J Immunol 1992;149:380–388.

882. Sharpe AH, Freeman G. The B7-CD28 superfamily. Nature Rev Immunol 2002;2:116–126.

883. Lenschow DJ, Walunes TL, Bluestone JA. CD28-B7 system of T cell costimulation. Annu Rev Immunol 1996;14;233–258.

884. Lanzavecchia A, Lezzi G, Viola A. From TCR engagement to T cell activation:a kinetic view of T cell behaviour. Cell 1999;96:1–4.

885. Durandy A, De Saint Basile G Lisowska-Grospierre B Gauchet JF Foreville M Kozczek RA Bonnefoy JY Fischer A. Undectable CD40 ligand on T cells and low B cell responses to CD40 binding agonists in human newborns. J Immunol 1995;154:1560–1568.

886. Nonoyamma S, Penix LA, Edwards CP, et al. Diminished expression of CD40 ligand by activated neonatal T cells. J Clin Invest 1995;95:66–75.

887. Splawski JB, Nishioka J, Nishioka Y, et al. CD40 ligand is expressed and functional on activated neonatal T cells. J Immunol 1996;156;119–127.

888. Ramsdell F, Seaman MS, Clifford KN, et al. CD40 ligand acts as a costimulatory signal for neonatal thymic gamma delta T cells. J Immunol 1994;152:2190–2197.

889. Wyss DF, Choi JS, Li J, et al. Conformation and function of the N-linked glycan in the adhesion domain of human CD2. Science 1995;269:1273–1278.

890. Haynes BF, Singer KH, Denning SM, et al. Analysis of expression of CD2, CD3, and T cell antigen receptor molecules during early human thymic development. J Immunol 1988;141:3776–3784.

891. Barcena A, Galy AH, Punomen J, et al. Myeloid and lymphoid differentiation of fetal liver CD34$^+$ lineage cells in human thymic organ culture. J Exp Med 1994;180:123–132.

892. Denning SM, Kurtzberg J, Leslie DS, et al. Human postnatal CD4$^-$ CD8$^-$ CD3$^-$ thymic T cell precursors differentiate in vitro into T cell receptor (-bearing cells. J Immunol 1989;142:2988–2997.

893. Galy A, Verma S, Barcena A, et al. Precursors of CD3$^+$ CD4$^+$ CD8$^+$ in the human thymus are defined by expression of CD35. J Exp Med 1993;178:391–401.

894. Ahearn JM, Fearon DT. Structure and function of the complemet receptors CR1(CD35) and CR2 (CD21). Adv Immunol 1989;46:183–203.

895. Thornton CA, Holloway JA, Warner JO. Expresssion of CD21 and CD23 during human T cell development. Pediatr Res 2002;52:245–250.

896. Hurley TR, Hyman R, Sefton BM. Differential effect of expression of the CD45 tyrosine protein phosphatase on the tyrosine phosphorylation of the lck, fyn, and c-src tyrosine protein kinases. Mol Cell Biol 1993;13:1651–1656.

897. Pani G, Fischer K-D, Mlinaric-Rascan I, et al. Signaling capacity of the T cell antigen receptor is negatively regulated by the PTP1C tyrosine phosphatase. J Exp Med 1996;184:839–852.

898. Pingel JT, Thomas ML. Evidence that the leukocyte-common antigen is required for antigen-induced T lymphocyte proliferation. Cell 1989;58:1055–1065.

899. Weaver CT, Pingel JT, Nelson GO, et al. CD8+ T-cell clones deficient in the expression of the CD45 protein tyrosine phosphatase have impaired responses to T-cell receptor stimuli. Mol Cell Biol 1991;11:4415–4422.

900. Koretzky G, Picus J, Schultz T, et al. Tyrosine phosphatase CD45 is required for both T cell antigen receptor and CD2 mediated activation of a protein tyrosine kinase and interleukin 2 production. Proc Natl Acad Sci USA 1991;88:2037–2041.

901. Shiroo M, Goff L, Biffen M, et al. CD45 tyrosine phosphatase-activated p59fyn couples the T cell antigen receptor to pathways of diacylglycerol production, protein kinase C activation and calcium influx. EMBO J 1992;11:4887–4897.

902. Ledbetter JA, Schieven GL, Uckun FM, et al. CD45 cross-linking regulates phospholipase C activation and tyrosine phosphorylation of specific substrates in CD3/Ti-stimulated T cells. J Immunol 1991;146:1577–1583.

903. Shivnan E, Biffen M, Shiroo M, et al. Does co-aggregation of the CD45 and CD3 antigens inhibit T cell antigen receptor complex-mediated activation of phospholipase C and protein kinase C? Eur J Immunol 1992;22:1055–1062.

904. Ostergaard HL, Trowbridge IS. Coclustering CD45 with CD4 or CD8 alters the phosphorylation and kinase activity of p56lck. J Exp Med 1990;172:347–350.

905. Jackman JK, Motto DG, Sun Q, et al. Molecular cloning of SLP-76, a 76-kDa tyrosine phosphoprotein associated with Grb-2 in T cells. J Biol Chem 1995;270:7079–7032.

906. Bergman M, Mustelin T, Ockten C, et al. The human p50csk tyrosine kinase phosphorylates p56lck at Tyr-505 and down regulates its catalytic activity. EMBO J 1992;11:2919–2924.

907. Sondhi D, Xu W, Songyang Z, et al. Peptide and protein phosphorylation by protein tyrosine kinase Csk: insights into specificity and mechanism. Biochemistry 1998;37:165–172.

908. Lind EF, Prockop SE, Poritt HE, et al. Mapping precursor movement through the postnatal thymus reveals specific microenvironments supporting defined stages of development. J Exp Med 2001;194:127–134.

909. Oerry SS, Pierce JL, Slayton WB, et al. Characterization of thymic progenitors in adult mouse bone marrow. J Immunol 2003;170:1877–1886.

910. Wilson A, Capone M, McDonald HR. Unexpectedly late expression of intracellular CD3(and TCR γ/δ proteins during T cell development. Int Immunol 1999;11:1641–1650.

911. Feheling HJ, von Boehmer H, Earlt AB. T cell development on the thymus of normal and genetically altered mice. Curr Opin Immunol 1997;9:263–275.

912. Renno T, Wilson AQ, Dunkel C, et al. A role for CD147 in thymic development. J Immunol 2002;168:4946–4950.

913. Scollay R, Godfrey DI. Thymic emigration: conveyor belts or lucky dips? Immunol Today 1995;16:268–274.

914. Anderson G, Hare KJ, Jenikson EJ. Positive selection of thymocytes: the long and widing road. Immunol Today 1999;20:463–468.

915. Starr TK, Jameson SC, Hogquist KA. Positive and negative selection of T cells. Annu Rev Immunol 2003;21:139–176.

916. Moel PJ, Alegre ML, Reiner SL, et al. Impaired negative selection in CD28-deficient mice. Cell Immunol 1998;187:131–138.

917. Foy TM, Page DM, Waldschmidt TJ, et al. An essentail role for gp39 ligand for CD40, in thymic selection. J Exp Med 1995;182:1377–1388.

918. Page DM, Roberts EM, Peschon JJ, et al. TNF receptor-deficient mice reveal striking diffeneces between several models of negative selection. J Immunol 1998;160:120–133.

919. Calman BJ, Szychowski S, Chan FK, et al. A role for the orphan receptor Nur77 in apoptosis accompanying antigen-induced negative selection. Immunity 1995;3:272–282.

920. Zhou T, Cheng J, Yang P, et al. Inhibition of Nurr 77/Nurr1 leads to inefficient clonal deletion of self reactive T cells. J Exp Med 1996;183:1879–1892.

921. Gong Q, Cheng AM, Akk AM, et al. Disruption of T cell signaling networks and development by Grb2 haploid insufficiency. Nat Immunol 2001;2:29–36.

922. McMahan CJ, Fink PJ. RAG re-expression and DNA recombination of T cell receptor loci in peripheral CD40⁻ T cells. Immunity 1998;9:637–647.

923. Gargill MA, Derbinski JM, Hogquist KA. Receptor editing in developing T cells. Nat Immunol 2000;1:336–341.

924. Hansen JD, Kaatari SL. The receombination activation gene 2 (RAG) of rainbow trout Onchrhynchus mykiss. Immunogenetics 1956;44:203–211.

925. Hansen JD. Characterization of rainbow trout terminal deoxynucleotdyl transferase (TdT) and RAG 1coexpression define the trout primary lymphoid organs. Immunogenetics 1997;46:367–375.

926. Willett CE, Zapata AG, Hopkins N, et al. Expression of zebrafish rag gene during early development of thymus nurse cells. Dev Biol 1997;182:17–24.

927. Jurgens JB, Gartland LA, Du Pasquier L, et al. Identification of a candidate CD5 homologue in the amphibian Xenopos laevis. J Immunol 155:4218–4223.

928. Chen-lo H, Chen R, Bucy P, et al. T cell differentiation in birds. Sem Immunol 1990;2:79–86.

929. Coltey M, Bucy RP, Chen CH, et al. Analysis of the first two waves of thymus homing stem cells and their T progeny in chick-quail chimeras. J Exp Med 1989;170:543–557.

930. Havran WL, Alisson JP. Developmentally ordered appearance of thymocytes expressing different T cell antigen receptors. Nature 1988;335:443–445.

931. Sowder JT, Chen CH, Chak J, et al. T cell ontogeny:suppressive effects of embryonic treatment with monoclonal antibodies to T3, TCR1 or TCR2. FASEB J 1988;2:A466.

932. Washington EA, Kimpton WG, Cahill RN. Changes in the distribution of alpha beta and gamma delta T cells in blood and lymph nodes from fetal and postnatal lambs. Dev Comp Immunol 1992;16:493–501.

933. Witherden DA, Abernethy NJ, Kimpton WG, et al. Antigen-independent maturation of CD2, CD11a/CD18, CD44 and CD58 expression on thymic emigrants in fetal and postnatal sheep. Dev Immunol 1995;4:199–209.

934. Cunningham CP, Cahill RN, Washington EA, et al. Regulation of T cell homeostasis during fetal and early postnatal life. Vet Immunol Immunopathol 1999;72:175–181.

935. Sinkora M, Sinkora J, Rehakova Z, et al. Early ontogeny of thymocytes in pigs: sequential colonization of the thymus with T cell progenitors. J Immunol 2000;165:1832–1839.

936. Goldman M, Van der Vost P, Lambert P, et al. Persistance of anti-donor helper T cells secreting interleukin 4 after neonatal induction of transplanation tolerance. Transplant Proc 1989;21:238–239.

937. Bosing-Schneider R. Functional maturation of neonatal spleen cells. Immunology 1979;36:527–532.

938. Haines KA, Siskind GW. Omtogeny of T cell function. J Immunol 1980;124:1878–1882.

939. Adkins B, Bu Y, Cepero E, et al. Exclusive Th2 primary effector function in spleen but mixed Th1/Th2 function in lymph nodes of murine neonates. J Immunol 2000;164:2347–2353.

940. Min B, Legge KL, Pack C, et al. Neonatal exposure to self-peptide-immunoglobulin chimera circumvents the use of adjuvant and confere resistance to autoimmune disease by a novel mechanism involving IL-4 lymph node deviation and interferon gamma-mediated splenic anergy. J Exp Med 1998;188:2007–2018.

941. Pack CD, Cestra AE, Min B, et al. Neonatal exposure to antigen primes the immune system to develop responses in various lymphoid organs and promotes bystander regulation of diverse T cell specificities. J Immunol 2001;167:4187–4195.

942. Adkins BA, Ghanei A, Hamilton K. Develpmental regulation of IL-4, IL-2 and INF-γ production by murine peripheral T lymphocytes. J Immunol 1993;151:6177–6183.

943. Adkins B, Chun K, Hamilton K, et al. Naïve nurine neonatal T cells undergo apoptosi in response to primary stimulation J Immunol 1996;157:1343–1349.

944. Adkins BA, Ghanei A, Hamilton K. Upregulation of murine neonatal helper cell function by accessory cell factors. J Immunol 1994;153:3378–3385.

945. Donckier V, Flamand V, Desalle F, et al. IL-12 prevents neonatal inductioon of transplantation tolerance in mice. Eur J Immunol 1998;28:1426–1430.

946. Flamand V, Donckier V, Demoor F, et al. CD40 ligation prevents neonatal induction of transplantation tolerance J Immunol 1998;160:4666–4669.

947. Forstthuber T, Yip HC, Lehmann PV. Induction of Th1 and Th2 immunity in neonatal mice. Science 1996;271:1728–1730.

948. Radu DL, Brumeanu T-D, McEnvoy RC, et al. Escape from self-tolerance leads to neonatal insulin-dependent diabetes mellitus. Autoimmunity 1999;30:199–207.

949. Tung KSK, Agerborg SS, Alard P, et al. Regulatory T-cells, endogenous antigen and neonatal enviromennt in the prevenytion and induction of autoimmune diease. Immunol Rev 2001;182:135–148.

950. Adkins B, Du RQ. Newborn mice develop balanced Th1/Th2 primary effector responses in vivo but are biased to Th2 secondary response. J Immunol 1998;160:4271–4224.

951. Bot A, Bot S, Bona C. Enhanced protection against influenza virus of mice immunized as newborns with a mixture of plasmids expresing hemagglutinin and nucleoprotein. Vaccine 1998;16:1675–1682.

952. Li L, Lee H-H, Bell JJ, et al. IL-4 utilizes an alternative receptor to drive apoptosis of Th1 T cells and skwees neonatal immunity toward Th2. Immunity (in press).

953. Delespesse G, Yang LP, Ohishima Y, et al. Maturation of human neonatal CD4$^+$ and CD8$^+$ T lymphocytes into Th1/Th2 effectors. Vaccine 1998;16:1415–1419.

954. Morein B, Abusugra I, Blomqvist G. Immunity in neonates. Vet Immunol Immunopathol 2002;87:207–213.

955. Kasahara M, Flajnik MF, Ishibash T, et al. Evolution of the major histocompatibility complex: a current overview. Transplant Immunol 1995;3:1–23.

956. Flajnik MF, Kaufman JF, Hsu E, et al. Major histocompatibility complex-encoded class I molecules are absent in immunologically immunocompetent Xenopous before metamorphosis. J Immunol 1986;137:3891–3899.

957. Salter-Cid L, Nonoka M, Flajnik MF. Expression of class Ia and class Ib during ontogeny: high expression in epithelia and coregulation of class Ia and lmp7 genes. J Immunol 1998;160:2853–2861.

958. Jaffe L, Robertson EJ, Bikoff L. Distinct patterns of expression of MHC and class I and (2-microglobulin trnascripts at early stages of mouse development. J Immunol 1991;157:2740–2749.

959. Landsbereger N, Wolffe PA. Chromatin and transcriptional activity in early Xcnopous development. Cell Biol 1995;6:191–207.

960. Dadaglio G, Sun C-M, Lo-Man R, et al. Efficient in vivo priming of specific cytotoxic T cell responses by neonatal dendritic cells. J Immunol 2002;168:2219–2224.

961. Herzenberg LA, Bianchi DW, Schroder J, et al. Fetal cells in the blood of pregnant women's detection and enrichment by fluorescence-activated cell sorting. Proc Natl Acad Sci USA 1979;76:1453–1455.

962. Houlihan JM, Biro PA, Fergar-Payne A, et al. Evidence for the expression of non-HLA-A-B-C class I genes in the fetal human liver. J Immunol 1992;149:668–675.

963. Wood GW. Is restricted antigen presentation the explanation for fetal allograft survival? Immunol Today 1994;15:15–18.

964. Hermann E, Truyens C, Alonso-Vega C, et al. Human fetuses are able to mount an adult-like CD8 T-cell response. Blood 2002;100:2153–2158.

965. Braciale TJ, Braciale VL. Antigen presentation: structural themes and functional variations. Immunol Today 1991;12:124–130.

966. Bona C. Processing and presentation of self-antigens. In: The Molecular Pathology of Autoimmune Diseases (Theofilopoulos AN, Bona CA, eds.) Taylor and Francis London, New York 2002 pp. 184–192.

967. Stan AC, Casares S, Brumeanu T-D, et al. CpG motifs of DNA vaccines induce the expression of chemokines and MHC class II molecules on myocytes. Eur J Immunol 2001;31:301-310.

968. Hagerty DT, Allen PM. Processing and presentation of self and foreign antigens by the renal proximal tubules. J Immunol 1992;148:2324–2330.

969. Frei K, Lins H, Schwerdel C, et al. Antigen presentation in the central nervous system. J Immunol 1994;152:2720–2728.

970. Rott O, Tontsch U, Fleischer B. Dissociation of antigen-presenting capacity of astrocytes for peptides-antigens versus superantigens. J Immunol 1993;150:87–95.

971. So AL, Small G, Sperber K, et al. Factors affecting antigen uptake by human intestinal epithelial cell lines. Dig Dis Sci 2000;45:1130–1137.

972. Kitaura M, Kato T, Inaba K, et al. Ontogeny of macrophage function. VI. Down regualtion for Ia-exexpression in newborn mice macrophages by endogenous beta-interferon. Dev Comp Immunol 1988;12:645–655.

973. Lu CY, Calamai EG, Unanue ER. A defect in the antigen presenting function of macrophages from neonatal mice. Nature 1979;282:327–329.

974. Lee PT, Holt PG, McWilliam AS. Failure of MHC calss II expression in neonatal alveolar macrophages: potential role of class Ii transactivator. Eur J Immunol 2001;31:2347–2356.

975. Cristau B, Schafer PH, Pierce SK. Heat shock enhances antigen processing and accelerates the formation of compact class II dimers. J Immunol 1994;152:1546–1556.

976. Gosselin EJ, Wardwell K, Gosselin DR, et al. Enhanced antigen presentation using human Fc(receptor-specific immunogens. J Immunol 1992;149:3477–3483.

977. Thornton BP, Vetvicka V, Ross GD. Natural antibody and complement-mediated antigen processing and presentation by B lymphocytes. J Immunol 1994;152:1727–1736.

978. Liu K-J, Parikh VS, Tucker PW, et al. Role of the B cell antigen receptor in antigen processing and presentation. J Immunol 1993;151:6143–6154.

979. Hayakawa K, Tartilion D, Hardy RR. Absence of MHC class II expression distinguish fetal from adult B lymphopoiesis in mice. J Immunol 1994;152:4081–4087.

980. Tarlion D. Direct demonstration of MHC class II surface expression on murine pre-B cells. Int Immunol 1993;5:1629–1635.

981. Kearney JF, Cooper MD, Klein ER, et al. Ontogeny of Ia and IgD on IgM-bearing B lymphocytes in mice. J Exp Med 1977;146:297–305.

982. Sproul TW, Cheng PC, Dykstra ML, et al. A role of MHC class II antigen processing in B cell development. Intern Rev Immunol 2000;19:139–157.

983. Tasker L, Marshall-Clarke S. Immature B cells from neonatal mice show a selective inability to up-regulate MHC class II expression in response to antigen receptor ligation. Intern Immunol 1997;9:474–484.

984. Muthukkumar S, Goldstein J, Stein KE. The ability of B cells and dendritic cells to present antigen increases during ontogeny. J Immunol 2000;165:4803–4813.

985. Petty RE, Hunt DWC. Neonatal dendritic cells. Vaccine 1998;16:1378–1382.

986. Romani N, Schuler G, Frisch P. Ontogeny of Ia-positive and Thy-1 positive leucocytes in epidermis. J Invest Dermatol 1986;86:129–133.

987. Kobayashi M, Asano H, Fujita Y, et al. Development of ATPase-positive, immature Langerhans cells in fetal epidermis and their maturation during early postnatal period. J Immunol 1987:143:2431–2438.

988. Dewar AL, Doherty KV, Woods GM, et al. Acquisition of immune function during the neonatal development of the Langerhans cell network in neonatal mice. Immunology 2001;103:61–69.

989. Bona CA. Structure and direction of message in the immune network circuits. In: The Semiotics of Cellular Communication in the Immune System. (Sercaz EE, Celada F, Mitchison NA, Tada T, eds.), Springer Verlag. Berlin: 1988, pp. 105–116.

990. Henderson B, Seymour RM. Microbial modulation of cytokine networks. In: Bacterial Evasion of Host Immune Response. (Henderson B, Oyston PCF, eds.), Cambridge University Press. Cambridge: 2003 pp. 223–243.

991. Wilson CB, Lewis DB. Basis and implications of selectively diminished cytokine production in neonatal susceptibility to infections. Rev Infect Dis 1990;12:S410.

992. Miller ME. Current topics in host defence of the newborns. In: Advances in Pediatrics. (Barness LA, ed.), Year book Medical Publisher. Chicago:1978, pp. 25–34.

993. Clement LT, Yamashita N, Martin AM. The functionality distinct subpopulation of human CD4+ helper/inducer T lymphocytes defined by anti-CD45R antibodies derive sequentially from differentiation pathway that is regulated by activation-dependent post-thymic differentation. J Immunol 1988;141:1464–1475.

994. Pirenne H, Ajuard Y, Eljaafari A, et al. Comparison of T cell function change during childhood with ontogeny CDw29 and CD45RA expression on CD4+ T cells. Pediatr Res 1992;32:81–93.

995. Schibler KR, Trautman MS, Liechty KW, et al. Diminished transcription of interleukin-8 by monocytes from preterm neonates. J Leukoc Biol 1993;53:399–403.

996. Dammann O, Leviton A. Maternal intrauterine infection, cytokines and brain damage in preterm newborn. Pediatr Res 1997;42:1–8.

997. Heinikkinen J, Mottonen M, Komi J, et al. Phenotypic characterization of human decidual macrophages. Clin Expl Immunol 2003;131:498–505.

998. Benett WA, Lagoo-Deenadayalan S, Whitworth NS, et al. First-trimester human chorionic villi express both immunoregulatory an inflammatory cytokines: a role for interleukin-10 in regulating the cytokine network during pregnancy. Am J Reprod Immunol 1999;41:70–78.

999. Von Rango U, Classen-Linke I, Raven G, et al. Cytokine microenvironments in human first trimester decidua are dependent on trophoblast cells. Fert Ster 2003;79:1176–1186.

1000. Williams TJ, Jones CA, Miles EA, et al. Fetal and neonatal IL-13 production during pregnancy and at birth and subsequent development of atopic symptoms. J Allergy Clin Immunol 2000;105:951–959.

1001. Hebra A, Strange P, Egbert JM, et al. Intracellular cytokine production by fetal and adult monocytes. J Pediatr Surg 2001;36:1321–1326.
1002. Han P, Hodge G. Intracellular cytokine production and cytokine receptor interaction of cord mononuclear cells: relevance to cord blood transplantation. Br J Hematol 1999;107:450–457.
1003. Zhao Y, Dai P-Z, Gao X-M. Phenotypic and functional analysis of human T lymphocytes in early second and third-trimester fetuses. Clin Exp Immunol 2002;129:302–308.
1004. Daikoku NH, Kaltreider DF, Khouzami VA, et al. Premature rupture of membranes and preterm labor: maternal endrometric risk. Obstet Gynecol 1982;59:13–20.
1005. Nesein M, Cunningham-Rudles S. Cytokines and neonates. A. J Perinat 2000;17:393–403.
1006. Schultz C, Rott C, Temming P, et al. Enhanced interleukin-6 and interleukin-8 synthesis in term and preterm infants. Pediatr Res 2002;51:317–322.
1007. Dembiski J, Behrendt D, Heep A, et al. Cell-associated interleukin-8 in cord blood of term and preterm infants. Clin Diag Lab Immunol 2002;9:320–323.
1008. Kashlan F, Smulian J, Shen-Schwartz S, et al. Umbilical vein interleukin-6 and tumor necrosis factor alpha plasma concentrations in the very preterm infants. Pediatr Inf Dis 2000;19:238–243.
1009. Brener R, Niemeyer CM, Letititis JU. Plasma levels and gene expression of granulocyte colony-stimulating factor, tumor necrosis factor alpha, interleukin 1-beta, IL-6, IL-8 and soluble intercellular adhesion molecules-1 in neonatal early sepsis. Pediatr Res 1998;44:469–477.
1010. Mc Cloy MP, Roberts IAG, Horwath LJ, et al. Interleukin-11 levels in healthy and thrombocytopenic neonates. Pediatr Res 2002;51:756–760.
1011. Michie C, Harvey D. Can expression of CD45RO, A T-cell molecule, be used to detect congenital infection? Lancet 1994;343:1259–1260.
1012. Matsuoka T, Matsubara T, Katayama K, et al. Increase of cord bloodd cytokine-producing T cells in intrauterine infection. Pediatr Intern 2001;43:453–457.
1013. Weeks JW, Reynolds L, Taylor D, et al. Umbilical cord blood interleukin-6 and neonatal morbidity. Obstet Gynecol 1997;80:815–818.
1014. Malhotra. I, Ouma J, Wamachi A, et al. *In utero* exposure to helminth and mycobacterialantigens generates cytokine responses similar to that obseved in adults. J Clin Invest 1997;99:1759–1766.
1015. Sodora DL, Douek DC, Silvestri G, et al. Quantification of thymic function by measuring T cell receptor excision circles within peripheral blood of monkey. Eur J Immunol 2000;30:1145–1153.
1016. Shiratsuchi H, Tsyuiguchi I. Tuberculin PPD reactive T cells in cord blood lymphocytes. Infect Immun 1981;33:651–658.
1017. Munk ME, Kaufmann SHE. Human cord blood receptor cell response to protein antigens of *Paracoccidoides braziliensis*. Immunology 1995;84:98–105.
1018. Miles EA, Warner JA, Jones AC, et al. Peripheral blood mononuclear cells proliferative response in the first year of life in babies born to allergic parents. Clin Exp Allergy 1996;26:780–789.

1019. Holt PG. Primary allergic sensitization to environmental antigens:Perinatal T cell priming as a determinant of responder phenotype in adulthood. J Exp Med 1996;182:1297–1306.

1020. Zola H, Fusco M, Marcardle PJ, et al. Expression of cytokine receptors by human cord blood lymphocytes: comparison with adult blood lymphocytes. Pediatr Res 1995;38:397–403.

1021. Marodi L. Defiecient interferon-γ receptor-mediated signaling in neonatal macrophages. Acta Pediatr 2002;438:117–119.

1022. Hodge S, Hodge G, Flower R, et al. Cord blood leukcocyte expressionn of functionally significant molecules involved in the regulation of cellular immunity. Scan J Immunol 2110;53:72–78.

1023. Sautois B, Fillet G, Beguin Y. Comparative cytokine production by in vitro stimulated mononuclear cells from cord and adult blood. Exp Hematol 1997;25:103–108.

1024. Chalmers IMH, Janossy G, Contreras M, et al. Intracellular cytokine profile of cord and adult lymphocytes. Blood 1998;92:11–18.

1025. Schilber KR, Liechty KW, White WL, et al. Defective production of IL-6 by monocytes; a possible mechanism underlying several host deficiencies in neonates. Pediatr Res 1992;31:18–21.

1026. Yachie A, Takano N, Yokoi T. The capacity of neonatal leucocytes to produce IL-6 on stimulation assessed by whole blood culture. Pediatr Res 1990;27:227–233.

1027. Cohen SBA, Perez-Cruz I, Fallen E, et al. Analysis of the cytokine production by cord and adult blood. Hum Immunol 1999;60:331–336.

1028. Upham JW, Lee PT, Holt BJ, et al. Development of interleukin-12-producing capacity throughout childhood. Inf Immun 2002;70:6583–6588.

1029. Lee S, Suen Y, Chang L, et al. Decreased interleukin-12 from activated cord versus adult pripheral blood mononuclear cells. Blood 1996;88:945–954.

1030. La Pine TR, Joyner JL, Augustine NH, et al. Defective production of IL-18 and IL-12 by cord blood mononuclear cells influences the T-helper-1 interferon gamma response to group B streptococci. Pediatr Res 2003;54:1–6.

1031. Joyner JL, Augustine NH, Taylor KA, et al. Effects of group B streptococci on cord and adult mononuclear cell interleukin-12 and interferon-γ mRNA accumulation and protein secretion. J Inf Dis 2000;182:974–977.

1032. Wilson CB, Westall J, Johnson L, et al. Decreased production of interferon gamma by human neonatal cells. Intrinsic and regulatory deficiencies. J Clin Invest 1986;77:860–867.

1033. Chalmers IMH, Janossy G, Contreras M, et al. Intracellular cytokine profile of cord and adult blood lymphocytes. Blood 1998;92:11–18.

1034. Trivedi HN, HayGlass KT, Gangur JE, et al. Analysis of neonatal T cell and antigen presenting functions. Hum Immunol 1997;57:69–79.

1035. Wakasugi N, Virelizier JL, Seisdedos A, et al. Defective IFNγ production by the human neonate. J Immunol 1985;134:167–175.

1036. Rainford E, Reen DJ. Interleukin 10, produced in abundance by human newborn T cells, may be the regulator of increased tolerance associated with cord blood stem cell transplantation. Brit J Haematol 2002;116:702–709.

1037. Ribiero-do-Couto LM, Boeije LCM, Kroon JK, et al. High IL-13 production by human neonatal T cells: neonate immune system regulator. Eur J Immunol 2001;31:3394–3402.

1038. Kotiranta-Ainamo A, Rautonen J, Rautonen N. Interleukin-10 production by cord blood mononuclear cells. Pediatr Res 1997;41:110–113.

1039. Chheda S, Palkowetz KH, Garofalo R, et al. Decreased interleukin-10 production by neonatal monocytes and T cells: relationship to decreased production and expression of tumor necrosis factor-alpha and its receptors. Pediatr Res 1996;40:475–483.

1040. Krampera M, Tavecchia L, Benedetti F, et al. Intracellular cytokine profile of cord blood T- and NK-cells and monocytes. Haematologica 2000;85:675–679.

1041. Hoshino T, Winkler-Pickett RT, Mason AT, et al. IL-13 production by NK cells. J Immunol 1999;162:51–59.

1042. Warren HS, Kinnear BF, Phillips JH, et al. Production of IL-5 by human NK cells and IL-5 secretion by IL-4, IL-10 and IL-12. J Immunol 1995;154:5144–5152.

1043. Loza MJ, Zamai L, Azzoni L, et al. Expression of type 1 (interferon gamma) and type 2 (interleukin-13, interleukin-5) cytokines at distinct stages of natural killer cell differentiation. Blood 2002;99:1273–1281.

1044. Nomura A, Takada H, Jim C-H, et al. Functional analyses of cord blood natural killer cells and T cells: a distinctive interleukin-18 response. Exp Haematol 2001;29:1169–1176.

1045. Dominguez E, Madrigal JA, Laryse Z, et al. Foetal natural killer function is suppressed. Immunology 1998;94:109–114.

1046. Gaddy J, Ridsson G, Broxmeyer HE. Cord blood natural killer cells are functionally and phenotypically immature but readly respond to interleukin 2 and interleukin-12. Cytokine Res 1995;15:527–536.

1047. Kawano T, Tanaka Y, Shimizu E, et al. A novel recognition motif of human NKT antigen receptor for a glycolipid ligant. Int Immunol 1999;11:881–887.

1048. Van Der Vilet HJ, Nishi N, de Gruijl TD, et al. Human natural killer T cells acquire a memory-activated phenotype before birth. Blood 2000;95:2440–2442.

1049. D'Andrea A, Goux D, De Lalla C, et al. Neonatal invariant Vα24$^+$ NKT lymphocytes are memory cells. Eur J Immunol 2000;30:1544–1550.

1050. Kadowaki N, Antonenko S, Ho S, et al. Distinct cytokine profiles of neonatal killer T cells after expansion with subsets of dendritic cells. J Exp Med 2001;193:1221–1226.

1051. Adkins B, Hamilton K. Freshly isolated, murine neonatal T cells produce IL-4 in response to anti-CD3 stimulation. J Immunol 1992;149:3448–3455.

1052. Widmer MB, Cooper EL. Ontogeny of cell-mediated cytotoxicity:induction of CTL in early postnatal thymocytes. J Immunol 1979;122:291–295.

1053. Schwartz DH, Doherty PC. Virus-immune and alloraective response characteristics of thymocytes and spleen cells from young mice. J Immunol 1981;127:1411–1414.

1054. Ridge JP, Fuchs EJ, Matzinger P. Neonatal tolerance revisited: turning on newborn T cells with dendritic cells. Science 1996;271:1723–1726.

1055. Langrish CL, Buddle JC, Thrasher AJ, et al. Neonatal dendritic cells are intrinsically biased against Th-1 immune response. Clin Exp Immunol 2002;128:118–123.

1056. Barff LJ, Leake RD, Burstyn DG. Immunologic responses to early and routine DTP immunization in infants. Pediatrics 1984;73:37–42.

1057. Holocombe CBA, Omotura J, Eldridge J, et al. *H. pylori* the most common bacterial infection in Africa; random serological study. Am. J Gastroenterol 1992;87;28–39.

1058. Thomas JE, Dale A, Harding M, et al. *Helicobacter pylori* colonization in early life. Pediatr Res 1999;45:218–223.

1059. Eisenberg JC, Czinn SJ, Garhart C, et al. Protective efficay of anti-*Helicobacter pylori* immunity following systemic immunization of neonatal mice. Inf Immun 2003;71:1820–1827.

1060. Franchini M, Abril C, Schwerdel C, et al. Protective T-Cell-based immunity induced in neonatal mice by a single replicative cycle herpes simplex virus. J Virol 2001;75:83–89.

1061. Siegrist C-A, Saddallah F, Tougne C, et al. Induction of neonatal Th1 and CTL response by live viral vaccines: a role for replication patterns within antigen presenting cells? Vaccine 1998;16:1473–1478

1062. Brazolot Millan CL, Weeratna R, Krieg AM, et al. CpG DNA can induce strong Th1 humoral and cell-mediated immune responses against hepatitis B surface antigen in young mice. Proc Natl Acad Sci USA 1998;95:15,553–15,558.

1063. Pertmer T, Oran AE, Mandorin CA, et al. Th1 genetic adjuvants modulate immune response in neonates. Vaccine 2001;19:1764–1771.

1064. Bryston YJ, Winter HS, Gard SE, et al. Deficiency of immune interferon production by leukocytes of normal newborns. Cell Immunol 1980;55:191–197.

1065. Lewis DB, Wilson A, Wilson CB. Reduced interferon-γ mRNA levels in human neonates. J Exp Med 1986;163:1018–1024.

1066. Frenkel L, Bryston YLJ. Ontogeny of phytohemagglutinin-induce γ intreferon by leukocytes of healthy and infants and children:evidence for decreased production in infants then 2 month of age. J Pediatr 1987:119:97–106.

1067. Corinti S, Albanesi C, La Sala A, et al. Regulatory activity of autocrine IL-10 on dendritic cell functions. J Immunol .2001;166:4312–4318.

1068. Yu HR, Chang JC, Chuang H, et al. Different antigens trigger different Th1/Th2 reaction sin neonatal mononuclerar cells realting to T-bet/Gata-3 expression. J Leukoc Biol 2003;74(5):952–958.

1069. Marchant A, Goetghebuer T, Ota MO, et al. Newborns develop a Th1-type immune response to *Mycobacterium bovis Bacillus* Calmatte–Guerin vaccination. J Immunol 1999;163:2249–2255.

1070. Vekemans J, Amedei A, Ota MO, et al. Neonatal bacillus Calmette-Guerin vaccination induces adult-like IFNg production by CD4+ T lymphocytes. Eur J Immunol 2001;31:1531–1535.

1071. Mascart F, Verscheure V, Malfroot A, et al. *Bordetella pertussis* infection in 2-month-old infants promotes typeI T cell responses. J Immunol 2003;170:1504–1509.

1072. Zaghouani H, Krystal M, Kuzu H, et al. Cells expressing a heavy chain immunoglobulin gene carrying a viral T cell epitope are lysed by specific cytolytic T cells. J Immunol 1992;140:3604–3609.

1073. Kuzu Y, Kuzu H, Zaghouani H, et al. Priming of CTL at various stages of ontogeny with transfectoma cells expressing a chimeric Ig heavy chain gene bearing an influenza virus nucleoprotein peptide. Int Imm 1993;5:1301–1307.

1074. Sarzotti M, Robbins DS, Hoffman PM. Induction of protective CTL responses in newborn mice by murine retrovirus. Science 1996;271:1726–1728.

1075. Moser JM, Altman JD, Lukacher AE. Antiviral CD8 T cell responses in neonatal mice: susceptibility to polyoma virus-induced tumors is associated with lack of cytotoxic function by viral antigen-specific T cells. J Exp Med 2001;193:595–605.

1076. Bot A, Bot S, Garcia-Sastre A, et al. Protective cellular immunity against influenza virus induced by plasmid inoculation of newborn mice. Dev Immunol 1998;5:197–210.

1077. Sarzotti M, Dean TA, Temington MP, et al. Induction of cytotoxic T cell responses in newborn mice by genetic immunization. Vaccine 1997;15:795–797.

1078. Hassett DE, Zang J, Silfka M, et al. Immune responses following neonatal DNA vaccination are long-lived, abundent and qualitatively similar to those induced by conventional immunization. J Virol 2000;74:2620–2647.

1079. Zang J, Silvestri N, Whitton JL, et al. Neonates mount robust and protective adult-like CD8$^+$-T-cell response to DNA vaccination. J Virol 2002;76:11:911–11,919.

1080. Gray D, Matzinger P. T cell memory is short-lived in the absence of antigen. J Exp Med 1991;174:965–974.

1081. Brander C, Goulder PJR, Luzuriaga K, et al. Persistant HIV-1-specific CTL clonal expansion despite high viral burden post *in utero* HIV-1 infection. J Immunol 1999;162:4796–4800.

1082. Luzuriaga K, Holmes D, Hereema A, et al. HIV-1-specific cytotoxic T lymphocytes responses in the first year of life. J Immunol 1995;154:433–443.

1083. Isaacs D, Bangham CRM, McMichael AJ. Cell-mediated cytotoxic response to respiratory syncitial virus in infants with bronchiolitis. Lancet 1987;2:769–772.

1084. Mbawuike IN, Piedra PA, Cate TR, et al. Cytotoxic T lymphocytes responses of infants after natural infection or immunization with cold-live recombinant or inactivated influenza A virus vaccine. J Med Virol 1998;50:105–111.

1085. Nossal GJV. Cellular mechanisms of immunological tolerance. Annu Rev Immunol 1994;1:33–62.

1086. Bretscher P, Cohn M. A theory of self–nonself discrimination. Science 1970;169:1042–1044.

1087. Ohashi PS, Oehen S, Buerki K, et al. Ablation of "tolerance" and induction of diabetes by virus infection in viral antigen transgenic mice. Cell 1991;65:305–317.

1088. Oldstone MB, Nerenberg M, Southern P, et al. Virus infection triggers insulin-dependent diabetes mellitus in a transgenic model: role of anti-self (virus) immune response. Cell 1991;65:319–31.

1089. Gershon RK, Kondo K. Infectious immunological tolerance. Immunology 1971;21:903–912.

1090. Fakaura H, Kent SC, Pietrusewicz MJ, et al. Induction of circulating myelin basic protein and proteolipid protein-specific transforming growth factor beta1-secreting Th3 T cells by oral administration of myelin in multiple sclerosis patients. J Clin Invest 1996;98:70–77.

1091. Abbas AK, Murphy KM, Sher A. Functional diversity of helper T lymphocytes. Nature 1996;383:787–793.

1092. Powrie F, Leach MW, Mauze S, et al. Inhibition of Th1 responses prevents inflammatory bowel disease in SCID mice reconstituted with CD45RBhi CD4 T cells. Immunity 1994;1:553–5562.

1093. Powrie F, Correa-Oliveira R, Mauze S, et al. Regulatory interactions between CD45RBhigh and CD45RBlow CD4 T cells are important for the balance between protective and pathogenic cell-mediated immunity. J Exp Med 1994;179:589–600.

1094. Powrie F, Carlino J, Leach MW, et al. A critical role for transforming growth factor-beta but not interleukin 4 in the suppression of T helper type 1-mediated colitis by CD45RB(low) CD4 T cells. J Exp Med 1996;183:2669–2674.

1095. Groux H, Bigler M, de Vries JE, et al. Interleukin-10 induces a long-term antigen-specific anergic state in human CD4 T cells. J Exp Med 1996;184:19–29.

1096. Groux H, O'Gara A, Bigler MA. CD4 T-cell subset inhibits antigen specific T-cell responses and prevents colitis. Nature 1997;389:737–742.

1097. Lepault F, Gagnerault MC. Characterization of peripheral regulatory CD4+ T cells that prevent diabetes onset in nonobese diabetic mice. J Immunol 2000;164:240–247.

1098. Kuniashu Y, Takahashi T, Itoh M, et al. Naturally anergic and suppressive CD25+CD4+ T cells as a functionally and phenotypically distinct immunoregulatory T cell population. Int Immunol 2000;12:1145–1155.

1099. Nishizuka Y, Sakakura T. Thymus and reproduction: sex-linked dysgenesis of the gonad after neonatal thymectomy in mice. Science 1969;166:753–755.

1100. Seddon B, Mason D. Regulatory T cells in the control of autoimmunity: the essential role of transforming growth factor beta and interleukin 4 in the prevention of autoimmune thyroiditis in rats by peripheral CD4+CD45RC− cells and CD4+ CD8− thymocytes. J Exp Med 1999;189:279–288.

1101. Honey K, Cobbold SP, Waldmann H. Dominant tolerance and linked suppression induced by therapeutic antibodies do not depend on FAS-FASL interactions. Transplantation 2000;69:1683–1689.

1102. Osmond DG. Proliferation kinetics and the life span of B cells in central and peripheral lymphoid organs. Curr Opin Immunol 1991;3:179–185.

1103. Wang H, Shlomchik MJ. High affinity rheumatoid factor transgenic B cells are eliminated in normal mice. J Immunol 1997;1125–1134.

1104. Carsetti R, Kohler G, Lamers MC. Transitional B cells as target of negative selection in B cell compartment. J Exp Med 1995;181:2129–2140.

1105. Fulcher DA, Basten A. B-cell activation versus tolerance. The central role of immunoglobulin receptor engagement and T-cell help. Intern Rev Immunol 1997;15:33–53.

1106. Wang H, Shlomchik MJ. Maternal Ig mediates neonatal tolerance in rheumatoid factor transgenic mice but tolerance breaks down in adult mice. J Immunol 1998;160:2263–2271.

1107. Braun C, Mahouy G, Bona C, et al. Failure to suppress theta antigen expression in progeny derived from pre-immunized maternal recipients. J Immunogenet 1976;3:307–314.

1108. Owen RD. Immunogenetic consequences of vascular anastomoses between bovine twins. Science 1945;102:400–404.

1109. Hasek M, Hraba T. Immunological effects of experimental embryonal parabiossis. Nature 1995;175:764–767.

1110. Waters CA, Pilarski LM, Wegman TG, et al. Tolerance induced during ontogeny. J Exp Med 1979;149:1134–1151.

1111. Chiller JM, Habicht GS, Weigle WO. Cellular sites of immunological unresponsiveness. Proc Natl Acad Sci USA. 1970;65:551–555.

1112. Lazizi Y, Badur S, Perk Y, et al. Selective unresponsiveness to HbsAg vaccine in newborns related with an in utero passage of hepatatis virus DNA. Vaccine 1997;15:1095–1100.

1113. Dent PB, Rawls WE. Human congenital rubella: the relationship of immunologic aberration to viral persistence. Ann NY Acad Sci 1971;181:209–221.

1114. Gehrtz RC, Li Y, Echardt Y-NC, et al. Relevance of immune responses to pathogensis of cytomegalovirus-associated diseases. Transplant Proc 1991;23(suppl);75–84.

1115. Melsom R, Harbo M, Duncan ME, et al. IgA and IgM antibodies against Mycobacerium leprae in cord sera of patients with leprosy; an indicator of intrauterine infection in leprosy. Scand J Immunol 1981;14:343–352.

1116. Arnold LW, Pennell CA, McCray SK, et al. Development of B-1 cells: segregation of phosphatidyl choline-specific B cells to the B-1 population occurs after immunoglobulin gene expression. J Exp Med 1994;179:1585–1595.

1117. Kawaguchi S. Induction of tolerance in B-1 cells for bromelain-treated mouse red blood cells by a transient presence of anti-idiotype antibodies in neonatal and adult mice. J Immunol 1998;160:4796–4800.

1118. Lawton AD. Suppression of immunoglobulin synthesis in mice. I. Effects of treatment with antibody to μ-chain. J Exp Med 1972, 139:277–297.

1119. Sidman CL, Unanue ER. Receptor-mediated inactivation of early B lymphocytes. Nature 1975;257:149–151.

1120. Felton LD, Ottinger B. Pneumococcus polysaccharides as a paralysing agent on the mechanism of immunity in white mice. J Immunol 1942;74:17–29.

1121. Feldmann M, Howard JG, Desmayard C. Role of antigen structure in the discrimination between tolerance and immunity in B cells. Transplant Rev 1975;23;78–97.

1122. Hanna MG, Oyama J. Inhibition of antibody formation in mature rabbits by contact with antigen at an early age. J Immunol 1954;73:49–61.

1123. Dixon FJ, Maurer PH. Immunological unresponsivness induced by protein antigens. J Exp Med 1955;101:833–849.

1124. Cambier JC, Kettman JR, Vitetta ES, et al. Differential susceptibility of neonatal and adult murine spleen cells to in vitro induction of B-cell tolerance. J Exp Med 1976;144:293–297.

1125. Klimann NR. The clonal selection hypothesis and current concepts of B cell tolerance. Immunity 1996;5:189–195.

1126. Metcalf ES, Klinman NR. In vitro tolerance induction in neonatal immune B cells. J Exp Med 1976;143:1327–1338.

1127. Aifanis I, Piviniouk VI, Gartner F, et al. Allelic exclusion of T cells receptor beta locus requires the SH2 domain containing leukocyte protein (S9SLP)-adaptor protein. J Exp Med 1999;190:1093–1102.

1128. Del Porto P, Bruno L, Matei MG, et al. Cloning and comparative anlysis of the human pre-T-cell receptor alpha-chain gene. Proc Natl Acad Sci USA 1995;92:12,105–12,109.

1129. Mitchison NA. Induction of immune paralysis in two zones of dosage. Proc Roy Soc Lond B 1964:161:275–282.

1130. Schwartz RH, Mueller DL, Jenkins MK, et al. T-cell clonal anergy. Cold Spring Harbor Symp Quant Biol 1989;54:605–610.

1131. Schwartz RH. Reversal of in vitro T-cell clone anergy by IL-2 stimulation. Intern Immunol 1992;4:661–671.

1132. Marrack P, Kappler J. T cells can distinguish between allogeneic mmajor histocompatibility complex of different cell type. Nature 1988;332:840–843.

1133. Festenstein H. Immunogenetics and biological aspects of in vitro allotransformation (MLR) in the mouse. Transplant Rev 1973;15:62–88.

1134. Simpson E. Positive and negative selection of the T cell repertoire: role of MHC and other ligands. Int Rev Immunol 1992;8:269–277.

1135. Beutner U, Rudy C, Huber BT. Molecular characterization of Mls-1 Int Rev Immunol 1992;8:279–288.

1136. Tomonari K, Fairchild O, Rosenwasser OA, et al. Endogenous ligands selecting Y cells expressing particular Vβ elememts. Int. Rev Immunol 1992;8:289–310.

1137. MacDonald HR, Pedrazzini T, Schneider R, et al. Intrathymic eliminatiom of Mls^a-reactive (Vβ6$^+$) cells during neonatal tolerance induction to Mls^a-encoded antigens. J Exp Med 1988;167:2005–2010.

1138. Mazda O, Watanabe Y, Gyotoku J-I, et al. Requirment of dendritic cells and B cells in the clonal deletion of Mls-reactive T cells in thymus. J Exp Med 1991;173:539–547.

1139. Kieselow P, Bluthmann H, Stearz UD, et al. Tolerance in T-cell receptor transgenic mice involves deletion of nonmature CD4$^+$ CD8$^+$ thymocytes Nature 1988;333:742–746.

1140. von Boehmer H, Kieselow P. Self–nonself discrimination by T cells. Science 1990;248:1369–1373.

1141. Zang M, Cacchio MS, Vitica BP, et al. I. T cell tolerance to a neo-self antigen expressed by thymic epithelial cells. J Immunol 2003;170:3954–3962.

1142. Antonia S, Geiger T, Miller J, et al. Mechanisms of immune tolerance induction through thymic expression of a peripheral tissue-specific protein. Int Immunol 1995;7:715–725.

1143. Legge KL, Min B, Pack C, et al H. Differential presentation of an alterd peptide within fetal central and peripheral organs supports an avidity model for thymic cell development and implies a peripheral readjustment for activation. J Immunol 1999;162:5738–5746.

1144. Kuzu H, KuzuY, Zaghouani H, et al. In vivo priming effect during various stages of ontogeny of an influenza A virus nucleoprotein peptide. Eur J Immunol 1993;23:1397–1400.

1145. Lamb JR, Feldman M. Essential requirment for major histocompatibility complex recognition in T-cell tolerance induction. Nature 1984;308:72–74.

1146. Rammensee H-G, Bevan MJ. Evidence from in vitro studies that tolerance to self-antigens is MHC-restricted. Nature 1984;308:741–742.

1147. Schonrich G, Alferink J, Klevenz A, et al. Tolerance induction as a multi-step process. Eur J Immunol 1994;24:285–293.

1148. Alferink J, Tafuri A, Vesweber D, et al. Control of neonatal tolerance to tissue antigens by peripheral T cell trafficking. Proc Natl Acad Sci USA 1998;282:1338–1341.

1149. Morgan DJ, Kurts C, Kreuwel HTC, et al. Ontogeny of T cell tolerance to peripherally expressed antigens. Proc Natl Acad Sci USA 1999;96:3854–3858.

1150. Quin F, Sun D, Goto H, et al. Resistance to experimental autoimmune encephalomyelitis induced by neonatal tolererization to myelin basic protein: clonal deletion vs. regulation of autoreactive lymphocytes. Eur J Immunol 1989;19:372–380.

1151. Clayton JP, Gammon GM, Ando DG, et al. Peptide-specific preventation of experimental allergic encephalomyelitis. Neonatal tolerance induced to the dominant T cell determinant of myelin basic protein. J Exp Med 1989;169:1681–1691.

1152. Saegusa K, Ishimaru N, Haneji N, et al. Mechanisms of neonatal teolerance induced in an animal model for primary Sojgren's syndrome by intravenous administration of autoantigen. Scand J Immunol 2000;52:264–270.

1153. Billingham RE, Lampkin GH, Medawar PB, et al. Tolerance to homografts diagnosis and the free martin conditions in cattle. Heredity 1999;6:201–211.

1154. Allard P, Matriano JA, Socarras S, et al. Detection of donor-derived cells by polymerase chain reaction in neonatally tolerant mice. Transplantation 1995:60:1198–

1155. Kawamura H, Kameyama H, Kosaka T, et al. Association of CD8+ natural killer T cells in the liver with neonatal tolerance phenomenon. Transplantation 2002;73:978–994.

1156. Chen N, Gao Q, Field EH. Prevention of Th1 response is critical for tolerance. Transplantation 1996;61:1076–1083.

1157. Weigle WO. Immunological unresponsiveness. Adv Immunol 1973;16:61–83.

1158. Reylandt M, De Wit D, van Mechelen M, et al. Lack of T cell tolerance in mice exposed to a protein antigen through lactation. Cell Immunol 1995:162:89–96.

1159. Gammon GM, Dunn K, Shhastri N, et al. Neonatal T-cell tolerance to minimal immunogenic peptides is caused by clonal inactivation. Nature 1986;312:413–415.

1160. Shenoy M, Oshima M, Atassi MZ, et al. Suppression of experimental autoimmune myasthenia gravis by epitope-specific neonatal tolerance to synthetic region α146-160 of acetyl choline receptor. Clin Immunol Immunopathol 1993;66:230–238.

1161. Simpson CC, Woods GM, Muller HK. Impaired CD40-signalling in Langerhans' cells from murine neonatal draining lymph nodes:implication for neonatally induced cutaneous tolerance. Clin Exp Immunol 2003;132:201–208.

1162. Legge KL, Gregg RK, Maldonado-Lopez R, et al. On the role of dendritic cells in peripheral T cell tolerance and modulation of autoimmunity. J Exp Med 2002;196;217–227.

1163. Chang H-C, Zhang S, Kaplan MH. Neonatal tolerance in absence of Stat4- and Stat6-dependent Th cell differentiation. J Immunol 2002;169:4124–4128.
1164. Field AC, Caccavelli L, Fillion J, et al. Neonatal toleance and maintennance of tolerance to Th2-induced immune manifestation in rats. Transpl Proc 2001;33:2275–2276.
1165. Zinkernagel RM. On natural and artificial vaccination. Annu Rev Immunol 2003;21:515–546.
1166. Reharmann B, Farrari C, Pasquinelli C, et al. The hepatitis B virus persists decades after patients'recovery from acut hepatitis despite active maintenance of a cytotoxic T-lymphocyte response. Nat Med 1996;2:1–6.
1167. Enders JF, Weller TH, Robbins FC. Cultivation of Lansing strain of poliomyelitis virus in culture of various human embryonic tissues. Science 1949;109:85–87.
1168. Stienlauf S, Shoresh M, Solomon A, et al. Kinetics of formation of neutralizing antibodies against vaccinia virus following re-vaccination. Vaccine 1999;17:201–204.
1169. Cono J, Casey CG, Bell DM. Smallpox vaccination and adverse reactions. Guidance for clinicians. MMWR Recomm Rep 2003;52:1–28.
1170. Thayyil-Sudhan S, Kumar A, Singh M, et al. Safety and effficiveness of BCG vaccination in preterm babies. Arch Dis Child Fetal Neonatal Ed 1999;81:F64–F66.
1171. Ferreira AA, Bunn-Moreno MM, Sant'Anna CCS, et al. BCG vaccinationn in low birth weight new borns:analysis of lymphocyte proliferation, IL-2 generation and intradermal reaction to PPD. Tuber Lung Dis 1996:77:476–481.
1172. Inaba K, Inaba M, Naito M, et al. Dendritic cell progenitors phagocytize particulates including bacillus Calmette–Guerin organism and sensitized mice to mycobacterial antigens in vivo. J Exp Med 1993;178:479–456.
1173. Henderson RA, Watkins SC, Flynn JL. Activation of human dendritic cells following infection with Mycobacteriuim tuberculosis. J Immunol 1997;159:635–642.
1174. Ota MOC, Vekarmans J, Schegel-Hauueter S, et al. Influence of Mycobacterium bovis Calmette-Guerin on antibody and cytokine response to human neonatal vaccination. J Immunol 2002;168:919–925.
1175. Belshe RB, Mendelman PM, Treanor J, et al. The efficacy of live attenuated cold-adapted, trivalent, intranasal influenza virus vaccine in children. N Engl J Med 1998;338:1405–1412.
1176. Brisson M, Edmunds WJ, Gay NJ. Varicella vaccination: impact of vaccine efficacy on the epidemiology of VZV. Med Virol 2003:70:S31–S37.
1177. Habermehl P, Lignitz A, Knuf M, et al. Cellular immune response of a varicella vaccine following simultaneous DTaP and VZV vaccination. Vaccine 1999:17:669–674.
1178. Hope-Simpson R. The nature of varicella-zoster virus in immunocompromised children. Proc Roy Soc Lond 1965;58:9–20.
1179. Krause PR, Klinman DM. Varicella vaccination: evidence for frequent reactivation of the vaccine strain in healty children. Nat Med 2000;6:451–454.
1180. Seward JF, Watson BM, Peterson CL, et al. Varicella disease after introduction of varicella vaccine in USA. JAMA 2002;287:606–611.

1181. Shinnefield HR, Black SB, Staehle BO, et al. Vaccination with measles, mumps and rubella vaccine and varicella vaccine: safety, tolerability, immunogenicity, persistence of antibody and duration of protection agianst varicella in health children. Pediatr Infec Dis J 2002;21:555–561.

1182. Gans H, Yasukawa L, Rinki M, et al. Immune response to measles and mumps vaccination of infants at 6, 9, and 12 months. J Inf Dis 2001;184:817–826.

1183. Dorig RE, Marcil A, Richardson CD. CD46, a primate-specific receptor for measles virus. Trends Microbiol 1994;2:312–323.

1184. Karp CL. Measles: immunosuppression, interleukin-12 and complement receptors. Immunol Rev 1999;168:91–101.

1185. Orenstein WA, Markowitz LE, Atkinson WL, et al. Worldwide measles pervention. Isr J Med Sci 1994;30:469–481.

1186. Peltla H, Heinonen OP, Valle M, et al. Th elimination of indigenous measles, mumps, rubella from Finland by a 12-year, two dose vaccination program. N Engl J Med 1994;331:1398–1402.

1187. Cherry JD. Measles. In: Textbook of Pediatric Infectious Diseases (Feigin R, Cherry JD, eds.) Philadelphia Saunders 1997.

1188. Tischer A, Gerike E. Immune response after primary and re-vaccination with different vaccines against measles, mumps, rubella. Vaccine 2000;18:1382–1392.

1189. Poland GA, Ovsyannikova IG, Jacobson RM, et al. Identification of an association between HLA class II alleles and low antibody levels after measles immunization. Vaccine 2001;20:430–408.

1190. Gans H, Maldonado Y, Yasukawa LL, et al. IL-12, IFN-Pγ and T-cell proliferation to measles in immunized infants. J Immunol 1999;162:5569–5575.

1191. Auwaerter PG, Hussey GGD, Goddard EA, et al. Changes within T cell receptor Vβ subsets in infants following measles vaccination. Clin Immunol Immunopatol 1996; 79:163–170.

1192. Ura Y, Hara T, Nagata M, et al. T cell activation and T cell receptor varaible usage gene in measles. Acta Pediatr Jpn 1992;34:273–277.

1193. Jaye A, Magnusen AF, Sadiq AD, et al. Ex vivo analysis of cytotoxic T lymphocytes to measles antigens during infection and after vaccination in Gambian children. J Clin Invest 1998;102:1111969–1977.

1194. Carlsson R-M, Claedon BA, Fagerlund E, et al. Antibody persistence in five-year-old children who received a pentavalent combination vaccine in infancy. Pediatr Inf Dis J 2002;21:535–541.

1195. Kirmani KI, Lofthus G, Pichichero ME, et al. Seven year follow-up vaccine response in extremely premature infants. Pediatrics 2002;109:498–504.

1196. Hoberman A, Greenberg DP, Paradise JL, et al. Effectiveness of inactivated influenza vaccine in preventing acute otitis media in young children. JAMA 2003;290:1608–1620.

1197. Maeda T, Shintani Y, Miyamoto H, et al. Prophylactic effect of inactivated vaccine on young children. Pediatr Int 2002;44:43–46.

1198. Quach C, Piche-Walker L, Platt R, et al. Riskk factors associated with severe influenza infections in chilhood: implication for vaccine strategy. Pediatrics 2003;112:197–201.

1199. Esposito S, Faldella G, Giammanco A, et al. Long-term pertussis-specific immun eresponse to a combined diphtheria, tetanus tricomponent acellular pertussis and hepatitis B vaccine in pre-term infants. Vaccine 2002;20:2928–2932.

1200. Goldblatt D, Richmond P, Millard E, et al. The inductuion of immunological memory after vaccination with Haemophilus influenzae type b conjugate and accelular pertussis containing diphtheria, tetanus and pertussis vaccine combination. J Inf Dis 1999;180:538–541.

1201. Rowe J, Macaubas C, Monger TM, et al. Antigen-specific resposnes to diphtheria, -tetanus-acelullar pertussis vaccine in human infants are initially Th2 polarized. Inf Immun 2000;68:3873–3877.

1202. Mahon BP, Ryan MS, Griffin F, et al. Interleukine-12 is produced by macrophages in respons to live or killed Bordetella pertussis and enhances the efficacy of an acellular perussis vaccine by promoting of Th1 cells. Infect Immun 1996;64:5295–5301.

1203. Ryan MS, Murphy G, Gotherfors L, et al. *Bordetella pertussis* respiratory infection in children is associated with preferntial activation of type 1 T helper cells. J Inf Dis 1997;175:1246–1250.

1204. Zhao YL, Meng ZD, Xu ZY, et al. H2 strain attenuated lived hepatitis A vaccines: protective efficacy in a hepatitis A outbreak. World J Gastroenterol 2000;6:829–832.

1205. Piazza M, Safary A, Vegnente A, ct al. Safety and immunogenicity of hepatatis A vaccine in infants. Vaccine 1999;17:585–588.

1206. Bell BP. Hepatitis A vaccine. Rev Pediatr Inf Dis 2000;1:1187–1188.

1207. Lagardere B. Vaccination contre l'hepatite A. Arch Pediatr 1998;5:321–325.

1208. Ambrosch F, Wiedermann H, Jonas S, et al. Immunogenicity and protectivity of a new liposomal hepatitis A vaccine. Vaccine 1997;15:1209–1213.

1209. Chavez A, Pujol M, Alsina MA, et al. Membrane fusion induced by a lipopeptidic epitpe from VP3 capside protein of hepatatis A virus. Luminiscence 2001;16:135–143.

1210. Eskola J, Kayhty H, Takala AK, et al. A randomized, prosepective, field trial of conjugated vaccine in the protection of infants and young children against Haemophilus influenzae type b disease. N Engl J Med 1990;323:1381–1386.

1211. Adderson EE. Antibody repertoires in infants and adults: effects of T-independent and T-dependent immunizations. Springer Semin Imunnopathol 2001;23:387–403.

1212. Finn A, Blondeau C, Bell F. Haemophilus influenzae type b antibody responses in children given containing diphteria, tetanus acellular pertussis-Hib vaccine combination. J Inf Dis 2000;181:217–218.

1213. Insel RA, Kittelberg A, Anderson PW. Oligosaccharide-protein conjugate vaccine induce and prime for oligoclonal IgG response to Haemophilus influenzae type b capsular polysaccharide restricted and identical spectrotype in adults. J Immunol 1985:135:2810–2816.

1214. Lucas AH. Expression of crossreactive idiotypes by human antibodies specific for the capsular polysaccharide of Haemophilus influenzae B. J Clin Invest1988;81:480–486.

1215. Scott MJ, Tarrand JJ, Crimmins DL, et al. Clonal characterization of human IgG antibody repertoire to Haemophilus influenzae type b capsular polysaccharide. J Immunol 1989;143:293–298.

1216. Lucas AH, Moulton KD, Reason DC. Role of kappa II-A2 light chain CDR-3 junctional residues in human antibody binding to Haemophilus influenzae type b capsular polysaccharide. J Immunol 1998;162:3776–3783.

1217. McIntosh EDG, Paradiso PR. Recent progress in the development of vaccines for infants and children. Vaccine 2003;21:601–604.

1218. Veenhoven R, Bogaert D, Uiterwaal C, et al. Effect of conjugate pneumococcal vaccine followed by polysaccharide pneumococcal vaccine on recurrent acute otitis media: a randomized study. Lancet 2003;361:2189–2195.

1219. MacDonald NE, Hborrow R, Fox AJ, et al. Salivary antibodies following parenertal immunization of infants with a memingococcal serogroup A and C conjugated vaccine. Epidimiol Infect 1999;123:201–208.

1220. Halperin SA, Law BJ, Forrest B, et al. Induction of immunological memory by conjuagted vs plain meningococcal C polysaccharide vaccine in toddlers. JAMA 1998;280:1685–1689.

1221. Zhang Q, Pattitt E, Burkinshaw R, et al. Mucosal immune response to meningococcal conjugate polysacchride vaccines in infants. Pediatr Infect Dis J 2002;21:209–213.

1222. Gotschlich DM, Goldschneider I, Arenstein MS. Human immunity to the meningococcus. J Exp Med 1969;129:1385–1395.

1223. Mac Lennan J, Obaro S, Deeks J, et al. Immunologic memory 5 year after meningococcal A/C conjugate vaccination in infancy. J Inf Dis 2001;183:97–104.

1224. Zuckerman JN, ZuckermanAJ, Symington I, et al. Evaluation of a new hhepatitis B triple-antigen vaccine in inadequate responders to current vaccines. Hepatology 2001;34:798–802.

1225. Koff RS. Hepatatis vaccines: recent advances. Int J Parasitol 2003;33:517–523.

1226. Gupta I, Ratho RK. Immunogenicity and safety of two schedules of hepatitis B vaccination during pregnancy. J Obstet Gynececol Res 2003;29:84–86.

1227. Sood A, Singh D, Mehta S, et al. Response to hepatatis B vaccine in preterm babies. Indian J Gastroenterol 2002;21:52–54.

1228. Bona CA, Bot A. Genetic Immunization. Kluwer Academic/Plenum Publishers. New York: 2000.

1229. Brumeanu T-D, Casares S, Harris PE, et al. Imunopotency of viral peptides assembled on the carbohydrate moieties of self immunoglobulins. Nat Biotechnol 1996;14:722–725.

1230. Bona CA, Casares S, Brumeanu T-D. Towards development of T-cell vaccines. Immunol Today 1998;19:126–133.

1231. Casares S, Bot A, Brumeanu T-D, et al. Foreign peptides expressed in engineered chimeric self-molecules. Biotechnol Genetic Eng Rev 1998;15:159–198.

1232. Zaghouani H, Steinman R, Nonacs R, et al. Presentation of a viral T cell epitope expreseed in the CDR 3 region of a self-immunoglobulin molecule. Science 1993;259:224–227.

1233. Ogawa M, Maruyama T, Hasegawa T, et al. The inhibitory effect of neonatal thymectomy on the incidence of insulitis in non-obese diabetic (NOD) mice. Biomed Res 1985;6:103–109.

1234. Bowman MA, Leiter EH, Atkinson MA. Prevention of diabetes in NOD mouse: implications for therapeutic interventions in human disease. Immunol Today 1994;15:115–120.

1235. Miyakazi A, Hanafusa T, Yamada K, et al. Predominance of T lymphocytes in pancreatic islets and spleen of pre-diabetic non-obese diabetic (NOD) mice: a longitudinal study. Clin Exp Immunol 1985;60:622–629.

1236. Serreze DV, Leiter EH, Worthen SM, et al. NOD marrow stem cells adoptively transfer diabetes to resistant (NOD × NON) F1 mice. Diabetes 1988;37:252–255.

1237. Wicker LS, Miller BJ, Muller Y. Transfer of autoimmune diabetes mellitus with splenocytes from nonobese diabetic (NOD) mice. Diabetes 1986;35:855–860.

1238. Peterson JD, Pike B, McDuffie M, et al. Islet-specific T cell clones transfer diabetes to nonobese diabetic (NOD) F1 mice. J Immunol 1994;153:2800–2806.

1239. Elias D, Cohen IR. Peptide therapy for diabetes in NOD mice. Lancet 2002;343:704–706.

1240. Herold KC, Montag AG, Buckingham. F. Induction of tolerance to autoimmune diabetes with islet antigens. J Exp Med 1994176:1107–1114.

1241. Shizuku JA, Taylor-Edwards C, Banks BA, et al. Immunotherapy of the non obese diabetic mouse:treatment with an antibody to T-helper lymphocytes. Science 1998;240:659–662.

1242. Koikc T, Itoh Y, Ishi T, et al. Preventive effect of monoclonal anti-L3T4 antibody on development of diabetes in NOD mice. Diabetes 1987;36:539–541.

1243. Atkinson MA, Kaufman DL, Campbell L, et al. Response of peripheral-blood mononuclear cells to glutamate decarboxylase in insulin-dependent diabetes. Lancet 1992;339:458–459.

1244. Miller GG, Pollack MS, Nell LJ, et al. Insulin-specific human T cells. Epitope specificity of major histocompatibility complex restriction, and alloreactivity to a diabetes-associated haplotype. J Immunol 1987;139:3622–3629.

1245. Passini N, Larigan JD, Genovese S, et al. The 37/40-kilodalton autoantigen in insulin-dependent diabetes mellitus is the putative tyrosine phosphatase IA-2. Proc Natl Acad Sci USA 1995;92:9412–9416.

1246. Elias D, Reshef T, Birk OS, et al. Vaccination against autoimmune diabetes with a T-cell epitope of the human 65-kDa heat shock protein. Proc Natl Acad Sci USA 1991;88:3088–3091.

1247. Roep BO, Duinkerken G, Schreuder GMT, et al. HLA-associated inverse correlation between T cell and antibody responsiveness to islet autoantigen in recent-onset insulin-dependent diabetes mellitus. Eur J Immunol 1996;26:1285–1289.

1248. Miyazaki T, Uno M, Uehira M, et al. Direct evidence for the contribution of the unique I-ANOD to the development of insulitis in non-obese diabetic mice. Nature 1990;345:722–723.

1249. Slattery RM, Kjer-Nielsen L, Allison J, et al. Prevention of diabetes in nonobese diabetic I-Ak transgenic mice. Nature 1990;345:724–726.

1250. Lund T, O'Reilly L, Hutchings P, et al. Prevention of insulin-dependent diabetes mellitus in non-obese diabetic mice by transgenes encoding modified I-A beta-chain or normal I-E alpha-chain. Nature 1990;345:727–729.

1251. Tisch R, McDevitt HO. Insulin-dependent diabetes mellitus. Cell 1996;85:291–297.

1252. Fox CJ, Danska JS. IL-4 expression at the onset of islet inflammation predicts nondestructive insulitis in nonobese diabetic mice. J Immunol 1997;158:2414–2424.

1253. Tisch R, Yang XD, Singer SM, et al. Immune response to glutamic acid decarboxylase correlates with insulitis in non-obese diabetic mice. Nature 1993;366:72–75.

1254. Katz JD, Benoist C, Mathis D. T helper cell subsets in insulin-dependent diabetes. Science 1995;268:1185–1188.
1255. Trembleau S, Penna G, Bosi E, et al. Interleukin 12 administration induces T helper type 1 cells and accelerates autoimmune diabetes in NOD mice. J Exp Med 1995;181:817–821.
1256. Wang Y, Hao L, Gill RG, et al. Autoimmune diabetes in NOD mouse is L3T4 T-lymphocyte dependent. Diabetes 1987;36:535–538.
1257. Debray-Sachs M, Carnaud C, Boitard C, et al. Prevention of diabetes in NOD mice treated with antibody to murine IFN gamma. J Autoimmun 1991;4:237–248.
1258. Peterson LD, van der Keur M, de Vries RRP, et al. Autoreactive and immunoregulatory T-cell subsets in insulin-dependent diabetes mellitus. Diabetologia 1999;42:443–449.
1259. Han HS, Jun HS, Utsugi T, et al. A new type of CD4+ T cells completely prevents spontaneous autoimmune diabetes ands recurrent diabetes in syngeneic islet-transplanted NOD mice. J Autoimmun 1996;9:331–339.
1260. Pankewycz OG, Guan JX, Benedict JF. A protective NOD islet-infiltrating CD8+ T cell clone, I.S.2.15, has in vitro immunosuppressive properties. Eur J Immunol 1992;22:2017–2023.
1261. Han HS, Jun HS, Utsugi T, et al. Molecular role of TGF-beta, secreted from a new type of CD4+ suppressor T cell, NY4.2, in the prevention of autoimmune IDDM in NOD mice. J Autoimmun 1997;10:299–307.
1262. Sumida T, Furukawa M, Sakamoto A, et al. Prevention of insulitis and diabetes in beta 2-microglobulin-deficient non-obese diabetic mice. Int Immunol 1994;6:1445–1449.
1263. Katz J, Benoist C, Mathis D. Major histocompatibility complex class I molecules are required for the development of insulitis in non-obese diabetic mice. Eur J Immunol 1993;23:3358–3360.
1264. Skyler JS. The winds of change. Diabetes 1993;45:637–642.
1265. Song YH, Li Y, McLaren N. The nature of autoantigens targeted in autoimmune endocrine diseases. Immunol Today 1996; 17:232–238.
1266. Petersen JS, Karlsen AE, Markholst H, et al. Neonatal tolerization with glutamicacid decarboxylase but not with bovine serum albumin delays the onset of diabetes in NOD Mice. Diabetes 1994;43:1478–1484.
1267. Bot A, Smith D, Bot S, et al. Plasmid vaccination with insulin B chain prevents autoimmun edibetes in nonobese diabetic mice. J Immunnol. 2001;167:2950–2955.
1268. Casares S, Zong CS, Radu D, et al. Antigen specific signaling by a soluble, dimeric peptide MHC class/Fc chimera leading to T helper cell type 2 differentiation. J Exp Med 1999;190:543–553.
1269. Casares S, Hurtado A, Mc Envoy RC, et al. Down regulation of diabetogenic CD4+ T cells by a soluble dimeric peptide-MHC class II chimera. Nature Immunol 2002;3(4):383–391.

Index